Practical Guide to Abdominal and Pelvic MRI

Practical Guide to Abdominal and Pelvic MRI

John R. Leyendecker, M.D.

Assistant Professor
Director, Body Magnetic Resonance Imaging
University of Texas Health Science Center at San Antonio
San Antonio, Texas

Jeffrey J. Brown, M.D.

Associate Professor
Co-Director, Magnetic Resonance Imaging
Mallinckrodt Institute of Radiology
Washington University School of Medicine
St. Louis, Missouri

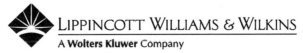

LIPPINCOTT WILLIAMS & WILKINS
A **Wolters Kluwer** Company

Philadelphia • Baltimore • New York • London
Buenos Aires • Hong Kong • Sydney • Tokyo

Acquisitions Editor: Lisa McAllister
Developmental Editor: Lisa Consoli
Production Editor: Frank Aversa
Manufacturing Manager: Colin J. Warnock
Compositor: TechBooks
Printer: Maple-Press

Library of Congress Cataloging-in-Publication Data

Leyendecker, John R.
    Practical guide to abdominal and pelvic magnetic resonance imaging/John R.
Leyendecker, Jeffrey J. Brown.
      p. ; cm.
    Includes bibliographical references and index.
    ISBN 0-7817-4295-1
    1. Abdomen—Magnetic resonance imaging—Handbooks, manuals, etc.   2. Pelvis—Magnetic resonance imaging—Handbooks, manuals, etc.   I. Brown, Jeffrey J.   II. Title.
    [DNLM: 1. Abdomen—pathology—Handbooks.   2. Magnetic Resonance
Imaging—methods—Handbooks.   3. Digestive System Diseases—diagnosis—Handbooks.
4. Pelvis—pathology—Handbooks. WI 39 L683p 2004]
    RC944.L394   2004
    617.5′507548—dc22

                 2003061929

To Mary, Michael, and Bridget,
my source of academic time during the writing of this book.
JRL

For my wife, Ann,
and my children, Preston, Nathan and Kalli.
JJB

Contents

Preface

Magnetic resonance imaging (MRI) applications in the abdomen and pelvis have traditionally lagged behind neurological and musculoskeletal applications. Among the factors contributing to this relatively slow growth are the physiologic motion inherent to abdominal imaging and the unique and separate physiologies of the various abdominal and pelvic organs. Now, with improved hardware, faster imaging sequences, newer contrast agents, and greater clinical experience, MRI of the abdomen and pelvis is finally ready for prime time. However, the very advances responsible for the recent growth of abdominal and pelvic MRI have dramatically increased the complexity of this field. These complexities are further compounded by the proliferation of confusing acronyms and vendor-specific terminology, which have plagued MRI since its clinical debut.

During the course of educating others about this exciting and dynamic field, it became clear to us that many individuals would benefit from a practical guide to imaging the abdomen and pelvis with magnetic resonance. Our aims for this guide were twofold: 1) to produce a concise reference for improving image quality and optimizing MR imaging protocols; and 2) to provide a distillate of clinically useful information to help with the interpretation of abdominal and pelvic MR examinations. In this endeavor, we have focused our efforts on the most common clinical scenarios encountered in daily practice. To maintain flexibility, we chose to abandon a "cookbook" approach in favor of providing the necessary tools to help individuals develop and implement protocols to fit most practice environments.

This book is divided into four sections. The first section introduces essential physical principles and provides necessary tools for successful data acquisition, image optimization, and protocol development. The next section reviews specific abdominal and pelvic MRI techniques, such as MR angiography, that have recently come into the mainstream. The third section provides a concise description of the MRI appearance of a broad range of abdominal and pelvic entities, covers many common differential diagnoses, and provides aids for the interpretation of preoperative imaging studies. The final section reviews abdominal and pelvic MRI anatomy, demystifies MR acronyms and terminology, and answers many frequently asked questions regarding the performance and interpretation of abdominal and pelvic MR examinations.

Throughout this text, we have made every effort to ensure that the material presented is up-to-date. We avoided lengthy discussions of techniques that can be performed at only a few centers worldwide. In other words, we have attempted to produce a "see what *you* can do" rather than a "see what *we* can do" type of book. We sincerely hope that our combination of concise explanations and concentrated clinical information satisfies the needs of practicing radiologists in need of a handy reference, radiology residents preparing for board examinations, and technologists performing MR studies of the abdomen and pelvis.

John R. Leyendecker, M.D.
Jeffrey J. Brown, M.D.

Acknowledgments

First, I acknowledge Dr. Roderic I. Pettigrew for stimulating my interest in the field of magnetic resonance imaging (MRI) when I was a resident. This project would not have been possible without the guidance and encouragement of my co-author, mentor, and friend, Dr. Jeffrey J. Brown, at the Mallinckrodt Institute of Radiology. I also express my sincere appreciation to Drs. Carlos F. Aquino, Kyongtae T. Bae, Jay P. Heiken, and Cary L. Siegel, for always being available to help with those really tough cases, and giving me a standard to strive for in my own career.

I acknowledge the following individuals for their superb textbooks, which comprised the core readings during my MRI training, and which I now recommend to my own fellows: Drs. Allen D. Elster and Jonathan H. Burdette, Ray H. Hashemi and William G. Bradley, Robert B. Lufkin, Donald G. Mitchell, Richard C. Semelka, and David D. Stark.

I am indebted to the following individuals for their invaluable observations and comments regarding portions of the manuscript: Drs. Markus Lämmle, Geoffrey D. Clarke, Robert Kadner, Dacia H. Napier, W. Kenneth Washburn, and Morton S. Kahlenberg. I also thank my former MRI fellow, Dr. Lin Xiong, my former MRI co-fellow (who wishes to remain anonymous), and all of the former MRI fellows at the Mallinckrodt Institute of Radiology for expertly monitoring many of the cases presented in this book. Of course, the images contained within this text would not have been possible without the dedication of the MR technologists at University Hospital and the Audie Murphy VA Medical Center in San Antonio and Barnes-Jewish Hospital in St. Louis, and the photographic expertise of Jonathon Sumner.

John R. Leyendecker

First and foremost, I thank John Leyendecker, whose intelligence, clarity, and vision were the driving forces behind this book. Thanks also to Vamsidhar Narra for sharing his passion for excellence in MR imaging. We owe gratitude to Michael Crowley for reviewing the physics portions of the book. Eric Schallen, Vladislav Gorengaut, and Jeffrey Brent provided useful comments on the manuscript. A special note of appreciation to my mother, Esther Brown, for her expert proofreading. Finally, I thank my wife, Ann, for tolerating my long hours away from home.

Jeffrey J. Brown

SECTION 1

Imaging the Abdomen and Pelvis

SECTION 1.1

Basic Magnetic Resonance Imaging Principles for the Abdomen and Pelvis

A basic understanding of a limited number of physical principles is essential to performing and interpreting abdominal and pelvic magnetic resonance imaging (MRI) examinations. However, it is not necessary, or even advisable, for most radiologists to understand MRI physics at the quantum level to perform high-quality clinical MRI studies. Few of us fully understand Einstein's general theory of relativity, but none of us would willingly vacate an airplane at 15,000 feet without a parachute. In other words, a full understanding of the physics or mathematics of gravity is unnecessary to predict the behavior of an object within a gravitational field. Similarly, an in-depth understanding of MR physics remains a luxury for most radiologists, most of whom need more practical knowledge. Therefore, this discussion on abdominal and pelvic MRI is focused on the principles that are most relevant to the needs of practicing radiologists.

Disclaimer: Most of the discussions of MR physics in this text are based on Newtonian approximations. An understanding of the behavior of individual protons requires knowledge of quantum mechanics beyond the normal scope of working knowledge of most practicing radiologists. However, because MRI measures the signal of large populations of protons rather than individual protons themselves, these approximations are sufficient to predict behavior, which is really what interests clinical imagers. Attempts to explain all MRI phenomena using only Newtonian models may eventually result in frustration and confusion. Therefore, our simplistic explanations should be viewed not so much as statements of ultimate truth but rather as practical mnemonic devices beneficial to the clinical application of MR.

T1 AND T2

Most abdominal and pelvic MR images fall into one of two categories: T1-weighted or T2-weighted. Differences in T1 relaxation times between tissues determine the image contrast in a T1-weighted image, and differences in T2 relaxation times between tissues determine the image contrast in a T2-weighted image. MR images are referred to as *weighted*, because no image represents only differences in T1 or T2 relaxation times. There is always some T2 contrast in a T1-weighted image and some T1 contrast in a T2-weighted image. Figure 1.1 illustrates the differences between these two types of images.

The source of the signal measured by MRI is the hydrogen nucleus or proton. To understand T1 and T2, it is helpful to imagine what happens to these protons when placed in a magnetic field and exposed to radiofrequency (RF) pulses. Because protons may be thought of as spinning charged particles, they are associated with a small magnetic field (magnetic dipole moment). This magnetic field may be represented as a vector along the axis of the spinning proton. Normally, the magnetic field vectors of all of the body's protons are randomly aligned. When placed in a strong external magnetic field (such as an MRI scanner), these vectors align parallel or antiparallel to the main magnetic field. Because slightly more proton vectors align in the parallel direction than the antiparallel direction, a net magnetization vector results, representing the sum of all the individual magnetization vectors of the protons. This net magnetization vector is referred to as *longitudinal magnetization*. The net magnetization vector is the one of interest.

The individual magnetic field vectors of protons placed in the MRI scanner do not actually align perfectly with the external field. Instead, they precess about the external magnetic field vector much like the earth precesses in space or a top precesses under the influence of gravity. In addition, the individual protons precess out-of-phase with one another much like a random assortment of spinning tops would be tilted slightly in different directions at any moment in time. Even though a group of hydrogen protons placed in an external magnetic field does not initially spin in-phase, protons

3

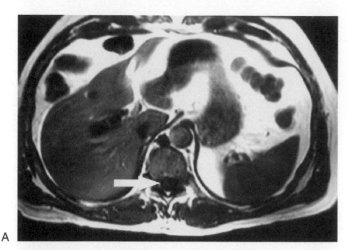

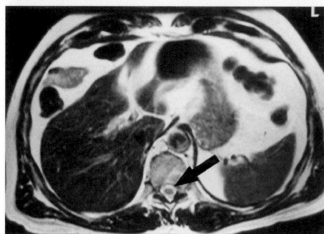

FIG. 1.1. T1-weighted image versus T2-weighted image. **A:** Axial T1-weighted spin echo image. Bright fat and dark fluid (cerebrospinal fluid [CSF]) (*arrow*) are characteristic of T1-weighted images. Signal intensity of liver is normally slightly greater than that of spleen. **B:** Axial T2-weighted fast spin echo image. Bright fluid (CSF) (*arrow*) is characteristic of T2-weighted images. Fat is also bright on fast spin echo images. Signal intensity of spleen is normally slightly greater than that of liver, a difference that is considerably more apparent on fat-suppressed images.

existing in a similar chemical environment precess at the same frequency according to the Larmor equation:

Resonant frequency (MHz)
= [42.6 MHz/tesla][magnetic field strength (in tesla)]

The Larmor equation indicates that the precessional frequency of protons is directly proportional to the strength of the external magnetic field. In other words, hydrogen protons precess slower at 0.5 T than they do at 1.5 T. This has important implications for how signal from protons is localized in space and for techniques such as fat suppression.

To generate signal from protons placed within a magnet, two things must be accomplished. First, the protons must be made to precess in-phase (i.e., their magnetic field vectors point in the same direction) to yield maximal signal. Second, the net magnetic field vector must be tipped from the longitudinal axis (aligned with the external magnetic field) into the transverse plane (aligned perpendicular to the external magnetic field). This latter condition results from the need to create an oscillating magnetic field in the patient, which generates a current (the echo) in the receiver coil. These two conditions (creation of transverse magnetization and phase coherence) are accomplished with the application of an RF pulse at the resonant frequency of hydrogen protons.

The application of the RF pulse (which is actually an oscillating magnetic field) causes the longitudinal magnetization vector to spiral down into the transverse plane so it can be measured. This initial RF pulse is commonly referred to as an *excitation pulse*. The amount of transverse magnetization created depends on the amplitude and duration of the RF pulse. The angle between the original longitudinal magnetization and the new net magnetization vector created by the RF pulse is referred to as the *flip angle*.

Once the RF pulse is shut off, the protons begin to realign themselves with the external magnetic field. As this occurs, the net longitudinal magnetization vector regrows in a logarithmic fashion. The time it takes for approximately two thirds (63%) of the original longitudinal magnetization to regrow is referred to as the *T1 relaxation time* (longitudinal relaxation time) (Fig. 1.2). As longitudinal magnetization regrows, transverse magnetization diminishes (decays). This loss of transverse magnetization (an exponential decay function) not only results from the conversion of transverse magnetization back into longitudinal magnetization, but also from an energy exchange between protons (referred to as *spin-spin interaction*). The loss of transverse magnetization resulting from the interaction between hydrogen nuclei is an irreversible process. The time it takes for transverse magnetization to decay to approximately one third (37%) of its maximum value (as a result of irreversible causes) is referred to as the *T2 relaxation time* (Fig. 1.3).

In a perfect world, the discussion of T1 and T2 would end here; however, no magnetic field is perfect. Subtle differences in the local magnetic field strength around individual protons are caused by imperfections in the scanner itself or the material (e.g., metal, air, tissue) placed within the scanner. This magnetic field heterogeneity increases the rate of loss of transverse magnetization. This occurs because protons precess at slightly different rates when exposed to slightly different local magnetic field strengths. Therefore, decay of transverse magnetization occurs more rapidly than would be predicted based on a perfect magnetic field. Unlike spin-spin interactions, loss of transverse magnetization resulting from static variations in local magnetic field strength is a reversible process. This more rapid loss and decay of transverse magnetization is referred to as $T2^*$. In other words, T2* reflects

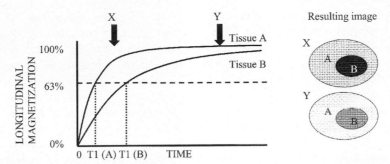

FIG. 1.2. T1 relaxation and T1 contrast. At time = 0, tissue A and tissue B are subjected to a 90 degree RF pulse, eliminating longitudinal magnetization. Tissue A recovers its longitudinal magnetization quicker than tissue B and, therefore, has shorter T1 relaxation time (when it recovers approximately 63% of its initial longitudinal magnetization). At time X (*arrow X*), there is a relatively large difference in longitudinal magnetization between tissue A and tissue B. Therefore, an image based on this difference (upper oval to right of graph) would have excellent T1 contrast. An image based on the difference in longitudinal magnetization at time Y (*arrow Y*) would have considerably less image contrast (lower oval to right of graph).

loss of transverse magnetization from both reversible (due to static magnetic field heterogeneity) and irreversible (due to spin-spin relaxation) causes. T2* is always shorter than T2, and T2 is always shorter than T1.

Different tissues in the body have different T1 and T2 values. For example, water has relatively long T1 and T2 values, whereas the T1 and T2 values of fat are considerably shorter. A tissue with a short T1 recovers full longitudinal magnetization faster than a tissue with a long T1, and therefore appears relatively brighter on a sequence designed to bring out the differences in T1 relaxation (a T1-weighted scan). A tissue with a short T2 loses transverse magnetization quicker than a tissue with a long T2, and therefore appears relatively darker on a sequence designed to bring out differences in T2 relaxation (a T2-weighted scan). These differences in T1

and T2 values give rise to most of the tissue contrast seen in abdominal and pelvic MRI.

SPIN ECHO VERSUS GRADIENT ECHO

One of the major components of the MRI pulse sequence is the RF excitation pulse, which is used to convert net longitudinal magnetization into net transverse magnetization. For a spin echo sequence, this pulse is 90 degrees, which means that all of the initial longitudinal magnetization is converted into transverse magnetization. However, the initial net transverse magnetization decays too rapidly to be of much use in generating an image. This is because the transverse magnetization vectors of the individual protons rapidly lose their phase coherence (they become out-of-phase with each other

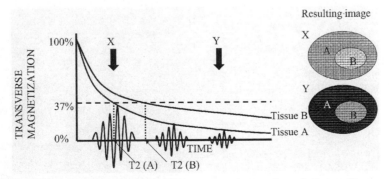

FIG. 1.3. T2 relaxation and T2 contrast. At time = 0, tissue A and tissue B are subjected to a 90 degree RF pulse, creating transverse magnetization. This excitation pulse is followed by three 180 degree refocusing pulses that result in three echoes (*wavy lines*). Only echoes for tissue A are shown on the diagram. The T2 relaxation curve follows echo peaks. Note that tissue A loses its transverse magnetization more rapidly than tissue B and, therefore, has shorter T2 relaxation time (when it decays to approximately 37% of its initial value). At time X (*arrow X*), there is a relatively small difference in transverse magnetization between tissue A and tissue B. Therefore, an image based on this difference (upper oval to right of graph) would have poor T2 contrast. An image based on the difference in transverse magnetization at time Y (*arrow Y*) would have considerably more image contrast (lower oval to right of graph).

due to variations in the local magnetic field), resulting in loss of net magnetization. This initial rapid loss of signal is referred to as *free induction decay*, represented by T2*. To obtain a signal from which an MR image can be made, either RF refocusing or gradient refocusing must be done to bring the individual transverse magnetization vectors back into phase.

The spin echo family of pulse sequences makes use of a 180-degree RF pulse to bring the protons back into phase to create the echo, a process known as *RF refocusing*. The effect of the 180-degree pulse is to flip the individual transverse magnetization vectors so that the more rapidly precessing protons catch up with the slower protons, much like runners of different speeds realigning after their direction is reversed. The process of creating a spin echo is illustrated in Figure 1.4. A refocusing pulse of less than 180-degrees creates an echo, but a 180-degree pulse gives the maximum signal.

Because a 180-degree pulse results in the strongest echo, one might think that it is always desirable to use this type

of RF refocusing pulse. For a simple spin echo sequence, this is generally true. However, a 180-degree RF pulse is also associated with higher energy deposition in the patient (manifested as tissue heating) than a pulse with a lower flip angle,* because the higher flip angle requires increased amplitude or duration of the RF pulse. The use of a large number of 180-degree refocusing pulses (as may occur with fast spin echo or turbo spin echo imaging) can result in unacceptably high levels of energy deposition in the body, particularly if the RF pulses are spaced closely together. One way to prevent tissue heating and conform to Food and Drug Administration regulations is to reduce the refocusing pulses to less than 180-degrees (generally 150-degrees suffices).

In contrast to the spin echo family of sequences, gradient echo sequences make use of a gradient reversal to bring the protons back into phase to create the echo. In MRI, gradients are linear variations in magnetic field strength that are momentarily applied at specific times during a pulse sequence. A gradient applied along one axis of the body causes the protons along that gradient to precess at different frequencies according to the Larmor equation. Protons exposed to higher field strengths precess at a higher frequency than protons exposed to lower field strengths. The result of these different precessional frequencies is that the protons begin to dephase. By reversing this gradient, the protons can be made to rephase. One important difference between gradient refocusing and RF refocusing is that the former technique only corrects for dephasing induced by the initial gradient, whereas the latter technique also corrects for the effects of local magnetic field heterogeneities. Therefore, gradient echo pulse sequences are more susceptible to artifacts created by substances that alter the local magnetic environment of the proton, such as metal or air. Gradient echo sequences are preferred for the detection of iron (e.g., hemachromatosis) and spin echo sequences are preferred in the setting of implanted metallic prostheses. The initial RF excitation pulse is often less than 90 degrees for a gradient echo sequence, but any flip angle up to 90 degrees may be used. Examples of spin echo and gradient echo images are shown in Figure 1.5.

REPETITION TIME AND ECHO TIME

Two of the most frequently altered MRI parameters are the repetition time (TR) and the echo time (TE) (Fig. 1.6). To spatially encode MRI data, the tissue protons must undergo a series of steps referred to as *phase-encoding*. For most MRI sequences, the initial RF excitation pulse and the refocusing pulse (in the case of spin echo) or gradient reversal (in the case of gradient echo) must be repeated many times. Each time this series of events is repeated, a different strength gradient (referred to as the *phase-encoding gradient*) is applied

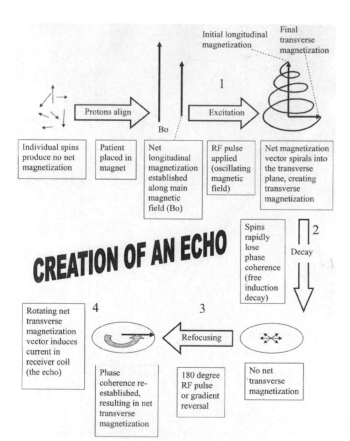

FIG. 1.4. Creation of a spin echo. Critical events in generation of an echo in MRI are (a) establishing longitudinal magnetization, (b) creating transverse magnetization through RF excitation, (c) decay of net transverse magnetization (loss of phase coherence), (d) refocusing of transverse magnetization (reestablishment of phase coherence), and (e) measurement of echo (induction of current in receiver coil). Large numbers correspond to time points in Figure 1.6, which are notated by the same numbers.

---

*The amount of energy deposited in a patient as a result of RF pulses is referred to as the *specific absorption rate* (SAR). Increases in flip angle, number and frequency of RF pulses, and main magnetic field strength all contribute to increases in SAR.

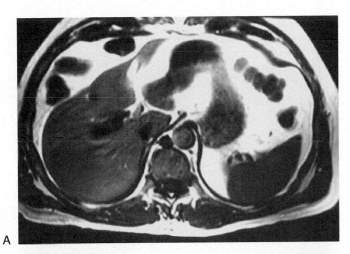

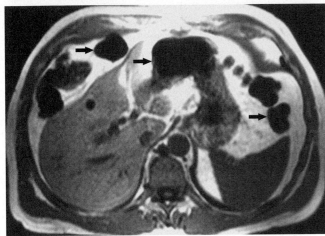

FIG. 1.5. Spin echo versus gradient echo. **A:** This axial spin echo T1-weighted image is the same as in Figure 1.1A. Acquisition time was approximately 2 minutes for the complete liver. Respiratory motion artifact was reduced by placement of a saturation band over anterior abdominal fat. **B:** Axial gradient echo T1-weighted image of the same patient. The entire liver was imaged in less than 30 seconds during breath-hold. The image has increased noise and more susceptibility artifact around bowel (*arrows*) than does the spin echo image.

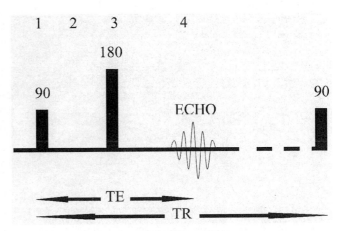

FIG. 1.6. Repetition time (TR) and echo time (TE) for spin echo sequence. TR represents elapsed time between successive 90-degree excitations. TE represents the time delay from the 90-degree excitation to the center of the echo. Note that 180-degree refocusing pulse occurs at time = ½ TE. Large numbers correspond to time points in Figure 1.4, which are notated by the same numbers.

to impart a phase difference upon the protons of interest. The time between one excitation pulse and the next is referred to as the *TR*. In other words, for a standard spin echo sequence, the TR is the time interval between consecutive 90-degree pulses. In general, a long TR allows for full recovery of longitudinal magnetization within tissues, regardless of their respective T1 values. Therefore, tissues cannot be differentiated on MR images based on their T1 values when a long TR is used. On the other hand, a short TR allows only enough time for tissues with a short T1 to recover a significant amount of longitudinal magnetization. Therefore, a short TR allows for differentiation of tissues on MR images based on their respective T1 values.

The time from the center of the excitation pulse to the center of the echo is known as the *TE*. The refocusing pulse

or refocusing gradient occurs halfway between the excitation pulse and the echo (at TE/2). A long TE allows more time for signal loss to occur from T2 decay. Therefore, a long TE allows for substantially greater signal loss from tissues with a short T2 than from tissues with a long T2 (Fig. 1.7). In other words, a long TE allows for differentiation of tissues based on their respective T2 values. Another important point is that a long TE allows more time for the effects of local magnetic field heterogeneities (T2* effects) to occur. As a result, magnetic susceptibility artifacts resulting from metal or air are exaggerated when imaging is performed with a longer TE (Fig. 1.8).

GRADIENTS

Producing a signal or echo is only the first step in creating an MR image. Equally important is localizing the signal in space. This may seem an impossible task, because the echo measured in MRI represents signal from the entire volume of tissue excited by the initial RF pulse, and this signal appears graphically like a wavy line. However, the data can be spatially encoded through the use of gradients. As mentioned earlier, a gradient is a linear variation in the magnetic field strength along an axis (although the term *gradient* is also commonly used to refer to the gradient coils that produce this variation in magnetic field strength). Because the MR signal must be localized in three dimensions, spatial encoding requires the use of three gradients.*

The *slice-select gradient* is the easiest gradient to understand. To produce signal from only one slice, a gradient is

---

*The slice-select gradient, frequency-encoding gradient, and phase-encoding gradient may be referred to as the Z, X, and Y gradients, respectively. To avoid confusion, we do not encourage the use of this terminology in the clinical setting, but rather favor the more descriptive terms.

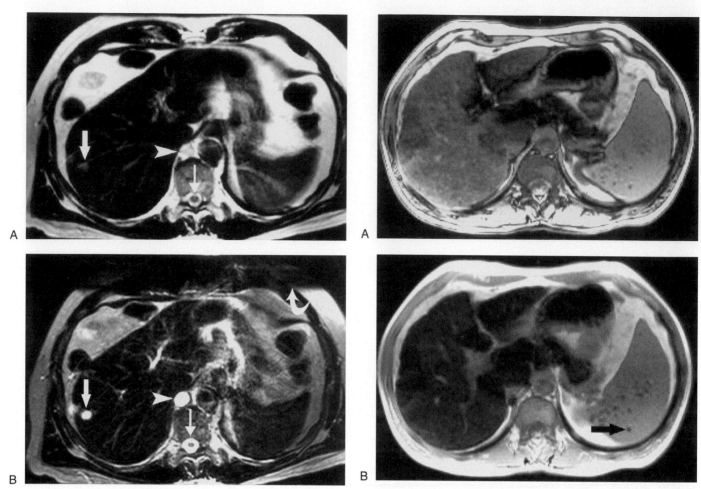

FIG. 1.7. Effect of TE on T2-weighted image. **A:** TE = 100 msec. Small hemangioma (*arrow*), cerebrospinal fluid (CSF) (*thin arrow*), and cisterna chyli (*arrowhead*) are not significantly different in signal intensity than fat. **B:** TE = 250 msec. Small hemangioma (*arrow*), CSF (*thin arrow*), and cisterna chyli (*arrowhead*) are significantly more conspicuous due to loss of signal intensity of background tissues having shorter T2. Note the use of a saturation band (*curved arrow*) over anterior subcutaneous fat to decrease respiratory artifact on this non–breath-hold examination.

FIG. 1.8. Effect of increasing echo time (TE) in a patient with hemochromatosis. **A:** Gradient echo T1-weighted image with TE = 2.7 msec. **B:** Gradient echo T1-weighted image in the same patient with TE = 5.3 msec. Note the lower signal intensity of liver relative to spleen with longer TE due to greater dephasing induced by the presence of parenchymal iron. Siderotic nodules within spleen (*arrow*) are also more conspicuous.

applied along an axis perpendicular to the desired slice. Because the magnetic field strength varies along this axis, the hydrogen protons precess at different rates based on their location relative to this gradient. A frequency-selective RF pulse (i.e., an RF pulse of a specific frequency) only excites those protons precessing at the same frequency as the RF pulse. Therefore, only protons at a specific location along the gradient are tipped into the transverse plane, and only these protons contribute to the final echo.

A second gradient (the *frequency-encoding gradient*) spatially localizes protons along an axis perpendicular to the slice-select gradient (i.e., in the plane of the slice) by causing the protons along this gradient to resonate at different frequencies at the time the echo is collected (or read out). This

gradient is often referred to as the *readout gradient*. During the application of the frequency-encoding gradient, the echo is detected by the receiver coil and digitally sampled to convert the analog signal into numeric data, which can be mathematically solved (via the Fourier transform) to create an image.

The slice-select and frequency-encoding gradients encode the signal in two dimensions. One might think that additional frequency-encoding gradients in the plane of the image slice would localize the signal in the third dimension. However, this approach has been largely abandoned in favor of a different approach called *phase-encoding*, which uses a third gradient to impart a phase difference along the direction of that gradient. In reality, this phase-encoding gradient must be applied many times (equal to the number of voxels one wishes to discriminate along the phase-encoding direction) to allow spatial localization. Each time the phase-encoding gradient is applied, its amplitude is varied slightly. In a traditional acquisition referred to as linear or sequential, the phase-encoding gradient is applied strongly in one direction and decreased with each repeat application until it reaches zero. This zero phase-encoding step imparts no phase shift but results in the strongest echo. Subsequently, the phase-encoding gradient is applied in the opposite direction, gradually increasing in strength with each application until the required number of phase-encoding steps is accomplished. The order in which the different phase-encoding gradients are applied can be varied. In one common variation, phase-encoding begins with the zero phase-encoding step and then alternates between negative and positive phase-encoding gradients of gradually increasing strength. This ordering of phase-encoding steps is referred to as *centric ordered* or a *low-high profile order*.

k-SPACE

The concept of *k-space* has confounded radiology trainees since MRI was first developed. Most of the confusion stems from its name, which provides no hint to the clinically inclined as to its meaning.* In fact, k-space can be better understood if it is thought of not as a space but rather as a digital representation of the multiple echoes produced during MRI.

When a population of spinning protons is flipped into the transverse plane, it has a net transverse magnetization vector that rotates in the transverse plane. This rotating vector induces a current in the receiver coil. This analog signal, or echo, consists of contributions from all the voxels in the image slice. Many echoes are collected to make an image—one for each application of the phase-encoding gradient. Each time an echo is produced (for each phase-encoding step), the echo is sampled multiple times and converted into digital data through the use of an analog-to-digital converter (the rate of sampling is determined by the receiver bandwidth). Once the echo is digitized, the mathematical technique of Fourier transformation is used to extract the spatial information from this digital data and create an image (Fig. 1.9).

Several properties of k-space are salient to the clinical practice of the MR practitioner. First, each data point in k-space contributes to the entire image, albeit in different ways. Data points close to the center of k-space (i.e., those obtained during the application of weak phase-encoding gradients and when maximum rephasing has occurred) have the highest amplitude and contribute most to image contrast. Data points near the periphery of k-space (i.e., those obtained during application of strong phase-encoding gradients and when the protons have only partially rephased) contribute most to spatial resolution and edge definition. Whereas an image can be

---

* The "k" in k-space refers to a mathematical term used by convention to define spatial frequency. This term appears in the mathematical description of the MR signal. Unfortunately, the term *k-space* has become entrenched in the MR lexicon and will not go away anytime soon.

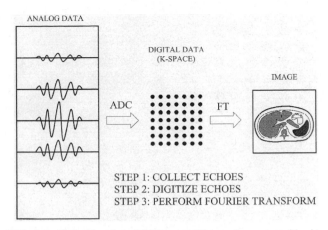

FIG. 1.9. Creation of an MR image. Three steps are critical to the creation of an MR image from spatially encoded signals: (a) the signal must be detected with receiver coil (echoes are in analog format when detected); (b) the analog signal must be digitized (ADC, analog-to-digital converter); and (c) Fourier transform (FT) must be performed.

made from only a portion of k-space, such an image may lack either image contrast or spatial detail. For most MR applications, the central lines of k-space are the most critical, particularly for a high-contrast technique such as MR angiography (MRA).

The relative position of the data points in k-space also controls image resolution and field of view. The overall size of k-space determines the image resolution. The spacing between data points in k-space determines the field of view. Increasing the overall size of k-space by adding data points, while maintaining the spacing between data points, improves spatial resolution without changing the field of view. Increasing the size of k-space by increasing the interval between the same number of data points improves resolution while decreasing field of view. Increasing the number of data points without increasing the overall size of k-space (by adding additional data points between the preexisting ones) increases the field of view without changing image resolution. Decreasing the interval between data points without adding additional ones contracts k-space, resulting in a larger field of view at the expense of decreased resolution. Figure 1.10 illustrates various manipulations of data in a simplified version of k-space and subsequent effects on the resulting images.

MULTIECHO ACQUISITIONS

Many strategies exist for shortening examination time in MRI. One of the simplest and most commonly implemented of such strategies involves collecting multiple echoes for each excitation pulse. For a standard spin echo sequence, one phase-encoding step is normally performed per TR (or per excitation pulse). This single phase-encoding step results in a single echo. However, a satisfactory MR image cannot be reconstructed based on a single echo. This process

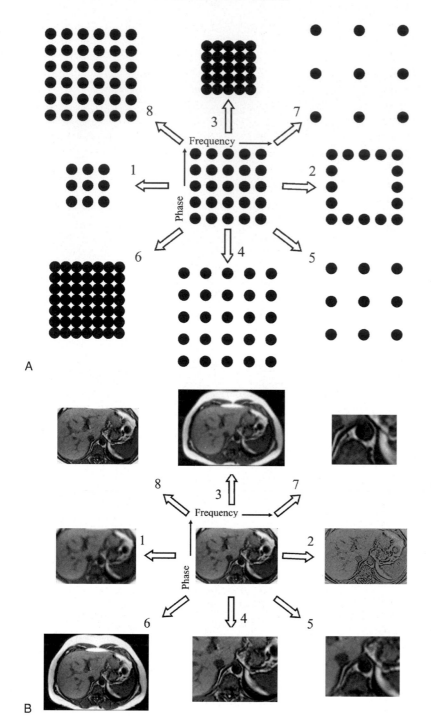

FIG. 1.10. Data manipulations in k-space. Each dot in **(A)** represents one data point in a simplified version of k-space. The pictures in **(B)** are modified to reflect the corresponding images resulting from the changes in **(A)**. The images in **(B)** do not actually represent separate acquisitions but were created from a single image using image processing software for illustrative purposes only. In reality, additional effects (such as truncation artifact) would be present on some images. The center grid represents the reference data. *1.* Failure to collect the peripheral (high spatial frequency) data points results in lower spatial resolution. *2.* Failure to collect the central data points results in reduced image contrast. *3.* The same number of data points occupying a smaller portion of k-space results in expanded field of view but lower spatial resolution. *4.* Expanding k-space with the same number of data points results in higher spatial resolution but smaller field of view. *5.* Fewer data points occupying the same area of k-space result in smaller field-of-view with comparable spatial resolution. *6.* Additional data points occupying the same area of k-space result in the same resolution with larger field of view. *7.* Expanding k-space with fewer data points results in higher spatial resolution but markedly reduced field of view. *8.* Expanding k-space with additional data points results in higher spatial resolution and same field of view.

must, therefore, be performed repeatedly (usually 128 or 256 times, depending on the matrix) for a typical abdominal or pelvic MRI study. One might conclude that the time to collect all the necessary data to make an image could be cut in half if two echoes were collected per TR and reduced further by collecting even more echoes per excitation. In fact, this strategy works extremely well and has essentially replaced standard T2-weighted spin echo imaging for abdominal and pelvic applications. To create multiple echoes, the 180-degree refocusing pulse must be reapplied many times

(once for each echo). The number of refocusing pulses applied per excitation pulse is referred to as the *echo train length* (also known as ETL or turbo factor). Typical ETLs for T2-weighted abdominal imaging range from 8 to 16. Some names for this multiecho spin echo technique are fast spin echo, turbo spin echo, or echo train spin echo. T1-weighted imaging is also possible with this technique, although the ETL needs to be shorter (due to the shorter TR), and the scan time reduction is not as dramatic as with T2-weighted imaging.

The multiecho spin echo technique can be taken to an extreme, applying the refocusing pulse enough times to make a complete image after a single excitation pulse. When all the necessary echoes to make an image are collected following a single excitation, the sequence is called *single shot*. In this situation, the TR is said to be infinite, because no further excitations follow the initial 90-degree pulse (although a number approximately equal to the scan duration typically appears with the scan data next to the TR on the resulting image).

When multiple echoes are collected per TR, each echo has a unique TE value. The order in which these echoes are collected can be modified on many scanners and affects image contrast. This means that the zero phase-encoding step representing the center of k-space can be performed at the middle of the acquisition, near the beginning of the acquisition, or near the end of the acquisition. Because most image contrast comes from the center of k-space, the effective TE is defined as the time interval between the excitation pulse and the peak of the echo created with a phase-encoding gradient strength of zero.

The single shot fast (or turbo) spin echo technique is often combined with another technique known as *half-Fourier imaging*. This technique takes advantage of the symmetry of k-space by collecting slightly more than half the necessary echoes to create an image and interpolating the rest. This option is also referred to as *HASTE* or *half scan*.

Despite the tremendous advantages of echo train spin echo techniques, which are henceforth referred to as *fast spin echo*, or FSE, there are some drawbacks resulting from long ETLs. For example, long ETLs are associated with image blurring. This blurring decreases with shorter inter-echo spacing.

As discussed earlier, there are two main families of pulse sequences: spin echo and gradient echo. Multiecho techniques can also be applied to gradient echo imaging, resulting in a technique referred to as *echo planar imaging*. As with spin echo techniques, echo planar imaging can be performed as a single shot. Images can be acquired extremely rapidly with echo planar techniques, although special high-performance gradients are required, and the images suffer from relatively poor signal-to-noise ratio, poor spatial resolution, and increased susceptibility artifact (because there are no 180-degree refocusing pulses to correct for magnetic field heterogeneity). Therefore, echo planar techniques are not widely used for abdominal and pelvic applications.

INVERSION RECOVERY SEQUENCES

One of the sequence variations commonly encountered in abdominal and pelvic MRI is inversion recovery. With this class of sequence, the part of the acquisition responsible for image creation is preceded by a 180-degree inversion pre-pulse. This 180-degree RF pulse inverts longitudinal magnetization, which then regrows according to the T1 of the tissue during the ensuing time period known as the *inversion time* (TI). The purpose of using an inversion pre-pulse is to control image contrast. As the longitudinal magnetizations of different tissues recover at different rates according to the T1 of those tissues, they pass through a point of zero longitudinal magnetization. If the data acquisition process is started at this point, tissues with no longitudinal magnetization produce no transverse magnetization and, therefore, no signal. In this manner, specific tissues such as fat, water, or even some liver metastases can be suppressed. Some MRI vendors have also used inversion pre-pulses as a means of improving image contrast for rapid imaging sequences (MP-RAGE, TFE, turboFLASH). The use of inversion recovery for fat suppression is discussed in the next section.

FAT SUPPRESSION

Fat suppression is one of the most frequently used options in abdominal and pelvic MR imaging. The use of fat suppression improves the conspicuity of enhancing tissues following the administration of intravenous paramagnetic contrast material (e.g., gadolinium chelates). It also aids in characterizing a variety of fat-containing lesions. Several methods of fat suppression have been described, although only a few are widely used for routine imaging. The term *fat suppression* is generic, encompassing a variety of techniques used to eliminate signal from fat. Most techniques used to suppress fat can also effectively be used to selectively eliminate signal from water, if desired.

Fat Saturation (Chemical Shift Selective Pulses)

Protons within fat precess at a slightly different frequency than protons within water. This difference in precessional frequency is referred to as *chemical shift*. At 1.5 T, water and fat protons differ in resonant frequency by approximately 220 Hz. At 0.5 T, this difference in frequency is only 72 Hz. As a result of this difference in resonant frequency, fat protons can be selectively excited (brought into the transverse plane with an RF pulse) and then spoiled through the application of a magnetic (spoiler or crusher) gradient.* This process of frequency selective excitation and spoiling effectively eliminates signal from fat. Because fat saturation relies on precisely applying a preparatory RF pulse at the resonant frequency of fat protons, fat suppression with this technique may be suboptimal when magnetic field heterogeneity causes the resonant frequency of fat protons to differ from the expected frequency. Therefore, fat saturation may not be the fat suppression technique of choice in patients with metallic

---

*The application of a gradient to destroy phase coherence is referred to as *gradient spoiling*. Spoiling is also commonly employed to destroy residual transverse magnetization between excitations during an MR acquisition. Most gradient echo pulse sequences for routine T1-weighted imaging apply this technique and are, therefore, referred to as *spoiled gradient echo sequences*. If the transverse magnetization was allowed to persist, it would be tipped into the longitudinal plane during the next excitation and would contribute to the image contrast.

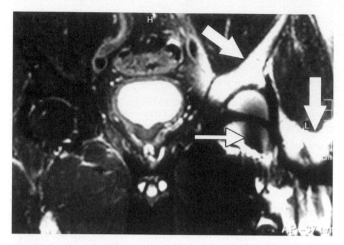

FIG. 1.11. Failure of fat suppression secondary to presence of a metallic foreign body. T2-weighted image of a patient with metallic orthopedic hardware in the left proximal femur shows adequate fat suppression in the right pelvis opposite the prosthesis, but subcutaneous and marrow fat are not suppressed (*arrow*) on the left side adjacent to the hardware (*thin arrow*).

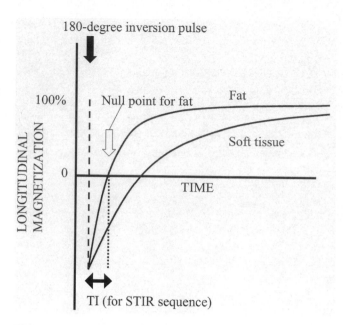

FIG. 1.12. Fat suppression by short tau inversion recovery (STIR). Following a 180-degree inversion pre-pulse (*solid arrow*), longitudinal magnetization vectors of fat and soft tissue invert. Because of its relatively short T1, fat recovers through point of zero longitudinal magnetization (null point) (*open arrow*) earlier than soft tissue. If the imaging cycle begins when fat passes through the null point, fat generates no signal. TI is time from inversion pulse to start of imaging cycle (for STIR, this occurs at null point for fat).

(e.g., hip) prostheses or for extremities that cannot be centered in the most homogeneous part of the magnetic field (Fig. 1.11). Because the application of the fat-selective RF pulse and spoiler gradient takes time, the use of fat saturation may increase scan time.

Short Tau Inversion Recovery

Water and fat protons recover longitudinal magnetization at different rates after an excitation (RF) pulse. This is another way of stating that fat and water have different T1 values. This difference can be exploited to eliminate or null the signal from fat (Fig. 1.12). This is accomplished through the use of a nonselective 180-degree inversion pre-pulse to invert both fat and water protons. As longitudinal magnetization regrows after the inversion pulse from −180 to +180 degrees, it passes through zero (referred to as the *null point*). Because fat and water have different T1 values, they pass through the null point at different times. If a subsequent imaging pulse sequence is begun when the longitudinal magnetization of fat is at zero (the null point), no signal is obtained from fat. This technique introduces a new sequence parameter known as the *inversion time* (TI). The TI is the time between application of the 180-degree inversion pulse and the start of the imaging sequence (e.g., the 90-degree excitation in a spin echo sequence). This parameter is less commonly referred to as *tau*. A relatively short TI (or tau) is used to null fat signal, due to the short T1 value of fat. Inversion recovery sequences that have been optimized to suppress fat signal are, therefore, often referred to as *short tau inversion recovery* (STIR) sequences.

Because the STIR technique relies on the T1 times of fat and water rather than a precisely (in terms of frequency) applied RF pulse, it is not as susceptible to magnetic field heterogeneity as fat saturation. Therefore, STIR works well in patients with metallic prostheses, for imaging the extremities, and at low field strength (when the difference in resonant frequency between fat and water is relatively small). However, STIR is not specific for fat and cannot distinguish between tissues or substances with similar T1 relaxation times. For example, gadolinium-enhanced tissues or hemorrhagic lesions may have short T1 values similar to fat. The use of a STIR sequence may eliminate signal from these substances along with fat signal. As a result, STIR should not be used to perform T1-weighted, fat-suppressed imaging following the administration of gadolinium chelates or for the detection of hemorrhage.

Specific anatomic structures may be difficult to delineate on a STIR image because of the near total and uniform nature of the fat suppression (Fig. 1.13). Some practitioners prefer to decrease the TI to produce slightly less fat suppression, allowing better delineation of anatomy. Alternatively, some individuals prefer to acquire an additional rapid non–fat-suppressed HASTE acquisition to provide anatomic correlation for the STIR image.

This technique can also be used to suppress the signal from water by using a TI corresponding to the null point for water. When an inversion recovery pulse is used in this manner, the sequence is commonly referred to as

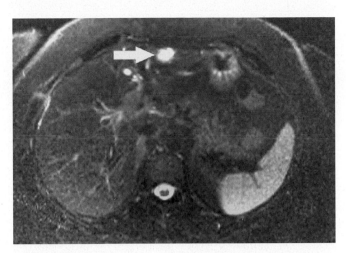

FIG. 1.13. Fat suppression using short tau inversion recovery (STIR). Near complete and uniform fat suppression characterize this axial turbo-STIR image through the upper abdomen. Lesion conspicuity is excellent (*arrow*), but anatomic borders are difficult to discern.

fluid-attenuated inversion recovery (FLAIR). FLAIR is rarely used in abdominal and pelvic imaging but is commonly used in neuroimaging.

Spectral Presaturation Inversion Recovery

Spectral presaturation inversion recovery (SPIR) is an inversion recovery technique that combines elements of fat saturation and STIR. With SPIR, a fat-selective, 180-degree RF pre-pulse precedes the standard pulse sequence. Imaging begins as longitudinal magnetization of the fat protons regrows through the null point. Because only fat protons are inverted, SPIR can be used successfully with sequences performed after the administration of paramagnetic contrast agents. However, because SPIR uses a frequency-selective RF inversion pre-pulse, it is sensitive to magnetic field heterogeneity much like fat saturation. The use of SPIR increases scan time for many sequences.

Water Excitation

As opposed to selectively eliminating signal from fat by actively suppressing it, fat signal can be selectively eliminated by not exciting it initially. In other words, images can be created by selectively exciting the water protons. Because none of the longitudinal magnetization of fat is converted into transverse magnetization, no signal is produced from fat. As with fat saturation, water excitation may be susceptible to magnetic field heterogeneity. One of the biggest advantages of this technique is that no preparatory RF pulses are required, minimizing the time penalty.

One form of water excitation uses a series of RF excitation pulses to separate the net magnetization vectors of fat and water by taking advantage of their different precessional frequencies. The sum of the flip angles of these individual excitation pulses equals 90 degrees, but with the exception of the first pulse, they are applied when water and fat are 180 degrees out-of-phase. By the end of the series of pulses, the net magnetization of the water is eventually flipped completely into the transverse plane, whereas the net magnetization of the fat ends up back in the longitudinal plane. For example, one permutation of this technique uses a combination of an initial 22.5-degree RF pulse followed by a 45-degree pulse applied when fat and water are completely out-of-phase. Once fat and water again become 180-degrees out-of-phase, another 22.5-degree pulse brings water completely into the transverse plane (therefore allowing creation of an echo) and fat completely into the longitudinal plane.

Unlike fat saturation, the series of initial RF pulses used with water excitation are spatially selective, because they essentially serve as the excitation pulse. This form of fat suppression has little relevance at low field strengths, because the time interval necessary to achieve a phase difference of 180 degrees between fat and water becomes unacceptably long.

In-Phase and Opposed-Phase Imaging

One of the important uses of fat suppression techniques in abdominal and pelvic MRI is to characterize fat-containing lesions. Any of the above techniques can be used to identify tissues consisting primarily of fat. However, most fat suppression techniques are not as successful at suppressing signal from tissues containing similar amounts of fat and water. The technique of in-phase and opposed-phase imaging (also referred to as *in-phase and out-of-phase*) is used to suppress signal from tissues containing similar amounts of fat and water.

The concept of in-phase and opposed-phase imaging is simple (Fig 1.14). The excitation pulse converts longitudinal

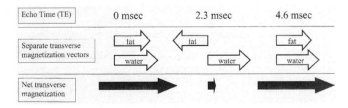

FIG. 1.14. Effect of echo time on a single voxel containing similar amounts of fat and water (slightly more water than fat) imaged with gradient echo sequence at 1.5 tesla. At time = 0 msec after creation of transverse magnetization by RF excitation pulse, fat and water protons precess in-phase. After 2.3 msec, the net magnetization vectors of fat and water protons are 180 degrees out-of-phase. Net transverse magnetization is minimal at this point. After 4.6 msec, fat and water protons again precess in-phase, resulting in maximal net transverse magnetization. An echo collected at 2.3 msec would yield little signal from the voxel. An echo collected at 4.6 msec would yield maximum signal from the voxel.

magnetization to transverse magnetization and makes all transverse magnetization vectors rotate in-phase. This means that water and fat protons begin spinning in-phase with one another immediately after an excitation pulse. Also, water protons and fat protons have slightly different precessional frequencies. Over time, they develop a phase difference as the slower precessing water protons lag behind the faster fat protons. At some point, the net magnetization vectors for fat and water become 180 degrees out-of-phase. If fat and water protons create net transverse magnetization vectors of similar amplitude within a voxel, the net magnetization vectors cancel each other out when fat and water protons are 180 degrees out-of-phase. Measuring an echo at this point results in very low signal. Again, cancellation of vectors only occurs if similar amounts of fat and water protons are present within a voxel. A predominately fat-containing structure in close proximity to a large water-containing structure only results in signal loss on an opposed-phase image at the border between the two structures, where fat and water are present together within the same voxels. Therefore, voxels that contain only fat, such as those within lipomas, intraabdominal fat, and subcutaneous fat, do not suppress on an opposed-phase image. In-phase and opposed-phase imaging is particularly useful for the diagnosis of fatty infiltration of abdominal organs such as the liver and pancreas, and some lipid containing tumors such as hepatic or adrenal adenomas.

After an excitation pulse, the net magnetization vectors for fat and water alternate between in-phase and out-of-phase. An in-phase image is acquired by selecting a TE resulting in a gradient echo that occurs when fat and water protons are in-phase. Opposed-phase images are acquired by adjusting the TE so that fat and water protons are out-of-phase during the echo. Many newer scanners can provide in-phase and opposed-phase images from a single dual echo acquisition with both an opposed-phase TE and in-phase TE. Table 1.1 provides the in-phase and opposed-phase echo times for various field strengths. As would be expected, the in-phase echo times are twice the opposed-phase echo times.

TABLE 1.1. *Approximate in-phase and opposed-phase echo times for various field strengths*

Field strength (T)	Opposed-phase TE (msec)	In-phase TE (msec)
0.5	6.9	13.8
1.0	3.4	6.8
1.5	2.3	4.6
3.0	1.2	2.3[a]

[a] The first echo time for an opposed-phase image is approximately 1.2 msec at 3 T. However, it is not technically feasible to perform a dual-phase acquisition with echo times of 1.2 msec (opposed-phase) and 2.3 msec (in-phase). Therefore, a dual-echo acquisition at 3 T may be performed using echo times of 2.3 msec (in-phase) and 5.7 msec (opposed-phase). The in-phase and opposed-phase acquisitions may be performed separately.

TE, echo time.

When interpreting in-phase and opposed-phase images, it is important to note which image is in-phase and which is opposed-phase. This can be determined by looking at the TE and referring to Table 1.1. Opposed phase images can also be readily identified by the characteristic dark borders at fat-water interfaces resulting from phase cancellation within the boundary voxels (Fig. 1.15).

Once the respective in-phase and opposed-phase images are correctly identified, it is important to know whether the images were obtained as a single acquisition for which two separate echoes were measured or whether two separate acquisitions with differing TE values were performed. When two echoes are measured for a single acquisition, all imaging and display parameters except TE are identical for both echoes. This allows direct comparison of regions of interest

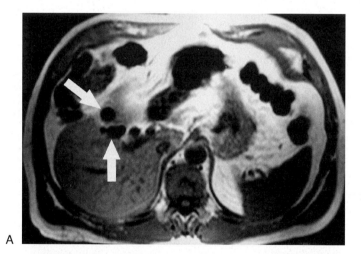

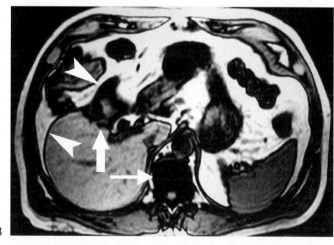

FIG. 1.15. In-phase and opposed-phase images. **A:** In-phase image (echo time [TE] = 4.6 msec). Susceptibility artifact from cholecystectomy clips (*arrows*) is greater with longer TE. **B:** Opposed-phase image (TE = 2.3 msec). Note the dark line around organs (*arrowheads*) due to phase cancellation at water-fat interfaces. Bone marrow is significantly darker due to presence of fat and water (*thin arrow*), and susceptibility artifacts are less conspicuous (*arrow*) on opposed-phase image.

(ROIs*) placed over pertinent structures. A loss of signal within the structure of interest on the opposed-phase image indicates substantial concentrations of lipid and water within each voxel. However, when two separate acquisitions are performed, the imaging parameters may not be the same and the signal intensity scale may differ between the two sets of images. In this situation, one cannot directly compare ROI measurements. Instead, the signal intensity of the structure of interest should be compared to a reference standard that is known not to contain intracytoplasmic lipid. One such readily available reference is the spleen. The liver is a poor choice, because it may be infiltrated with fat, resulting in substantial signal loss on opposed-phase images.

SATURATION AND SATURATION PULSES

The concept of saturation is important and relatively easy to understand. In the most basic sense, saturation refers to the loss of longitudinal magnetization resulting from repeated RF pulses, which are temporally spaced to prevent full recovery of longitudinal magnetization between successive pulses. In other words, as longitudinal magnetization recovers following an RF pulse, the protons are subjected to another RF pulse before full recovery. Each successive RF pulse applied in this manner further reduces longitudinal magnetization until a steady state is attained. As expected, substances with a relatively long T1 (e.g., fluid) are relatively easy to saturate. Substances with a short T1 (e.g., gadolinium chelates) are relatively resistant to saturation, because nearly full recovery of longitudinal magnetization occurs before application of the next RF pulse, unless the pulses are applied in very rapid succession. This concept has been exploited to create contrast-enhanced MRA images by adjusting the imaging parameters to saturate the background tissues while allowing the contrast agent within the vessels of interest to remain unsaturated (therefore appearing bright on the image).

An alternative method of eliminating signal from tissues is gradient spoiling. With this technique, application of a spoiling gradient in addition to a non–frequency-selective RF pulse eliminates signal from all tissues so treated. Spoiling is also frequently used to eliminate residual transverse magnetization between excitation pulses during a gradient echo acquisition.

Saturation techniques have many desirable applications and a few undesirable effects. Most commonly, saturation bands are used to eliminate artifacts resulting from moving tissues (e.g., respiratory phase ghosting) or to eliminate wraparound artifact during small field-of-view acquisitions.

---

*ROIs in MRI differ from those encountered in computed tomography. Whereas Hounsfield units can be standardized, MR signal intensity units are arbitrary and cannot be directly compared between two different acquisitions. For this reason, MR practitioners must rely on ratios for comparison purposes. One commonly used ratio compares the signal intensity of an adrenal mass to the signal intensity of the spleen on the in- and opposed-phase images.

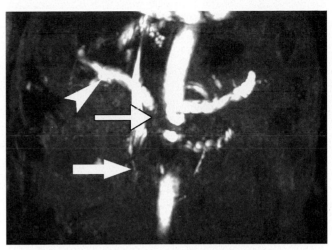

FIG. 1.16. In-plane saturation. Maximum intensity projection image from a two-dimensional time-of-flight MR angiogram of the abdomen acquired in the coronal plane. The lower inferior vena cava (*arrow*) and superior mesenteric vein (*thin arrow*) lack signal because they exactly parallel the imaging plane and have been exposed to repeated RF pulses. *Arrowhead* denotes portal vein.

Saturation bands are also used in time-of-flight MRA to selectively eliminate signal from arteries or veins or to determine direction of flow.

One of the most commonly encountered adverse effects of RF saturation is seen with MRA, particularly with time-of-flight. Any vessel running parallel to the imaging slice may encounter the same repetitive RF pulses that the stationary tissues experience. As a result, the signal of the flowing blood may progressively fade as the blood spends more time in the imaging slice. This phenomenon is known as *in-plane saturation* (Fig. 1.16). A similar problem arises with three-dimensional (3D) acquisitions due to the thickness of the acquisition volume.

FLOW

Flowing blood is responsible for a number of effects in MRI. The two most basic are the phenomena of flow-related signal void and flow-related enhancement. These effects are sometimes referred to as *dark blood* and *bright blood*, respectively.

On most spin echo images, blood vessels containing flowing blood are dark. To produce an echo on a spin echo image, the tissue within the imaging slice must experience both the 90-degree excitation pulse and the 180-degree refocusing pulse. These RF pulses only affect the protons within the imaging slice due to the application of magnetic field gradients. Flowing blood that experiences the 90-degree excitation pulse but leaves the image slice before the refocusing pulse does not rephase and, therefore, produces no signal. Similarly, blood flowing into the imaging slice after the 90-degree pulse has no transverse magnetization and, therefore, produces no signal.

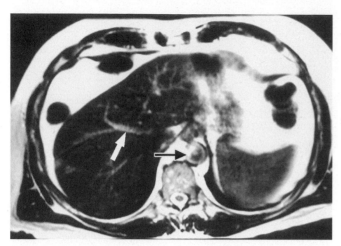

FIG. 1.17. Signal intensity of vessels. Hepatic vein (*arrow*) travels parallel to the imaging plane on this T2-weighted fast spin echo sequence, resulting in high signal intensity of blood similar to that of static fluid. This should not be confused with hepatic vein thrombosis or bile duct dilatation. Aorta (*thin arrow*) commonly has heterogeneous signal intensity on MR images.

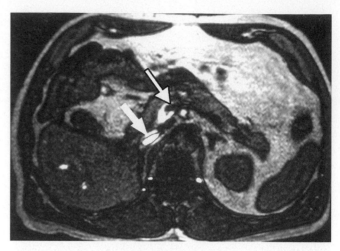

FIG. 1.18. Flow-related enhancement. Axial gradient echo image performed with a 60-degree flip angle and short repetition time in order to saturate stationary tissues. In addition, a superior saturation band was used to eliminate signal from aorta. The resulting image shows bright signal only in vessels flowing caudal to cranial inferior vena cava (*arrow*). Note the central low-signal area within the portal vein due to complex flow at the confluence (*thin arrow*). This latter finding may be confused with thrombus.

Not all blood is dark on spin echo images, however. For example, if blood travels within an image slice for a sufficiently long time to experience both the excitation pulse and the refocusing pulse in a T2-weighted acquisition, it will act as stationary fluid and appear bright on the image. This occurs when blood travels very slowly through the slice or when a vessel runs longitudinally within the image slice. This is why hepatic veins often appear bright and may be confused with bile ducts on T2-weighted images of the liver (Fig 1.17).

The phenomenon of flow-related enhancement is most commonly associated with gradient echo imaging and forms the basis for time-of-flight MRA. In a typical pulse sequence, stationary tissue is subjected to multiple RF pulses as all of the data (echoes) needed to create an image are collected. This causes the stationary tissues to become partially saturated, meaning that they no longer possess their full longitudinal magnetization. Less longitudinal magnetization means less subsequent transverse magnetization and, ultimately, less signal. However, blood flowing into the imaging slice from the outside has not been subjected to these RF pulses and, therefore, maintains its full longitudinal magnetization. This results in more subsequent transverse magnetization and, therefore, more signal. As a result, flowing blood appears relatively bright on this type of sequence (Fig. 1.18).

Signal within the vessels on an image created with a flow-related enhancement technique may not appear homogeneously bright, because protons in blood do not all flow at the same velocity. As the complexity of flow increases, so does the variation in phase accumulation between flowing spins (i.e., less phase coherence). This loss of phase coherence translates into lower signal. Loss of phase coherence may occur even in the setting of laminar flow, because protons experience a phase shift relative to background tissues in addition to the phase shift purposely induced for spatial encoding. Unless this dephasing is reversed, flowing blood within a vessel loses signal. This phase shift can be compensated for through the application of additional gradients, which serve to rephase constant velocity flow. This technique is referred to as gradient moment nulling or flow compensation. Higher orders of flow such as acceleration can theoretically be corrected for, although this is not practical given the increased complexity of the necessary gradients and resulting time penalty.

Flow-related enhancement is commonly seen in the slices at either end of a multislice spin echo sequence. End slices are involved, because blood flowing into these slices has not experienced any RF pulses and, unlike the surrounding stationary tissues, maintains full longitudinal magnetization. Once again, more longitudinal magnetization results in more transverse magnetization yielding greater signal. This effect is commonly referred to as *entry-slice phenomenon* and is essentially the same as flow-related enhancement. The best place to see this phenomenon is in the aorta on the uppermost images and in the inferior vena cava (IVC) on the lowermost images of a multislice axial scan of the abdomen (Fig. 1.19).

Another interesting phenomenon may result in variable signal intensity within vessels. If a patient's heart rate (in cycles per second) approximates some multiple of the TR, the data for each slice of a multislice acquisition are obtained during a particular part of the cardiac cycle. This results in high signal intensity in the aorta in some slices and low signal intensity in other slices depending on when during the cardiac cycle the slices were acquired. This phenomenon is referred to as *pseudogating*.

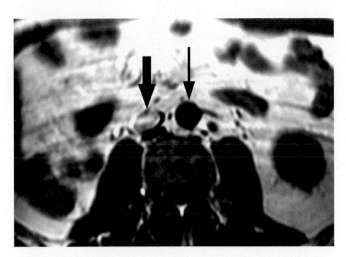

FIG. 1.19. Entry-slice phenomenon. Caudal-most slice of unenhanced spin echo T1-weighted scan shows high signal within the inferior vena cava (*arrow*) resulting from unsaturated blood entering the imaging volume. Blood within the aorta (*thin arrow*) is dark.

In summary, the signal intensity of flowing blood is affected by a multitude of factors, including the speed, direction, and type of flow (e.g., fast or slow, in-plane or through-plane, laminar or complex), the type of imaging sequence used (e.g., spin echo or gradient echo), the imaging parameters used (e.g., TR, TE, flip angle, and slice thickness), and the effects of entry-slice phenomenon and pseudogating. Therefore, a diagnosis of vascular thrombosis based on the signal intensity within a vessel alone should be made with caution.

TWO-DIMENSIONAL VERSUS THREE-DIMENSIONAL IMAGING

Most MR practitioners are familiar with the concept of a 2D acquisition. With 2D imaging, the images are acquired as a series of slices, which may be acquired in any order. With a three-dimensional (3D) technique, all of the data are acquired as a volume, and the slices that are subsequently viewed are actually partitions determined by a second phase-encoding gradient. A 3D acquisition allows thin contiguous partitions to be obtained during a single breath-hold. Therefore, 3D imaging is commonly used for high-resolution contrast-enhanced dynamic imaging of the liver, pancreas, and kidneys. The use of thin contiguous slices permits creation of high-quality multiplanar reformations and vascular reconstructions. However, because a 3D acquisition involves acquiring data from the entire volume of interest during the duration of the scan, any motion during the scan affects all images. Another drawback of 3D acquisitions is that flowing blood is in the acquisition volume longer, resulting in more saturation of the signal. Although this is not a problem for contrast-enhanced studies, saturation does limit slab thickness for time-of-flight MRA. As a result, it is common to

see a blood vessel such as the aorta or IVC progressively lose signal as it courses through the imaging volume of a 3D time-of-flight acquisition. This can be overcome through a technique available on some scanners (known as TONE), which gradually increases the flip angle along the direction of blood flow. Alternatively, multiple overlapping volumes may be acquired and combined (a technique referred to as *multiple overlapping thin slab acquisition* [MOTSA] or multi-chunk).

SECTION SUMMARY

1. Most MR images of the abdomen and pelvis are either T1- or T2-weighted.
2. T1-weighted images emphasize differences in the rate of recovery of longitudinal magnetization between tissues. T2-weighted images emphasize the differences in decay of transverse magnetization between tissues.
3. Longitudinal magnetization is necessary to produce transverse magnetization, and transverse magnetization is necessary to produce the MR signal.
4. Most MR sequences for the abdomen and pelvis are members of either the spin echo or gradient echo family.
5. TR represents the time between successive excitation pulses, whereas TE represents the time between an excitation pulse and the peak of the echo.
6. Spatial localization is accomplished in MR through the use of gradients. During an MR acquisition, the phase-encoding gradient must be applied multiple times at different amplitudes, thus generating multiple echoes of different amplitudes.
7. k-Space is the digital representation of all of the echoes collected to create an image. These echoes can be collected in any order.
8. More than one echo can be generated per TR, thus shortening scan time.
9. Inversion recovery sequences use a 180-degree pre-pulse to modify image contrast or selectively eliminate signal. Following an inversion pre-pulse, the time at which the longitudinal magnetization of a substance passes (recovers) through zero is referred to as the null point. The time between the inversion pre-pulse and the excitation pulse is referred to as the TI.
10. A variety of techniques can be used to suppress fat. Frequency-selective fat suppression techniques require a relatively uniform main magnetic field. Inversion recovery techniques should not be used to produce fat-suppressed T1-weighted images following administration of paramagnetic contrast agents. In-phase and opposed-phase gradient echo techniques are preferred for the characterization of fatty infiltration of organs or lipid-containing tumors (but not for suppressing adipose tissue).
11. Saturation of signal results from rapidly repeating RF pulses. Gradient spoiling eliminates residual net

transverse magnetization by destroying phase coherence. These techniques can effectively eliminate undesirable signal. Saturation may also result in loss of desirable signal such as that from blood flowing relatively slowly or within the imaging plane.

12. Depending on the pulse sequence, flowing blood may appear as dark or bright on MR images. Flow-related phase shifts result in artifacts that may be reduced with first order gradient moment nulling (flow compensation).

13. Three-dimensional imaging may allow for improved through-plane spatial resolution. As a result, 3D techniques are commonly used for contrast-enhanced dynamic imaging of the abdomen. However, motion occurring at any time during a 3D acquisition degrades the image quality of the entire data set.

SUGGESTED READINGS

Brown MA, Semelka RC. MR imaging abbreviations, definitions, and descriptions: a review. *Radiology* 1999;213:647–662.

Duerk JL. Principles of MR image formation and reconstruction. *Magn Reson Imaging Clin N Am* 1999;7:629–659.

Hennig J. K-space sampling strategies. *Eur Radiol* 1999;9:1020–1031.

Hood MN, Ho VB, Smirniotopoulos JG, et al. Chemical shift: the artifact and clinical tool revisited. *Radiographics* 1999;19:357–371.

Mezrich R. A perspective on k-space. *Radiology* 1995;195:297–315.

Pipe JG. Basic spin physics. *Magn Reson Imaging Clin N Am* 1999;7:607–627.

SECTION 1.2

Scan Optimization

The Art of Compromise

To be successful in magnetic resonance imaging (MRI), one must learn the art of compromise. With few exceptions, when attempting to optimize a scan, a positive change in one sequence parameter exacts a negative price elsewhere. In general, three key elements should be considered when planning and optimizing a scan: signal-to-noise ratio,* scan time, and image resolution. A beneficial change in one of these three elements usually results in an undesirable change in at least one of the other two elements (Figs. 1.20, 1.21).

Often, the MR clinician can control which elements to compromise when optimizing one particular aspect of a scan. For example, improvements in the signal-to-noise ratio can be attained by increasing the number of signal averages (which increases scan time) or by reducing the image matrix (which decreases resolution). Similarly, one can perform a quicker scan by reducing the number of phase-encoding steps (decreasing resolution) or by reducing the number of signal averages (decreasing the signal-to-noise ratio). In addition to these compromises, some attempts at image optimization result in artifacts. For example, switching from a breath-hold sequence to a non–breath-hold sequence to improve the signal-to-noise ratio not only increases scan time, but motion-related artifacts increase if additional steps are not taken to prevent them.

In this section, strategies to reduce acquisition time, improve spatial resolution, increase the signal-to-noise ratio, and reduce common artifacts in abdominal and pelvic MRI are discussed. Although most strategies require some form of compromise, there are new techniques that accomplish these improvements with minimal discernible penalty. However, the capacity to employ these latter techniques must be purchased from the manufacturer, often at considerable expense, resulting in a different form of compromise.

REDUCING SCAN TIME (IMPROVING TEMPORAL RESOLUTION)

One impediment to the success of abdominal and pelvic MRI has been the amount of time it takes to complete a study. At many institutions, appointment times of 1 hour or more are typical for even the most basic abdominal MRI protocols. As a result, many MR practices do not solicit abdominal and pelvic examinations. The benefits of reduced scan time, however, go beyond patient throughput. Quicker scans result in fewer artifacts from physiologic motion and reduced patient fatigue.

There are three primary approaches to shortening scan time. The first involves modifying the basic acquisition parameters for an existing sequence. This strategy is only effective to a limited extent, because modifying some parameters beyond certain limits results in undesirable changes in image contrast, resolution, or quality. The second strategy requires the use of a different sequence (e.g., substituting a gradient

---

*The signal-to-noise ratio, often referred to as *signal-to-noise* or *SNR*, is a measure of image quality referring to the amount of desirable signal contributing to the image compared with the undesirable background noise. Image noise may come from many sources and results in a random variation in signal intensity among the pixels in an image. A noisy image (see Fig. 1.21B) resembles a painting by the French impressionist Seurat. Noise is best appreciated in the air surrounding the body on an MR image. This noise has a speckled appearance when viewed with high level and wide window settings. Even though the signal-to-noise ratio is important, a more clinically relevant measure of the diagnostic utility of an image is the contrast-to-noise ratio. This ratio is a measure of how conspicuous a tissue or lesion is relative to another tissue or structure and is affected by the amount of background noise present. Figure 1.7A has a higher signal-to-noise ratio than Figure 1.7B. However, the contrast-to-noise ratio between the small hemangioma and liver parenchyma is higher in Figure 1.7B. Scan optimization is not a beauty contest; the prettiest images are not always the most diagnostically useful.

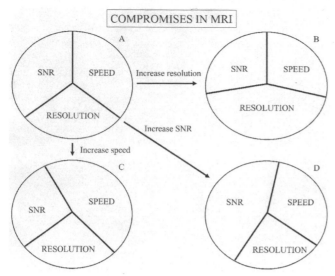

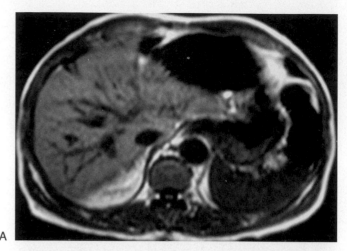

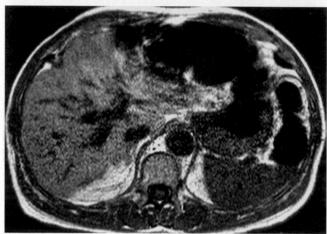

FIG. 1.20. Compromises in MRI. Any pulse sequence begins with potential signal-to-noise ratio (SNR), resolution, and scan time (speed) (A). Improvements in any of these three parameters results in decrement in one or both of other two parameters (B, C, D).

echo for a spin echo T1-weighted sequence). The success of the sequence-substitution approach depends on such factors as magnetic field strength, gradient strength, and available software. The third approach involves innovative shortcuts, most of which entail undersampling k-space and require special software or hardware. To optimize efficiency, more than one of the time-saving methods may be used in combination. However, one should not spend more time optimizing the sequence than it would take to complete the original sequence.

Parameter Modifications

Table 1.2 summarizes the parameter modifications most commonly used for reducing scan time. For a conventional spin echo or gradient echo sequence, acquisition time is given by the following equation:

Imaging time
= (repetition time [TR]) (number of phase-encoding steps)
(number of signal averages)

According to the above equation, steps that reduce the TR, number of phase-encoding steps, or number of signal averages will save time. MR technologists routinely vary the TR to reduce scan times. However, decreasing the TR beyond a certain point for a multislice acquisition actually increases scan time, because fewer slices can be acquired during the shorter TR. The rectangular field-of-view option saves time, because it allows fewer phase-encoding steps to be performed along one axis (usually anteroposterior for abdominal and pelvic examinations).

FIG. 1.21. Compromises in MRI. A: T1-weighted gradient echo image optimized for signal-to-noise ratio and time (10-second scan time) by using thick slices (10 mm) and fewer phase-encoding steps (112 × 256 matrix). Minimal background noise is present, but resolution is relatively poor and edges are blurred. B: Image optimized for resolution (246 × 512 matrix, 5-mm slice thickness) demonstrates considerably more noise and required 36-second scan time for same coverage.

TABLE 1.2. *Parameter modifications to reduce scan time*

Modification	Primary tradeoff
Shorten TR	Altered image contrast
Reduce number of signal averages	Reduced SNR
Increase slice thickness	Decreased through-plane spatial resolution
Decrease phase-encoding steps	Decreased in-plane spatial resolution; increased truncation artifact
Use of rectangular FOV	Reduced SNR
Increase sampling bandwidth	Reduced SNR
Increase echo train length	Increased image blurring; increased magnetization transfer effects

FOV, field of view; SNR, signal-to-noise ratio; TR, repetition time.

Other factors also play a role in acquisition time. The sampling bandwidth refers to the rate at which the echo is digitally sampled. More rapid sampling reduces acquisition time (and reduces chemical shift artifact) but increases image noise. Long echo train lengths reduce the number of excitations required to make an image. With sufficiently long echo train lengths, breath-hold T2-weighted imaging of the abdomen is possible. However, image blurring and magnetization transfer effects (which can affect solid lesion conspicuity) may become clinically significant with long echo train lengths. For this reason, the echo train length is generally kept below 16.

A more complete list of the various effects caused by changing MRI parameters is found in Section 4.3.

Sequence Substitutions

Table 1.3 demonstrates time-saving sequence substitutions. Extensive clinical experience suggests that T1-weighted spoiled gradient echo and T2-weighted fast spin echo can be routinely substituted for conventional spin echo sequences for most abdominal applications. Experience with single-shot (e.g., HASTE), gradient and spin echo hybrid (e.g., GRASE), and magnetization-prepared (e.g., MP-RAGE) techniques is considerably less. Therefore, these sequences are often used to supplement more traditional sequences or are reserved for uncooperative patients. These latter sequences are also continuously being improved by vendors. As a result, a scanner with state-of-the-art gradients and the most recent software release is more likely to yield clinically acceptable results with newer rapid imaging techniques than an older scanner. To determine the appropriateness of a particular sequence substitution in a particular practice, we recommend performing both the sequence to be replaced and the substitution under consideration until it is clear that important diagnostic information is not being lost.

TABLE 1.3. *Sequence substitutions to reduce scan time*

Substitution	Tradeoff
Gradient echo T1 for spin echo T1	Reduced SNR; increased susceptibility artifact
Fast spin echo for spin echo	Brighter fat may necessitate use of fat suppression
Single shot for multishot	Reduced SNR; loss of image sharpness; reduced conspicuity of solid lesions
GRASE for spin echo type sequences	Limited clinical experience
Magnetization prepared gradient echo for spoiled gradient echo (see MP-RAGE)	Limited clinical experience

GRASE, gradient and spin echo hybrid; SNR, signal-to-noise ratio.

Additional Techniques for Reducing Scan Times

Half-Fourier (1/2 NEX, Half Scan)

During MR data acquisition, the phase-encoding gradient is applied in equal increments on either side of the zero phase-encoding step. As a result, k-space is symmetric in the phase-encoding direction. It is therefore possible to create a clinically useful image from a fraction of k-space (slightly more than half). This technique is commonly applied with single shot acquisitions commonly referred to as HASTE, ssTSE, or ssFSE. Figures 1.41 and 1.43A are examples of HASTE images.

Partial or Fractional Echo Sampling

K-space is also symmetric in the frequency-encoding direction. Therefore, one can sample roughly half of each echo during application of the frequency-encoding gradient. This technique allows for a shorter minimum TE.

Zerofill Interpolation (ZIP, Reduced Acquisition)

Like the preceding techniques, zerofill interpolation involves collecting only a portion of the data necessary to fill k-space. In a common variation of this technique, the central lines of k-space are collected and the remaining peripheral portions of k-space are filled with zeros to allow a Fourier transform to be performed. Three-dimensional (3D) MR angiography (MRA) and gradient echo sequences used for dynamic contrast-enhanced imaging of the liver, pancreas, and kidneys often employ zero-fill interpolation. In this manner, high-resolution breath-hold imaging of the abdomen can be performed. Truncation artifacts are exacerbated with zero-filling, but this is rarely of clinical importance at the matrix sizes typically used. Fast 3D gradient echo imaging combined with zerofill interpolation is commonly referred to as *VIBE* (volumetric interpolated breath-hold examination). Many of the contrast-enhanced 3D gradient echo images found throughout this text were performed with zerofill interpolation.

Keyhole

Keyhole imaging is primarily applicable to dynamic contrast-enhanced scanning of a limited number of slices. Instead of filling only a portion of k-space for each image, the keyhole technique involves collecting a full set of image data at the beginning of the examination including both the high spatial resolution portions of k-space and the low spatial resolution portions responsible for image contrast. After the administration of an intravenous bolus of contrast material, subsequent acquisitions acquire only the central (high image contrast) portions of k-space. The peripheral, high spatial resolution portions of k-space are filled using data from the initial reference image. This dramatically reduces overall scan time, allowing for rapid dynamic contrast-enhanced imaging.

Parallel Imaging Techniques (SENSE, SMASH, ASSET)

Traditional MRI techniques rely on gradients to spatially encode information. This process of spatial encoding accounts for the majority of time required to complete an MR acquisition. Parallel imaging techniques represent a relatively new development in MR data acquisition that should have a dramatic impact on abdominal and pelvic MRI. These techniques take advantage of the differing sensitivities of the individual receiver coil elements of a multicoil array to spatially encode data. This allows multiple lines of k-space to be filled simultaneously (in parallel). In reality, the additional lines of data are not actually collected. Instead, k-space is undersampled in the phase-encoding direction, and the missing data are reconstructed by a variety of methods based on coil sensitivity patterns. For these techniques to work, the RF sensitivities of the individual coil elements must be determined through a calibration process before imaging. Parallel imaging works with most commercially available pulse sequences and can reduce scan times by an integer factor (e.g., a factor of 2 or 3). Figure 2.8 is an example of the use of SENSE to reduce acquisition time for an MRA study.

IMPROVING SPATIAL RESOLUTION

An MR image consists of *pixels*, the discrete units of any two-dimensional digital image. Each pixel represents a volume of tissue within the image slice known as a *voxel*. The brightness of each pixel is determined by the amount of MR signal produced by its corresponding voxel. Smaller voxels result in smaller pixels, which in turn create a higher resolution image. The slice thickness, field of view (which determines the amount of in-plane real estate to be divided into pixels), number of phase-encoding steps (determining the number of pixels along the phase-encoding axis), and number of frequency-encoding steps (determining the number of pixels along the frequency-encoding axis) determine voxel volume (Fig. 1.22).

Through-plane spatial resolution can be improved by reducing the slice thickness, whereas decreasing the field of view or increasing the number of phase- or frequency-encoding steps (matrix size) improves in-plane spatial resolution. In isolation, a reduction in slice thickness or field of view reduces anatomic coverage, whereas an increase in the number of phase-encoding steps increases scan time. Reducing the field of view can also result in wraparound artifact unless additional steps are taken. Any reduction in voxel volume reduces the amount of signal produced by each individual voxel, resulting in an overall decrease in the signal-to-noise ratio.

To avoid prolonging scan time during time-sensitive breath-hold or dynamic contrast-enhanced sequences, many MR practitioners rely on zerofill interpolation to improve spatial resolution. When scan time is not as critical, more signal rich sequences such as conventional spin echo or fast spin

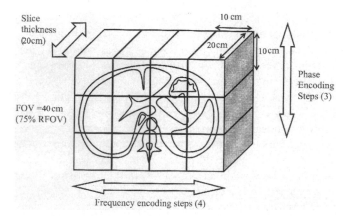

FIG. 1.22. Calculation of voxel volume. Simplified very low-resolution scan with 3 × 4 matrix and 20-cm slice thickness is presented. Field of view (FOV) is 40 cm, but 75% rectangular FOV (equivalent to 30 cm FOV in one direction) is applied in the phase-encoding direction to save time. Each voxel measures 10 × 10 × 20 cm. Each image pixel measures 10 × 10 cm.

echo are generally preferred over gradient echo or single-shot sequences for high-resolution imaging.

IMPROVING SIGNAL-TO-NOISE RATIO

The MRI signal is a measure of the net transverse magnetization created during a pulse sequence. More transverse magnetization translates into a greater signal induced in the receiver coil. In a perfect world, this signal would be perfectly smooth. However, there is a baseline random, low-amplitude variation in the signal known as *noise*. In the presence of a strong MR signal, this noise is barely perceptible. However, as the signal becomes weaker, the noise becomes increasingly conspicuous until image quality is compromised. The signal-to-noise ratio is, therefore, one measure of image quality. As

TABLE 1.4. *Methods of improving signal-to-noise ratio*

Method	Tradeoff
Increase slice thickness	Decreased spatial resolution
Decrease matrix	Decreased spatial resolution
Increase signal averages (NEX, NSA)	Increased scan time
Decrease receiver bandwidth (increase WFS)	Increased scan time; increased chemical shift artifact
Use surface coil	Reduced anatomic coverage
Increase field of view	Reduced spatial resolution
Increase field strength	Cannot be altered for a given scanner
Increase repetition time	Increased scan time; altered image contrast
Decrease TE (or effective TE)	Altered image contrast

NEX, number of excitations; NSA, number of signal averages; WFS, water-fat shift; TE, echo time.

a general rule, the signal-to-noise ratio can be improved by increasing the voxel size, using surface coils (instead of a circumferential body coil), and reducing the receiver bandwidth (sampling frequency). Strategies for improving the signal-to-noise ratio are listed in Table 1.4.

Whereas the signal-to-noise ratio is an important factor in determining image quality, the contrast-to-noise ratio is a more clinically important parameter. The signal-to-noise ratio determines whether an image is pleasant to look at, but the contrast-to-noise ratio helps determine whether the image is of diagnostic quality. In other words, the contrast-to-noise ratio helps determine lesion conspicuity.

IDENTIFYING AND ELIMINATING ARTIFACTS

Part of optimizing MR image quality involves elimination of undesirable artifacts, which can interfere with the diagnostic utility of an image. Some artifacts are unavoidable or inconsequential and do not justify the additional time necessary to prevent them. However, such artifacts may become clinically significant if they are not recognized as such and are misinterpreted as disease. This section discusses how to correctly identify common MR artifacts and presents some strategies for eliminating them (Table 1.5).

Chemical Shift Artifact

Chemical shift artifacts occur because water and fat protons precess at slightly different frequencies (a difference of 220 Hz at 1.5 T). Because MRI is based on the resonant frequency of water protons, fat protons are spatially misregistered on MR images. This results in bands of increased (on the high-frequency side) and decreased (on the low-frequency side) signal intensity on either side of a structure with a fat-water interface (Fig. 1.23). This misregistration occurs along the frequency encoding direction of the image.

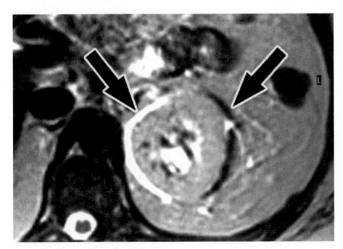

FIG. 1.23. Chemical shift artifact. T2-weighted image demonstrates chemical shift artifact (*arrows*) around the left kidney. The frequency-encoding direction is right to left.

TABLE 1.5. *Common magnetic resonance imaging artifacts*

Artifact	Eliminated or reduced by
Chemical shift	Increasing bandwidth; decreasing field strength
Wraparound	Phase oversampling; saturation bands
Susceptibility	Shortening TE; using spin echo; FSE; or HASTE
Truncation	Increasing spatial resolution in direction of artifact
Respiratory motion	Breath-hold imaging; respiratory triggering/ gating; retrospective k-space reordering; fast imaging; saturation bands
Vascular pulsation	Gradient moment nulling (flow compensation); change TR; saturation bands; cardiac gating
Zipper (extraneous RF)	Removing source of RF contamination

FSE, fast spin echo; RF, radiofrequency; TE, echo time; TR, repetition time.

Increasing the bandwidth (or as some vendors refer to it, decreasing the water-fat shift) reduces chemical shift artifact. This occurs because increasing the bandwidth expands the frequency range of each pixel. As a result, the chemical shift of 220 Hz occurs over fewer pixels, resulting in a thinner band of misregistration. However, increasing the bandwidth results in a lower signal-to-noise ratio. Chemical shift artifact is less conspicuous at lower field strengths, because the difference in precessional frequency between fat and water is smaller than at higher field strengths (according to the Larmor equation).

A different type of chemical shift artifact occurs at fat-water interfaces on gradient echo images acquired with certain echo times. On opposed-phase images, voxels that contain substantial concentrations of water and fat produce little or no signal. This results in a thin black line, sometimes referred to as *India ink etching*, at fat-water interfaces (Fig. 1.15B). This effect can be eliminated by choosing an in-phase echo time.

Wraparound

Wraparound (Fig. 1.24), sometimes referred to as *aliasing*, occurs when body parts are present outside of the field of view. The field of view of an image is defined in part by a range of frequencies determined by the sampling bandwidth. The frequency of precessing protons outside of the field of view exceeds or falls below this range of frequencies. The MR signal received from the image slice originates from all protons, even those outside the field of view. However, all protons contributing to the image are assumed to fall within the assigned range of frequencies. As a result, the body parts containing protons exceeding this frequency range will be

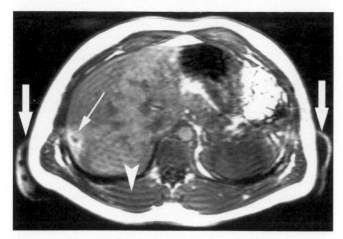

FIG. 1.24. Wraparound artifact. T1-weighted image of abdomen acquired with patient's arms at side and outside field of view. Note images of the arms overlying a portion of the abdomen (*arrows*). Artifact could simulate enhancing liver lesion in right hepatic lobe (*thin arrow*) on contrast-enhanced scan. Note also additional artifact (*arrowhead*) unrelated to field of view.

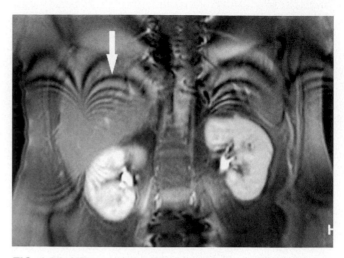

FIG. 1.25. Wraparound artifact with "zebra stripes." Coronal gradient echo image through kidneys shows wraparound artifact with zebra stripes (*arrow*). This artifact is common with large field-of-view gradient echo sequences.

incorrectly mapped to the low-frequency end of the image, and body parts containing protons precessing below this frequency range will be mismapped at the high-frequency end of the image. Wraparound in the frequency-encoding direction is no longer encountered clinically, because newer scanners filter the frequencies outside the established range or routinely use frequency oversampling.

Wraparound can also occur in the phase-encoding direction of the image. This occurs because an image is encoded for 360 degrees of phase shift. A phase shift greater than 360 degrees (e.g., 450 degrees) is interpreted as a lower phase shift within the established range (e.g., 90 degrees). The zebra stripes commonly encountered on coronal gradient echo images of the abdomen and pelvis are a result of wraparound combined with phase interference between tissues inside and outside the field of view occurring in the setting of magnetic field heterogeneity (created by air-tissue interfaces) (Fig. 1.25). A 3D acquisition has two phase-encoding directions, and wraparound artifact can occur along both of them.

Phase wraparound cannot be filtered out. Instead, additional phase-encoding steps must be performed outside the field-of-view to eliminate this artifact. Although these extra data are subsequently discarded, the additional phase-encoding steps add considerably to the scan time. This technique is referred to as *NPW* (no-phase-wrap), *phase oversampling*, or *foldover suppression*. Alternative methods of reducing wraparound include increasing the field of view or applying saturation bands outside of the field of view to eliminate signal from structures that might otherwise wrap into the image.

Magnetic Susceptibility Artifact

Substances with differing magnetic susceptibilities in close proximity distort the local magnetic field. Because magnetic

field strength determines precessional frequency, and frequency determines spatial localization, spatial misregistration occurs at these sites of field distortion. Susceptibility artifact (Fig. 1.26) is most problematic at air-tissue interfaces (e.g., bowel) and wherever metal is present. This artifact is also exacerbated at longer echo times, because more time is allowed for proton dephasing to occur as a result of field heterogeneity.

Because susceptibility differences cause magnetic field heterogeneity, the use of frequency-selective fat suppression techniques (e.g., fat saturation, spectral presaturation inversion recovery) may result in nonuniform fat suppression (Fig. 1.11). Short tau inversion recovery (STIR), on the other hand, is based on T1 relaxation, not precessional frequency. Therefore, STIR is the preferred technique for fat suppression when magnetic field homogeneity is suboptimal.

Susceptibility artifact can be reduced by shortening the TE, increasing receiver bandwidth, or substituting a spin echo or fast spin echo sequence for gradient echo. This sequence substitution is effective, because the 180-degree RF pulses found in spin echo type sequences largely correct for magnetic field heterogeneity (see Fig. 1.26B).

Truncation Artifact

Truncation artifact (Fig. 1.27) refers to truncation of the data (signal) used to create an MR image. The artifact occurs because an MR image is based on a finite number of data samples taken over a limited period of time. Fourier transform of this truncated data results in faint, closely spaced bands of alternating high and low signal that parallel high-contrast interfaces. Truncation artifact occurs most commonly in the phase-encoding direction, because this is typically the axis with the lowest resolution (i.e., fewest data samples). Truncation is often noticeable on 3D gradient echo images of the

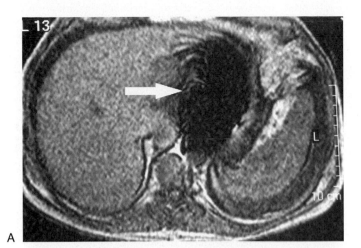

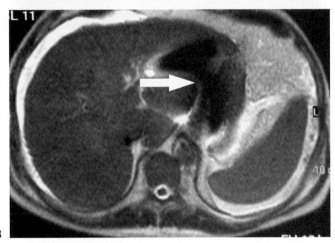

FIG. 1.26. Susceptibility artifact. **A:** Gradient echo image through stomach shows marked susceptibility artifact from metallic tip of feeding tube (*arrow*). **B:** Single-shot fast spin echo sequence shows marked reduction in susceptibility artifact (*arrow*) compared with gradient echo sequence.

abdomen and may be mistaken for phase-ghosting caused by respiratory motion.

Mild truncation artifact rarely interferes with interpretation of abdominal and pelvic MR examinations but can be reduced by increasing the spatial resolution in the phase-encoding direction (at the expense of a longer scan time).

Zipper Artifact

Zipper artifact (Fig. 1.28) gets its name from its alternating bright and dark signal occurring along a relatively thin line resembling a zipper. This artifact has several causes. For example, if the TE is sufficiently short, the sidelobes of the 180-degree refocusing pulse overlap the free induction decay signal causing a zipper to appear along the phase-encoding direction at zero frequency. This can be corrected by increasing the TE. A similar-appearing artifact can be seen when the excitation RF pulse is detected by the receiver coil (the receiver coil is only supposed to detect the echo created by the refocusing pulse). A zipper artifact along the frequency-encoding axis may result from stimulated echoes due to inadequate spoiling. However, the most commonly seen zipper artifact results from external sources of radiofrequency noise such as electronic equipment. This artifact differs from those discussed earlier in that it occurs along the phase-encoding axis at a location *away* from the point of zero frequency. In other words, the extraneous noise is mapped in the image according to its frequency.

Physiologic Motion Artifacts

The effects of physiologic motion go beyond the most mobile of the abdominal organs such as the liver, bowel, and kidneys,

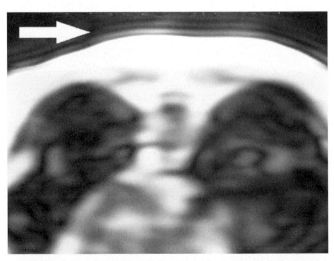

FIG. 1.27. Truncation artifact. Image performed with only 64 phase-encoding steps demonstrates multiple lines of alternating signal intensity (*arrow*) paralleling high-contrast interface at the skin surface.

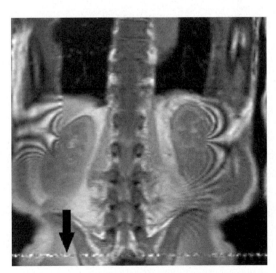

FIG. 1.28. Zipper artifact. T1-weighted spoiled gradient echo image with frequency-encoding axis from cranial to caudal. Note zipper artifact (*arrow*) occurs near bottom of image. Wraparound artifact with zebra stripes is also present on this image.

because any motion occurring during the image acquisition process results in phase misregistration. This manifests on the image as ghosting artifact, the conspicuity of which is related to the signal intensity of the offending structure (Figs. 1.29, 1.30). This common artifact can obscure important findings and distract or fool the reader.

A number of strategies exist for reducing motion artifact on MR images. The most obvious solution is to eliminate the problematic motion. In the case of respiratory motion, this can be accomplished through the use of breath-hold imaging. Similarly, bowel peristalsis can be reduced through the use of antispasmodics such as glucagon. The elimination of vascular pulsation is not recommended.

Frequently, the offending ghosts arise from structures not of particular interest to the imager such as subcutaneous fat (see Fig. 1.29) or the aorta (see Fig. 1.30) and inferior vena cava. In this case, the simple solution to the problem is to

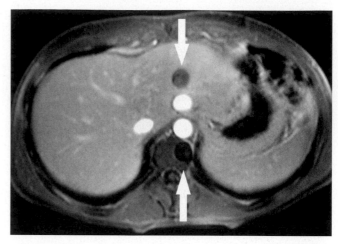

FIG. 1.30. Vascular pulsation artifact. Contrast-enhanced fat-suppressed T1-weighted gradient echo image shows multiple aortic phase ghosts along phase-encoding direction (*arrows*). Artifacts such as these could be mistaken for lesions of the left hepatic lobe or spine.

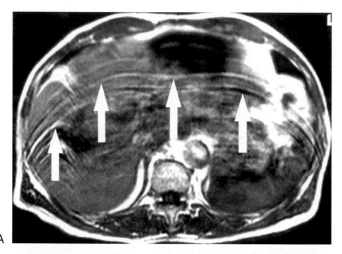

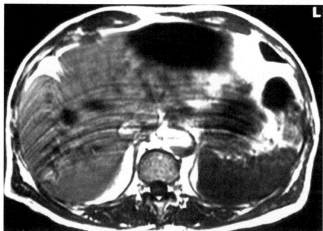

FIG. 1.29. Respiratory motion artifact. **A:** T1-weighted image through the upper abdomen obtained during free breathing. Image is severely degraded by respiratory motion. Note that ghosts (*arrows*) parallel the source of artifact (anterior abdominal fat). **B:** Modest reduction in respiratory artifact is achieved by increasing the number of signal averages from one to four (at the expense of scan time).

eliminate signal from the offending structure. This may be accomplished through the use of saturation bands applied over the anterior subcutaneous fat (see Fig. 1.7B) or, in the case of vascular artifact, applied cephalad and caudad to the imaging volume. Respiratory ghosting from anterior subcutaneous fat can also be limited by scanning with the patient prone, although this is unnecessary in most cases. In the case of peristalsis, elimination of signal from bowel requires the use of a negative oral contrast agent. Barium or iron-containing agents have been used successfully for this application, although few centers routinely administer bowel contrast.

A variety of hardware and software solutions to the problem of physiologic motion exist. By increasing the number of signal averages, the conspicuity of respiratory motion artifacts can be reduced (see Fig 1.29B). In a modification of this technique, the signal measurements to be averaged are separated in time to reduce the effects of low-frequency motion such as peristalsis. The techniques of respiratory triggering and gating require that a respiratory sensor be applied to the patient. This allows data acquisition to occur only when expiration is detected (in the case of triggering) or during a predefined end-expiratory period (in the case of gating). Because data are only acquired during part of the respiratory cycle, these techniques can significantly increase scan time (although the clear images produced often justify the additional time). One technique that does not increase scan time retrospectively reorders the echoes in k-space. The echoes acquired during the portion of the respiratory cycle having maximum motion are used to fill the outer lines of k-space. This technique improves image quality without increasing scan time, but still requires a respiratory sensor. It is important to be aware that not all respiratory artifact suppression techniques work with all pulse sequences.

Vascular pulsatile flow also results in phase errors that produce ghosts, the spacing of which decreases with increasing heart rate and decreasing TR. Vascular pulsation artifact differs from respiratory motion in that it affects less of the image and has a higher periodicity. Like respiratory motion, the resulting ghosts occur along the phase-encoding direction of the image (see Fig. 1.30). Typically, the phase-encoding direction for abdominal and pelvic imaging is anterior to posterior. This is done to allow for the use of a rectangular field of view that includes the entire abdomen. However, if vascular pulsation artifact is likely to obscure a structure of interest, such as the left lobe of the liver, the phase and frequency-encoding directions can be swapped, resulting in side-to-side artifacts that occur away from the area of interest. Vascular ghosts can be minimized by prescribing saturation bands parallel to the imaging plane to eliminate signal in the offending vessels or through the use of gradient moment nulling.

SECTION SUMMARY

1. Optimization of MR images requires compromises between the signal-to-noise ratio, scan time, and spatial resolution.

2. Scan time can be reduced through imaging parameter modifications, sequence substitutions, creative k-space sampling strategies, and parallel imaging techniques.

3. Improvements in spatial resolution result in smaller voxel size. Smaller voxel size results in a lower signal-to-noise ratio.

4. An increase in the signal-to-noise ratio may result in a prettier image, but an increase in the contrast-to-noise ratio is often more diagnostically relevant.

5. Abdominal and pelvic MR images may be degraded by a variety of artifacts. Not all artifacts must be eliminated, but they must be correctly identified to avoid confusion with genuine disease.

SUGGESTED READINGS

Hood MN, Ho VB, Smirniotopoulos JG, et al. Chemical shift: the artifact and clinical tool revisited. *Radiographics* 1999;19:357–371.

Ichikawa T, Araki T. Fast magnetic resonance imaging of the liver. *Eur J Radiol* 1999;29:186–210.

Mirowitz SA. MR imaging artifacts. Challenges and solutions. *Magn Reson Imaging Clin N Am* 1999;7:717–732.

Nitz WR. Fast and ultrafast non-echo-planar MR imaging techniques. *Eur Radiol* 2002;12:2866–2882.

van den Brink JS, Watanabe Y, Kuhl CK, et al. Implications of SENSE MR in routine clinical practice. *Eur J Radiol* 2003;46:3–27.

SECTION 1.3

Using Magnetic Resonance Contrast Agents in the Abdomen and Pelvis

INTRAVENOUS CONTRAST AGENTS

Intravenous magnetic resonance (MR) contrast agents are essential for the majority of abdominal and pelvic indications. Three main types of intravenous contrast agents are currently available for widespread clinical use: gadolinium chelates, manganese chelates, and superparamagnetic iron oxide. New agents are constantly being developed and tested, and new indications are being approved for existing agents. Therefore, one should always seek the most current information on approval status, indications, contraindications, and approved dosing. One should also be familiar with the package insert before administering any intravenous contrast agent.

Gadolinium Chelates

Four extracellular gadolinium-based agents have been approved for use in the United States. These agents are gadopentetate dimeglumine (Magnevist), gadodiamide (Omniscan), gadoteridol (ProHance), and gadoversetamide (OptiMARK). Of these agents, gadopentetate dimeglumine is ionic and the others are nonionic. Aside from this difference, the gadolinium chelates are very similar in most respects. After intravenous administration, these agents all equilibrate rapidly with the extracellular fluid space. They are all hyperosmolar to plasma, and none bind to serum proteins. All of the agents are eliminated almost entirely via renal excretion and are dialyzable. No clinically significant biliary excretion occurs with any of the gadolinium chelates listed. There are no significant differences in the imaging characteristics of these agents.

Other gadolinium chelates, none of which are currently approved for use in the United States, exhibit some hepatobiliary activity. These agents have the theoretical advantage for liver imaging of combining the benefits of an extracellular agent (e.g., vascular phase imaging) with the advantages of a hepatocyte-specific agent. One such agent, gadobenate dimeglumine (MultiHance), is currently available in Europe, but demonstrates only modest hepatic parenchymal retention and biliary excretion (5%). Another hepatobiliary agent under clinical development is gadolinium EOB-DTPA (Eovist). This agent has an ethoxybenzyl group that results in greater hepatocyte uptake and biliary excretion (roughly similar to its renal excretion) than achieved by gadobenate dimeglumine.

Mechanism of Action

Gadolinium chelates currently approved for use in the United States are paramagnetic extracellular agents. The paramagnetic nature of gadolinium causes shortening of the T1 relaxation time of nearby water protons, which results in increased signal intensity of tissues on T1-weighted images. In other words, the effect of gadolinium chelates on tissue is indirect. Because gadolinium chelates are extracellular agents, they do not cross cell membranes. Instead, these agents become distributed throughout the intravascular and interstitial spaces. In this respect, the extracellular gadolinium chelates behave in a similar manner to the iodinated contrast agents used for computed tomography (CT).

Imaging Appearance

Paramagnetic agents shorten the T1 relaxation time of nearby tissues, causing these tissues to appear brighter on T1-weighted MR images. Although paramagnetic agents also shorten T2 relaxation times, the T1 shortening effect predominates at typical tissue concentrations found after intravenous injection of a routine clinical dose. At higher concentrations, the T2 shortening effect predominates, resulting in signal loss (Figs. 1.31, 1.32). This effect is commonly seen in the renal collecting systems and bladder, where the gadolinium concentration increases markedly after contrast administration due to renal excretion of the contrast agent.

28

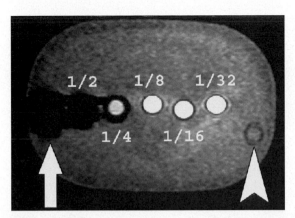

FIG. 1.31. Paramagnetic effects of gadolinium. A phantom consisting of varying concentrations of gadolinium chelate demonstrates relationship between gadolinium concentration and signal intensity on T1-weighted scan. Vial on far left is full-strength (0.5 mol/L) commercial preparation (*arrow*). Vial on far right of image is pure water (*arrowhead*). Each vial, from left to right, is half concentration of preceding vial. Note lack of signal from full-strength and half-strength preparations due to T2-shortening effect. T1-shortening effects predominate in less concentrated vials.

Indications

The indications for gadolinium-enhanced MR imaging (MRI) are similar to those for contrast-enhanced CT. In broad terms, the indications for intravenous contrast material include the detection and characterization of abdominal and pelvic pathology and the depiction of the abdominal and pelvic vasculature. Both sensitivity and specificity are improved for detection of most disease processes with the use of gadolinium chelates. We routinely use gadolinium for most

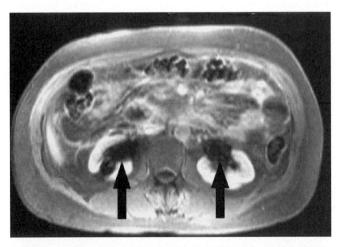

FIG. 1.32. Effect of concentrated gadolinium in renal collecting systems. Delayed fat suppressed T1-weighted gradient echo image shows dark, rather than bright, renal collecting systems (*arrows*) due to presence of concentrated gadolinium in urine. Earlier images with same sequence showed high signal intensity collecting systems due to lower gadolinium concentration in urine (not shown).

hepatic, renal, pancreatic, and vascular examinations. We selectively use gadolinium for adrenal and pelvic imaging. Not all gadolinium chelates are currently approved for all indications and age groups; refer to the appropriate package insert for the list of approved indications.

Contraindications and Special Clinical Scenarios

It is controversial whether cross-reactivity between gadolinium agents and iodinated contrast material exists. Therefore, caution should be exercised when administering gadolinium chelates to patients with a history of allergy or hypersensitivity to iodinated contrast. The use of prophylactic steroid treatment in patients allergic to iodinated contrast or gadolinium chelates before the administration of gadolinium chelates has not been thoroughly evaluated.

Significant nephrotoxicity has not been reported with the gadolinium chelates. Because these agents are dialyzable, they can be used safely in patients on renal dialysis. Multiple regularly scheduled dialysis sessions are required to clear the agent completely. The acceptable maximum duration between gadolinium administration and a patient's first dialysis session has not been established. Gadolinium chelates may be safely used in patients with hepatic dysfunction.

Gadolinium chelates are category C agents in the setting of pregnancy and should only be administered to pregnant women when the potential benefits clearly justify the potential risk to the fetus. Some preparations of gadolinium have been shown to cross the placenta and small amounts may be excreted in breast milk (1). However, gadolinium is poorly absorbed via the gastrointestinal tract, and there have been no reported adverse effects on an infant related to breast-feeding after maternal administration of an approved dose of gadolinium chelate. Despite the sparse data supporting this practice, many MR practitioners believe it may be prudent to temporarily interrupt breast-feeding for at least 24 hours following the administration of gadolinium to lactating women until more definitive safety data are available.

Intravenous gadolinium chelates pose a theoretical risk in patients with sickle cell anemia. Deoxygenated sickle erythrocytes align perpendicularly to an external magnetic field *in vitro*. It is feasible that paramagnetic contrast agents may potentiate this effect *in vivo*, possibly leading to vasoocclusive complications. Once again, no strong *in vivo* evidence exists to validate this concern.

Interestingly, gadodiamide and gadoversetamide have been shown to interfere with the colorimetric method of serum calcium measurement (2,3). As a result, serum calcium levels in patients who recently received these agents may falsely appear abnormally low.

Dose and Administration

The standard adult intravenous dose of currently available gadolinium chelates for abdominal and pelvic applications is 0.1 mmol/kg body weight administered at a rate of 1 to

2 mL/sec. A dose of 0.3 mmol/kg body weight should not be exceeded. The standard 0.1 mmol/kg dose also applies to pediatric patients for those agents approved for pediatric use. Not all intravenous gadolinium preparations have been approved for doses greater than 0.1 mmol/kg, rapid bolus injection, or multiple doses. Once again, we recommend checking the relevant package insert for more information before administering these agents.

Pitfalls

The goal of administering intravenous contrast agents for abdominal and pelvic MR applications is to increase the diagnostic efficacy of the examination. Contrast agents typically accomplish this goal by increasing lesion conspicuity. In many cases, the target lesion is a tumor within a solid organ, and tumors vary in enhancement characteristics based on their histologic properties and blood supply. Some tumors are most conspicuous during the arterial or venous phase of imaging, whereas other tumors are more conspicuous on precontrast images, becoming isointense to surrounding parenchyma after contrast administration. Therefore, an appropriately timed multiphase examination that includes precontrast images is critical to lesion detection in abdominal organs such as the liver and pancreas (Fig 1.33).

In most cases, fat suppression is recommended for postcontrast imaging with gadolinium. Fat suppression aids in improving image contrast between enhancing structures and the surrounding fat, particularly at the edges of organs. Keep in mind that non–radiofrequency (RF)-selective inversion recovery fat suppression techniques such as short tau inversion recovery (STIR) are not suitable for post-gadolinium imaging, because enhancing tissues can be suppressed along with other tissues having a short T1.

Some dynamic MR sequences are performed with an opposed-phase echo time (TE). In the setting of fatty infiltration of the liver, a nonenhancing lesion that is dark on precontrast in-phase T1-weighted images may exhibit pseudoenhancement when an opposed-phase dynamic contrast-enhanced scan is performed. The apparent enhancement of the lesion results from signal loss in the surrounding liver and not from contrast uptake by the cyst. Comparison to the precontrast images or subtracting the precontrast from postcontrast images usually resolves this issue (Fig 1.34).

Blood products may appear bright on a T1-weighted image due to the T1 shortening effects of methemoglobin. Therefore, a hematoma may be difficult to distinguish from an enhancing tumor if precontrast T1-weighted images are not obtained.

The T2 shortening effect of gadolinium may result in signal loss once gadolinium becomes sufficiently concentrated in a tissue. Therefore, for indications such as MR urography, it is important to reduce the dose of contrast administered, image quickly before the contrast becomes too concentrated, or hydrate the patient well to ensure dilution of the contrast within the renal collecting systems and ureters (Figs. 1.32, 1.35).

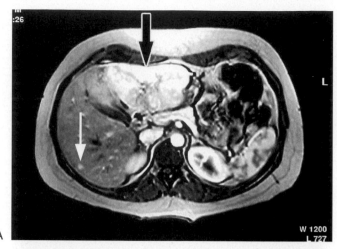

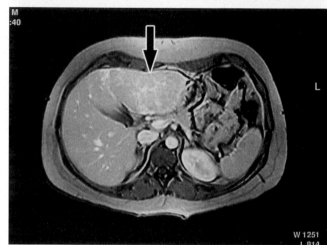

FIG. 1.33. Importance of multiphase imaging. **A:** Arterial phase gadolinium-enhanced T1-weighted image shows large focal nodular hyperplasia (FNH) in left lobe of liver (*arrow*) and second small hypervascular lesion in right lobe (*thin arrow*). **B:** More delayed image at same level only faintly shows large FNH (*arrow*) and fails to reveal smaller lesion in right lobe.

Similarly, gadolinium administered for *direct* MR venography must be diluted before administration.

Dynamic Imaging with Gadolinium Chelates

Indications

Rapid scanning techniques have ushered in the era of dynamic MRI of the abdomen and pelvis. As with CT, one can repeatedly image entire organs, achieving discrete temporal separation of vascular phases. In addition to increasing sensitivity for lesion detection, dynamic imaging improves the specificity of lesion characterization based on the pattern of contrast enhancement (4). In general, dynamic contrast-enhanced imaging is routinely recommended for the liver, pancreas, and kidneys. Evaluation and staging of neoplasms is often enhanced through the use of dynamic imaging. In addition, dynamic imaging provides "free" information about

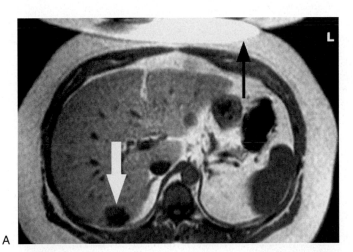

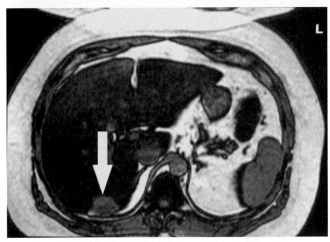

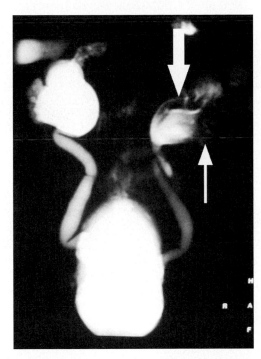

FIG. 1.35. Effect of gadolinium on MR urography. Static MR urogram performed in patient with bladder outlet obstruction using heavily T2-weighted sequence shows signal loss in left upper renal collecting system (*arrow*) and poor visualization of calyces due to presence of gadolinium (*thin arrow*).

FIG. 1.34. Pseudoenhancement of liver lesion due to hepatic steatosis. **A:** Cystic lesion of right hepatic lobe (*arrow*) has low signal intensity on in-phase gradient echo image. Note wraparound artifact from posterior subcutaneous fat (*thin arrow*). **B:** Lesion (*arrow*) appears relatively increased in signal intensity on opposed-phase image due to loss of hepatic parenchymal signal from hepatic steatosis. On postgadolinium images (not shown) performed with an opposed-phase echo time, this was misinterpreted by an inexperienced reader as enhancement.

the vascular anatomy. Because MRI does not involve the use of ionizing radiation, there is no increased risk associated with dynamic imaging other than the very small risk of administering an intravenous gadolinium chelate. Currently, dynamic contrast-enhanced MRI is only performed with gadolinium chelates, which can be injected rapidly. The currently approved manganese and iron-based contrast agents require a slower rate of administration.

Technique

For dynamic imaging to be performed, the gadolinium chelate must be injected rapidly. Favored injection rates vary, although a rate of 2 mL/sec works well for most applications. A mechanical injector is not critical for dynamic imaging,

but it is convenient and ensures uniformity and consistency. An experienced technologist can hand-inject contrast material and approximate the desired rate, although this requires the presence of a second person to initiate the scan at the appropriate time. Typically, injection of the contrast medium is followed by a saline flush of 15 to 20 mL. Successful dynamic imaging depends on adequate timing of the acquisition relative to the arrival of the contrast bolus. Typically, four sets of images are acquired: precontrast, arterial phase, portal venous phase, and equilibrium phase (Fig. 1.36). To achieve adequate temporal resolution and cover the entire organ of interest in a single breath-hold, the acquisition time for each phase should be kept as short as possible (while maintaining adequate spatial resolution and signal-to-noise ratio). On newer scanners, this can be easily achieved with acquisition times of less than 30 seconds per phase. Dynamic imaging can be performed with either a two-dimensional (2D) or a three-dimensional (3D) acquisition.

Timing

The benefits of dynamic imaging can only be reaped if the scans are performed when contrast enhancement of the organ of interest is optimal. This means that the data must be acquired at a specific time relative to the arrival of the contrast material. The appropriate scan delay varies depending on the information desired and the organ being imaged. Abdominal

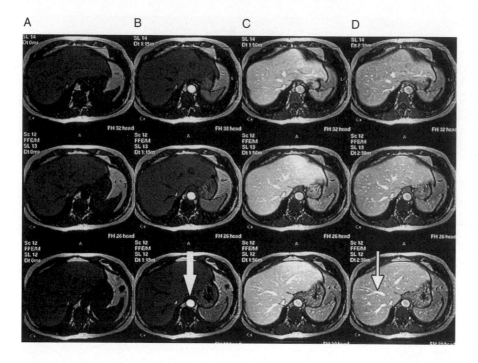

FIG. 1.36. Dynamic gadolinium-enhanced imaging. One precontrast **(A)** and three postcontrast **(B–D)** scans of upper abdomen were performed following bolus administration of intravenous gadolinium. Each T1-weighted gradient echo scan covered entire liver during breath-hold. Note varying signal intensity of hepatic parenchyma, aorta (*arrow*), and venous structures (*thin arrow*).

and pelvic organs do not enhance simultaneously, and peak parenchymal enhancement occurs at a slightly later time than peak arterial enhancement. Peak pancreatic enhancement occurs relatively early, approximately 15 seconds after the contrast agent arrives in the abdominal aorta (5). Like the pancreas, peak cortical enhancement of the kidneys occurs relatively soon after contrast injection. However, in many circumstances the corticomedullary phase is not as useful as the nephrogram phase obtained 90 seconds after contrast material injection. Maximal liver parenchymal enhancement occurs approximately 50 seconds after contrast injection; however, focal hepatic lesions may be more conspicuous at an earlier or later phase of enhancement (6).

In addition to differences between organs, there are considerable variations in optimal timing among patients. Peak hepatic enhancement in a young, healthy patient occurs sooner than in an older patient with poor cardiac function.

Adequate timing of a dynamic sequence can be achieved through the use of a timing bolus. This involves a 1- to 2-mL intravenous injection of contrast material while repeatedly imaging in a consistent location, most often at the level of the upper abdominal aorta. Typically, a gradient echo sequence is used, allowing rapid sequential imaging at approximately 1-second intervals. It is important that the timing bolus be injected at the same rate and with the same amount of saline flush as the actual diagnostic bolus. Even though the timing scan can be performed in any plane, some centers prefer the sagittal plane when timing the arrival of contrast material in the abdominal aorta, because this allows a larger portion of the vessel to be visualized and may reduce flow-related enhancement. Flow-related enhancement can result in increased signal in the vessel of interest that is not related to the arrival of the contrast bolus. This can mislead the technologist into

thinking that the contrast bolus has arrived, resulting in inaccurate timing. Flow-related enhancement is readily identified by its cyclic nature, resulting in alternating high and low signal intensity in the vessel occurring at regular intervals. The arrival of the timing bolus is marked by a relatively prolonged (over several cardiac cycles) and gradual increase in lumen signal intensity followed by a gradual decrease in signal. The disadvantage of using a sagittal scan plane for the timing run is that the technologist may confuse the inferior vena cava for the aorta or otherwise misplace the plane. This can be avoided with an axial imaging plane. A timing bolus may be difficult to visualize in vessels smaller than the aorta. Therefore, timing for a dynamic pelvic scan may be best performed using a timing scan centered over the lower aorta rather than over the iliac vessels.

Experienced radiologists or MR technologists may become adept at estimating the appropriate scan delay for a specific situation without the benefit of a timing bolus. Standard scan delay times can be implemented that result in successful dynamic imaging in most patients. This standard delay can then be modified in specific circumstances, or a timing run can be performed when a reasonable estimate cannot be made. However, such standard scan delay times are often not directly transferable between institutions because of scanner-specific variability in k-space ordering and acquisition times. Therefore, when instituting standard scan delays for abdominal and pelvic MRI, we suggest starting by timing each examination using a timing bolus until adequate experience is achieved. If a standard scan delay is chosen, take into account the cardiovascular status of the patient, location of the intravenous access (an intravenous line in the hand results in a later contrast arrival time than a central line), and injection rate.

Always check injector settings before injection. Common errors we have encountered include injection of the full diagnostic dose as a timing bolus, setting an injector delay instead of a scan delay (in this case, the injector will not inject until after the scan is initiated), and injection of an improper amount of contrast material due to errors in protocol selection or data entry.

Hepatobiliary Agents

Currently Available Agents

Of the hepatobiliary agents, only mangafodipir trisodium (Teslascan) has been approved for human intravenous use in the United States. Mangafodipir is a manganese-based paramagnetic contrast agent. Gadobenate dimeglumine (Multi-Hance) is a gadolinium-based agent currently approved for marketing in Europe. The following discussion pertains to the use of mangafodipir.

Mechanism of Action

Mangafodipir differs from the gadolinium chelates in several ways. Dissociation of the manganese ion from the fodipir moiety occurs relatively rapidly, as it is displaced by endogenous zinc. The fodipir is subsequently excreted in the urine, while much of the manganese is taken up by hepatocytes as well as the adrenal glands, pancreas, and kidneys. In the liver, the manganese is excreted in the bile and eliminated via the fecal route. For this reason, mangafodipir is classified as a hepatobiliary agent approved for liver imaging. Like gadolinium, manganese is paramagnetic and shortens the T1-relaxation time of surrounding tissue.

Imaging Appearance

Because of the T1 shortening properties of manganese, the liver parenchyma appears increased in signal intensity over baseline following the intravenous administration of mangafodipir. Tumors of hepatocellular origin, particularly if benign or well differentiated, may also take up this agent (Fig 1.37). Such lesions may demonstrate retention of the contrast agent relative to liver parenchyma on delayed images. With few exceptions, tumors not of hepatocellular origin (e.g., metastases) do not demonstrate appreciable uptake of manganese and appear dark compared to normal liver parenchyma (Fig. 1.38). Rim enhancement may occasionally occur in metastatic lesions, possibly due to bile stasis in the compressed or invaded liver parenchyma surrounding a metastatic mass.

Increased signal intensity of the liver can be appreciated on T1-weighted images up to 24 hours after injection. The adrenal glands, pancreas, and renal cortices also demonstrate increased signal intensity over baseline on mangafodipir-enhanced T1-weighted images. Because manganese is excreted in the bile, the bile ducts may also appear bright on delayed ($\geq$15 minutes) T1-weighted images (Fig 1.39).

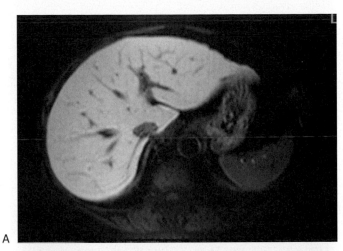

A

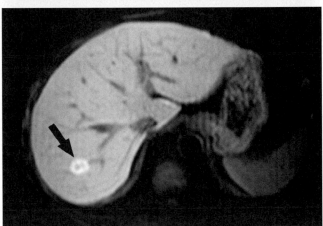

B

FIG. 1.37. Mangafodipir-enhanced image. **A:** Fat-suppressed T1-weighted image obtained 1 hour after administration of mangafodipir shows increased signal intensity of liver parenchyma. **B:** Seven hours after mangafodipir administration, a small lesion (presumed focal nodular hyperplasia faintly seen on the 1-hour scan) is quite conspicuous (*arrow*).

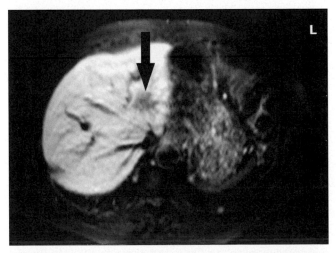

FIG. 1.38. Metastasis detected with mangafodipir. Fat-suppressed, post-mangafodipir T1-weighted image shows lesion (*arrow*) in left hepatic lobe that does not take up mangafodipir. Biopsy revealed metastatic pancreatic cancer.

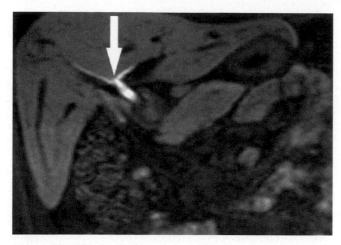

FIG. 1.39. Bile duct enhancement following intravenous administration of mangafodipir. Coronal image from fat-suppressed three-dimensional gradient echo sequence demonstrates high signal intensity of bile ducts (*arrow*) containing excreted manganese.

Indications

Mangafodipir is approved by the Food and Drug Administration (FDA) for liver imaging. Due to its hepatocyte uptake, it can help distinguish between lesions of hepatocellular and nonhepatocellular origin (7). Mangafodipir may also aid in determining the number and location of hepatic metastases as part of treatment planning. Mangafodipir has been investigated as a pancreatic imaging agent and as a means of performing contrast-enhanced magnetic resonance cholangiopancreatography.

Contraindications and Special Clinical Scenarios

Mangafodipir should be avoided in patients with known hypersensitivity to manganese or the ligand fodipir (dipyridoxyl diphosphate). As with all intravenous contrast agents, mangafodipir should be used with caution in patients with previous history of hypersensitivity or allergy of any type. Manganese has a prolonged half-life in patients with hepatic dysfunction. However mangafodipir is not contraindicated in this setting if a sufficiently compelling reason exists to administer this particular agent. No convincing evidence exists to suggest mangafodipir is unsafe in the setting of biliary obstruction, although the bulk of available data involves animal studies.

As with other intravenous MR contrast agents, mangafodipir is a category C substance and should not be administered to pregnant women except in extraordinary circumstances when the potential benefit to the patient justifies the potential risk to the fetus. Manganese has been shown to cross the placenta and may be excreted in breast milk. Therefore, the package insert for Teslascan recommends that nursing be temporarily discontinued following administration of this agent.

Dose and Administration

The approved intravenous dose of mangafodipir is 5 μmol/kg body weight administered over several minutes. Mangafodipir is not suitable for bolus injection, and a total dose of 15 mL should not be exceeded. Imaging may begin with fat-suppressed T1-weighted scans approximately 5 minutes after contrast administration. Tumors of hepatocellular origin tend to retain mangafodipir longer than surrounding liver. Therefore, delayed imaging may be helpful in demonstrating uptake of the contrast agent by lesions of hepatocellular origin. Diagnostically useful images may be obtained up to 24 hours after contrast administration. Repeated doses are unnecessary given the wide window of opportunity for imaging after injection.

Mangafodipir may have an increased association with nausea and vomiting compared to other intravenous MR contrast agents.

Pitfalls

Whereas mangafodipir helps categorize liver lesions as hepatocellular or nonhepatocellular in origin, it does not reliably distinguish between benign and malignant etiologies. Well-differentiated hepatocellular carcinoma, in addition to benign hepatic adenoma and focal nodular hyperplasia, may enhance with mangafodipir if they contain sufficient numbers of functioning hepatocytes. In other words, an enhancing lesion in the liver on a T1-weighted image obtained after administration of mangafodipir could be a benign primary hepatic tumor or a hepatocellular carcinoma. Furthermore, cysts and hemangiomas do not incorporate mangafodipir and may mimic metastases on postcontrast T1-weighted images. Therefore, the characteristics of a liver lesion on precontrast T1- and T2-weighted images must be taken into account when interpreting any MR examination of the liver performed with mangafodipir. Rarely, nonhepatocellular tumors may enhance with mangafodipir (8).

Superparamagnetic Iron Oxides

Currently Available Agents

Only one form of superparamagnetic iron oxides (SPIO) is currently approved for human use in the United States. This agent goes by the generic name ferumoxides and the trade name Feridex in the United States (Endorem in Europe). This agent consists of aggregates of small iron-based particles coated with dextran.

Mechanism of Action

SPIOs are phagocytosed in the hepatic sinusoids by Kupffer cells of the reticuloendothelial system (RES). The agent is also taken up by RES cells in the spleen and bone marrow. Eventually, the iron component enters the body's normal iron metabolic cycle. The dominant effect of SPIOs is to create distortions of the local magnetic field through susceptibility effects. This results in decreased signal intensity of the liver parenchyma, spleen, and bone marrow, best appreciated on T2 and T2*-weighted images.

Imaging Appearance

Following the injection of ferumoxides, the liver should be imaged with a T2 or T2*-weighted sequence. A T2*-weighted image may be produced using a spoiled gradient echo sequence with a relatively long TE. The decrease in hepatic signal intensity caused by SPIOs persists for many hours, allowing for repeat imaging hours after contrast administration. This effect may be less pronounced in the setting of cirrhosis. Liver lesions lacking Kupffer cells do not incorporate SPIOs and appear bright relative to liver parenchyma on T2 and T2*-weighted images after SPIO infusion. It is important to obtain precontrast T2 or T2*-weighted images in order to reliably determine whether a hepatic lesion (such as focal nodular hyperplasia) has taken up ferumoxides on postcontrast images.

Indications

SPIOs have been approved by the FDA for liver imaging and may increase the sensitivity and specificity of T2-weighted imaging of hepatic lesions. Therefore, SPIOs may be helpful in determining the number and location of liver metastases for treatment planning or in characterizing lesions containing significant numbers of active Kupffer cells such as focal nodular hyperplasia (Fig. 1.40).

Contraindications and Special Clinical Scenarios

Ferumoxides should be avoided in patients with known hypersensitivity to parenteral iron, dextran, or any other component of the commercially available product. A unique complication associated with ferumoxides is back, groin, or leg pain, which has been reported to be severe enough to cause interruption or discontinuation of contrast agent infusion in as many as 2.5% of patients according to the package insert. Symptoms generally develop within 15 minutes of starting the infusion and the incidence of back, leg, or groin pain is higher in patients with cirrhosis. SPIOs should not be administered to patients with systemic iron overload (i.e., hemochromatosis).

Dose and Administration

Feridex is administered as an intravenous infusion of 0.56 mg iron/kg body weight (0.05 mL of product/kg body weight) diluted in 100 mL 5% dextrose. The infusion should be administered over no less than 30 minutes through a 5-micron filter. Faster infusion rates may result in a higher incidence of severe back pain or vasodilation and hypotension. Imaging may begin immediately after completion of the infusion or

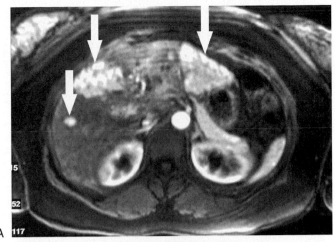

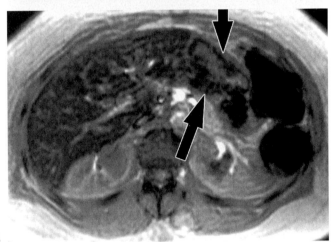

FIG. 1.40. Use of Feridex to characterize liver lesions. **A:** Multiple incidentally discovered lesions (*arrows*) within liver demonstrate brisk arterial enhancement on gadolinium-enhanced dynamic study suspicious for focal nodular hyperplasia (FNH). **B:** T2*-weighted gradient echo image after intravenous administration of ferumoxides shows uptake of agent by lesions, best demonstrated in the periphery of the left lateral segment lesion (*arrows*). This confirms Kupffer cell activity within the lesions, a finding compatible with diagnosis of FNH.

up to 3.5 hours after completion of the infusion. Repeated doses are unnecessary given the wide window of opportunity for imaging after injection.

Pitfalls

Any tumor containing sufficient numbers of Kupffer cells may decrease in signal intensity following administration of ferumoxides. Therefore, these agents cannot always distinguish between benign liver tumors having Kupffer cell activity, such as focal nodular hyperplasia, and some well-differentiated hepatocellular carcinomas. However, the signal loss seen with focal nodular hyperplasia tends to exceed that seen with other focal hepatic lesions (9). Similarly, benign lesions without Kupffer cell activity cannot be distinguished reliably from metastases based solely on the post-SPIO images.

Intravenous Contrast Agent Combinations

It may be advantageous to exploit the varying mechanisms of uptake and elimination of the different intravenous contrast agents available for hepatic imaging to improve lesion detection and characterization. This could be accomplished by administering different contrast agents to the same patient on different days, but this is inconvenient. Some investigators have explored the feasibility of administering two different liver agents sequentially during a single examination (10–14). In most cases, this involves a gadolinium chelate and either mangafodipir or ferumoxides. Although reports are limited, available data suggest that both mangafodipir and ferumoxides can be administered as part of a gadolinium-enhanced examination. Dynamic gadolinium-enhanced imaging can be performed immediately after imaging with a superparamagnetic iron oxide with no degradation of postgadolinium sequences. Ferumoxides or gadolinium can be administered in either order without significant loss of diagnostic information. Despite the feasibility of administering contrast agents with different mechanisms of action during a single imaging session, further study is needed to determine whether this approach increases the sensitivity of MRI for the detection of focal hepatic lesions. Therefore, we recommend that double contrast imaging be reserved for cases in which the expected benefit of adding a second agent justifies the resulting additional expense and prolonged examination time.

ENTERIC AGENTS

Enteric contrast agents are not used routinely in abdominal and pelvic MRI as they are with CT. Many MRI examinations of the abdomen and pelvis are performed to evaluate a specific finding in a solid organ of a patient who has had a previous cross-sectional imaging study. In this setting, enteric contrast agents contribute little to the clinical question, although they may improve image quality. As more MRI examinations are performed to evaluate specific symptoms rather than radiographic findings, the use of enteric contrast may increase.

There are two main categories of enteric MR contrast agents: those that eliminate signal from within bowel (negative contrast agents) and those that increase signal within the bowel lumen (positive contrast agents). By eliminating signal from bowel, artifacts from peristalsis or respiratory motion may be reduced. On MRCP images, high signal intensity within the stomach and duodenum, which can obscure the biliary tree and pancreatic duct, is eliminated with negative contrast agents. A dark bowel lumen is also advantageous when evaluating the bowel wall or organs such as the pancreas with intravenous contrast agents. In some cases, however, it is preferable to enhance visibility of the bowel lumen with a positive contrast agent to better delineate anatomy or evaluate bowel pathology. Some agents provide both low and high in-

traluminal signal, depending on the pulse sequence used. For example, water increases signal intensity within the bowel lumen on T2-weighted images while reducing signal intensity on T1-weighted images. Conversely, a paramagnetic contrast agent at the appropriate concentration may increase signal intensity within the bowel lumen on T1-weighted images while reducing signal intensity on T2-weighted images. Even though many enteric contrast agents have been proposed or investigated for use in abdominal and pelvic MRI, only a few agents are currently used to any degree in clinical practice (15–20).

Positive Oral Contrast Agents

The least expensive and simplest positive oral contrast agent to administer is water. Water within the bowel lumen appears bright on fat-suppressed T2-weighted images. When combined with HASTE imaging, water can provide excellent anatomic information and visualization of the bowel wall and lumen (Fig. 1.41). The utility of plain water as an oral contrast agent, however, only extends as far as the stomach and proximal small bowel. Other agents have been proposed as positive oral contrast agents to overcome the problem of water absorption, thereby permitting evaluation of the distal small bowel. In particular, polyethylene glycol appears to be significantly better than water for visualization of the distal small bowel (20). This agent is commonly used for bowel cleansing and, therefore, is readily available in most hospitals.

Paramagnetic contrast agents containing dilute gadolinium, ferric chloride, ferric ammonium citrate, or manganese chloride can be effective but are seldom used clinically. Blueberry juice is naturally high in manganese and has been used as a positive oral contrast agent (16). When used at the

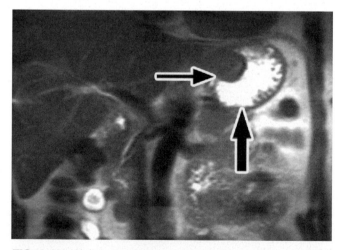

FIG. 1.41. Water as a positive oral contrast agent. Initial MR images (not shown) through upper abdomen suggested incidental mass in gastroesophageal region. Patient was removed from scanner and given several cups of water to drink. Repeat image performed with HASTE sequence clearly demonstrates high signal intensity water (*arrow*) outlining smoothly contoured mass (leiomyoma) (*thin arrow*).

appropriate concentration, paramagnetic agents result in T1 shortening of bowel contents, which appear bright on a fat-suppressed T1-weighted scan. Concentrated paramagnetic contrast agents also result in T2 shortening, resulting in a negative contrast effect on T2-weighted scans. Most paramagnetic positive oral contrast agents are limited by the effects of dilution as the contrast travels further along the bowel. In addition, because these agents increase the signal intensity of bowel on T1-weighted images, peristaltic motion artifact is exacerbated unless glucagon is administered.

In general, oral contrast agents provide limited utility in the colon, because they are either absorbed by the small bowel, diluted by the bowel contents, or do not mix well with bowel contents. Therefore, when colon imaging is of primary concern, it may be preferable to administer the contrast agent per rectum.

Negative Oral Contrast Agents

Negative oral contrast agents are used to suppress signal from the bowel lumen and are often combined with intravenous gadolinium for depiction of the bowel wall. In addition to its utility as a positive agent, water may also be an effective negative contrast agent when gadolinium-enhanced, fat-suppressed T1-weighted imaging is employed. Barium suspension is another effective, relatively inexpensive negative contrast agent for T1-weighted imaging. Barium has the advantage of not being significantly absorbed by the gastrointestinal tract and is readily available in radiology departments.

Superparamagnetic contrast agents consist of iron oxide particles in various types of inert material. They are more expensive than barium solutions, but are effective in reducing the intraluminal signal of bowel on many common MR sequences (Fig. 1.42). On fast 3D T1-weighted sequences with very short repetition and echo times, some superparam-

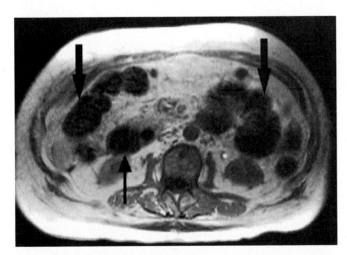

FIG. 1.42. Iron-based oral contrast. T1-weighted gradient echo image obtained after oral ingestion of iron-based contrast agent. Note the diminished signal intensity of small bowel (*arrows*). Such agents are particularly useful for eliminating signal from *duodenum* (*thin arrow*) for evaluation of pancreas.

agnetic contrast agents may increase the signal intensity of bowel contents.

Other Enteric Contrast Agents

Many other enteric contrast agents have been proposed or tested, such as perfluorochemicals, hyperpolarized noble gases, and oil emulsions. Because these compounds are either not widely available or are relatively expensive, they are seldom used clinically. Methylcellulose has been used successfully for MR enteroclysis but requires enteral intubation and cannot be administered orally.

SECTION SUMMARY

1. Three general categories of intravenous MR contrast agents are currently available—extracellular gadolinium chelates, hepatobiliary agents (e.g., mangafodipir trisodium), and reticuloendothelial agents (e.g., superparamagnetic iron oxide).
2. Extracellular gadolinium chelates are paramagnetic agents that shorten the T1 relaxation time of surrounding tissues.
3. Dynamic imaging after bolus administration of gadolinium chelates is indicated for the majority of contrast-enhanced MR examinations of the liver, pancreas, and kidneys as well as for many other abdominal and pelvic applications.
4. Selection of a scan delay appropriate for the organ of interest is essential to successful contrast-enhanced dynamic imaging.
5. Mangafodipir trisodium is a paramagnetic hepatobiliary agent. The manganese component is taken up by normal hepatocytes and excreted in the bile. Some well-differentiated tumors of hepatocellular origin may also accumulate this agent.
6. Superparamagnetic iron oxide particles (ferumoxides) are taken up by the reticuloendothelial system and decrease the signal intensity of the liver on T2 and T2*-weighted images. Liver tumors with sufficient numbers of Kupffer cells also accumulate ferumoxides.
7. Intravenous contrast agents can be used in combination when a single agent is insufficient for evaluation of the liver.
8. Many different enteric contrast agents have been tested, but few have found widespread application for abdominal and pelvic MRI. Water and barium are well-tolerated and cost-effective enteric agents.

REFERENCES

1. Kubik-Huch RA, Gottstein-Aalame NM, Frensel T, et al. Gadopentetate dimeglumine excretion into human breast milk during lactation. *Radiology* 2000;216:555–558.
2. Normann PT, Froysa A, Svaland M. Interference of gadodiamide injection (OMNISCAN) on the colorimetric determination of serum calcium. *Scand J Clin Lab Invest* 1995;55:421–426.

3. Lin J, Idee JM, Port M, et al. Interference of magnetic resonance imaging contrast agents with the serum calcium measurement technique using colorimetric reagents. *J Pharm Biomed Anal* 1999;21:931–943.
4. Quillin SP, Atilla S, Brown JJ, et al. Characterization of focal hepatic masses by dynamic contrast-enhanced MR imaging: findings in 311 lesions. *Magn Reson Imaging* 1997;15:275–285.
5. Kanematsu M, Shiratori Y, Hoshi H, et al. Pancreas and peripancreatic vessels: effect of imaging delay on gadolinium enhancement at dynamic gradient-recalled-echo MR imaging. *Radiology* 2000;215:95–102.
6. Coche EE, Bret PM, Reinhold C. Dynamic enhancement of upper abdominal organs in normal volunteers with MRI and effects of contrast dose reduction. *Abdom Imaging* 1999;24:604–609.
7. Liou J, Lee JK, Borrello JA, et al. Differentiation of hepatomas from non-hepatomatous masses: use of MnDPDP-enhanced MR images. *Magn Reson Imaging* 1994;12:71–79.
8. Mathieu D, Coffin C, Kobeiter H, et al. Unexpected MR-T1 enhancement of endocrine liver metastases with mangafodipir. *J Magn Reson Imaging* 1999;10:193–195.
9. Paley MR, Mergo PJ, Torres GM, et al. Characterization of focal hepatic lesions with ferumoxides-enhanced T2-weighted MR imaging. *AJR* 2000;175:159–163.
10. Halavaara J, Tervahartiala P, Isoniemi H, et al. Efficacy of sequential use of superparamagnetic iron oxide and gadolinium in liver MR imaging. *Acta Radiologica* 2002;43:180–185.
11. Kubaska S, Sahani DV, Saini S, et al. Dual contrast enhanced magnetic resonance imaging of the liver with superparamagnetic iron oxide followed by gadolinium for lesion detection and characterization. *Clin Radiol* 2001;56:410–415.
12. Martin DR, Semelka RC, Chung JJ, et al. Sequential use of gadolinium chelate and mangafodipir trisodium for the assessment of focal liver lesions: initial observations. *Magn Reson Imaging* 2000;18:955–963.
13. Semelka RC, Lee JK, Worrawattanakul S, et al. Sequential use of ferumoxide particles and gadolinium chelate for the evaluation of focal liver lesions on MRI. *J Magn Reson Imaging* 1998;8:670–674.
14. Ward J, Guthrie JA, Scott DJ, et al. Hepatocellular carcinoma in the cirrhotic liver: double-contrast MR imaging for diagnosis. *Radiology* 2000;216:154–162.
15. Grubnic S, Padhani AR, Revell PB, et al. Comparative efficacy of and sequence choice for two oral contrast agents used during MR imaging. *AJR* 1999;173:173–178.
16. Hiraishi K, Narabayashi I, Fujita O, et al. Blueberry juice: preliminary evaluation as an oral contrast agent in gastrointestinal MR imaging. *Radiology* 1995;194:119–123.
17. Kivelitz D, Gehl HB, Heuck A, et al. Ferric ammonium citrate as a positive bowel contrast agent for MR imaging of the upper abdomen. Safety and diagnostic efficacy. *Acta Radiol* 1999;40:429–435.
18. Laghi A, Carbone I, Catalano C, et al. Polyethylene glycol solution as an oral contrast agent for MR imaging of the small bowel. *AJR* 2001;177:1333–1334.
19. Malcolm PN, Brown JJ, Hahn PF, et al. The clinical value of ferric ammonium citrate: a positive oral contrast agent for T1-weighted MR imaging of the upper abdomen. *J Magn Reson Imaging* 2000;12:702–707.
20. Sood RR, Joubert I, Franklin H, et al. Small bowel MRI: comparison of a polyethylene glycol preparation and water as oral contrast media. *J Magn Reson Imaging* 2002;15:401–408.

SUGGESTED READINGS

Giovagnoni A, Fabbri A, Maccioni F. Oral contrast agents in MRI of the gastrointestinal tract. *Abdom Imaging* 2002;27:367–375.

Scheidler J, Reiser MF. MRI of the female and male pelvis: current and future applications of contrast enhancement. *Eur J Radiol* 2000;34:220–228.

Weinmann HJ, Ebert W, Misselwitz B, et al. Tissue-specific MR contrast agents. *Eur J Radiol* 2003;46:33–44.

SECTION 1.4

Abdominal and Pelvic Protocol Basics

All of the preceding information in this text serves primarily to provide the reader with the necessary tools to establish and understand magnetic resonance (MR) protocols for the abdomen and pelvis and to modify those protocols to ensure that diagnostically useful images are obtained within a reasonable amount of time. Due to hardware and software variations among different MR systems, no single textbook can provide detailed MR imaging (MRI) protocols that can be directly applied to every scanner. Individuals have their own tolerance or preferences for image noise, artifacts, scan time, and imaging planes. Any attempt to provide detailed vendor-specific protocols would please a few individuals while frustrating most others. Therefore, the following discussion provides generic versions of abdominal and pelvic protocols that can be used to develop specific protocols for unique practice situations. First, the most commonly used sequences for abdominal and pelvic imaging are reviewed, then a framework for specific clinical scenarios is provided to serve as a starting point for protocol development. We purposely omit parameters that must be individualized for each patient, such as field of view (FOV). Also note that specific parameters such as the repetition time (TR) and echo time (TE) vary according to personal preference, scanner type, desired imaging time, and field strength. The numbers provided herein should only serve as a starting point. We assume a field strength of 1.5 tesla (T) throughout, because this value is commonly used for abdominal and pelvic work. However, most of the principles presented herein are equally relevant to scanning at lower or higher clinically available field strengths.

We believe that many abdominal and pelvic MRI examinations require some degree of monitoring by a knowledgeable individual to ensure a diagnostically useful study is done. This monitoring allows additional sequences or imaging planes to be performed to best demonstrate pertinent anatomy or characterize lesions. In addition, because patient compliance varies considerably, protocol modifications may be necessary to accommodate a patient's clinical status.

COMMONLY USED SEQUENCES

Most MR protocols for the abdomen and pelvis contain a combination of T1- and T2-weighted sequences. The following discussion reviews the advantages and disadvantages of various T1- and T2-weighted techniques.

T1-Weighted Sequences

Spin Echo

Uses: T1-weighted non–breath-hold imaging of the abdomen and pelvis.

Strengths: High-resolution T1-weighted imaging is possible when motion is not a problem.

Weaknesses: Motion artifacts are difficult to completely eliminate. Sequences are time consuming.

Parameters: Most T1-weighted spin echo sequences use a TR of less than 500 msec and a TE as low as possible. Up to four signal averages are typically used. A rectangular FOV with anterior-posterior phase-encoding direction is most time efficient.

Echo Train Spin Echo (FSE, TSE)

Uses: T1-weighted imaging of the pelvis.

Strengths: A good compromise between spin echo and gradient echo in terms of image quality and scan time.

Weaknesses: Relatively few slices can be obtained during a single breath-hold.

Parameters: TR and TE should be kept as low as possible. A typical sequence has a TR of less than 500 msec and TE of 12 to 15 msec. The echo train length is commonly set at 3 but can be adjusted (with adjustments in the TR).

Two-Dimensional Spoiled Gradient Echo (FLASH, T1FFE, SPGR)

Uses: Breath-hold T1-weighted imaging of the abdomen and pelvis, often with in-phase and opposed-phase echo times.

Strengths: Breath-hold in-phase and opposed-phase imaging possible.

Weaknesses: Lower signal-to-noise ratio than spin echo techniques. Susceptibility artifact is more apparent.

Parameters: For in-phase imaging, the TR is usually 100 to 150 msec with the TE set at 4 to 4.5 msec. For opposed-phase imaging, the TE is set at 1.9 to 2.3 msec. Dual-echo sequences allow in-phase and opposed-phase echoes to be acquired during one TR and are usually preset for the appropriate echo times. The TR may be adjusted to accommodate modifications in other scan parameters. A flip angle of 70 to 80 degrees allows for adequate T1-weighted contrast and signal. Because these are breath-hold sequences, multiple signal averages are not used. The sampling bandwidth can be adjusted to alter scan time, image noise, or chemical shift artifact.

Three-Dimensional Spoiled Gradient Echo (VIBE)

Uses: Breath-hold dynamic contrast-enhanced imaging of the abdomen and pelvis.

Strengths: Allows rapid imaging with high through-plane spatial resolution. Isotropic voxel size can be achieved on some scanners, allowing high-quality vascular reconstructions in any plane.

Weaknesses: Motion causes degradation of entire data set.

Parameters: TR and TE should be minimized (TR < 5 msec, TE < 2 msec). A low flip angle (e.g., 15 degrees) allows for adequate T1 contrast. Zerofill interpolation is routinely used.

T2-Weighted Techniques

Half-Fourier Single-Shot Echo Train Spin Echo (HASTE, ssTSE, ssFSE)

Uses: Breath-hold localizer, rapid abdominal survey, fetal imaging, MR cholangiopancreatography (MRCP), bowel imaging, and MR urography.

Strengths: Very resistant to motion and susceptibility artifact. Cysts and hemangiomas appear very bright. Imaging times are brief (approximately 1 second or less per image).

Weaknesses: Images limited by relatively low signal-to-noise ratio and blurring. Malignant lesions within solid organs may be less conspicuous.

Parameters: The TR is infinite, because the excitation pulse is applied only once per image. The TE can be adjusted as desired. A short TE (40 to 60 msec) provides the best signal-to-noise ratio. A longer TE may be desirable in some cases for imaging fluid-filled structures. Flow artifacts may be accentuated with a longer TE. Generally, a single signal average and a flip angle of 150 to 180 degrees are used.

Echo Train Spin Echo (FSE, TSE)

Uses: Non–breath-hold imaging of the abdomen and pelvis.

Strengths: Good signal-to-noise ratio, good contrast-to-noise ratio.

Weaknesses: Time consuming. Image quality limited by motion unless some type of respiratory compensation (e.g., triggering) is used.

Parameters: For most abdominal and pelvic applications, the TR should be 2,000 to 5,000 msec and the TE should be 70 to 90 msec. The TR can be adjusted within this range to accommodate other parameter modifications. An echo train length of 8 to 16 with up to four signal averages is commonly used.

GraSE

Uses: General T2-weighted imaging of the abdomen.

Strengths: Relatively quick. Lower specific absorption rate than echo train spin echo techniques.

Weaknesses: Not widely available, limited clinical experience.

Parameters: A TR of 1,800 works well for most applications. Adjust the TE as for a fast spin echo sequence. Two signal averages, an echo train length of 14, and an EPI factor of 3 (i.e., the number of gradient echoes per spin echo) provide images similar to a standard echo train spin echo sequence.

TurboSTIR

Uses: Breath-hold fat-suppressed T2-weighted imaging of the abdomen.

Strengths: Covers most organs in one or two breath-holds. Uniform fat suppression can be achieved. Good lesion conspicuity in solid organs.

Weaknesses: Relatively low signal-to-noise ratio.

Parameters: A TR of 3,800 msec, TE of 70 to 80 msec, flip angle of 150 degrees, and an inversion time (TI) (for fat suppression) of 165 msec works well for most applications.

ABDOMINAL AND PELVIC PROTOCOLS

The following are examples of abdominal and pelvic protocols to serve as a starting point. We recommend using a phased-array surface coil whenever possible, although it is difficult to cover the entire abdomen and pelvis in a single FOV with most commercially available surface coils. For this reason, it is usually not possible to perform high-quality, contrast-enhanced dynamic MRI of both the abdomen and pelvis in the axial plane with a phased-array surface coil. If contrast-enhanced imaging of both the abdomen and pelvis is desired during a single session, one must determine where dynamic imaging will be most useful. In addition, each time a different anatomic region is examined, the surface coil must be repositioned and new localizer images obtained. In the rare case when high-quality dynamic imaging of both the abdomen and pelvis is required, it may be necessary to schedule the patient for examinations on two different days, because persistent enhancement of some anatomic structures from the first dynamic study may impact the quality of a second contrast-enhanced examination performed without sufficient delay.

Basic Abdominal Protocol

General comments: Many abdominal protocols are slight variations of a simple protocol (Fig. 1.43) such as that below. We have found this protocol to be effective for the majority of liver, pancreas, adrenal, and renal examinations. When developing a protocol, it may be helpful to start with this one, modifying it to suit the specific clinical scenario. Additional information on specific techniques such as MR angiography (MRA), MRCP, and MR urography is provided in Section 2.

Breath-hold localizer: HASTE/ssFSE/ ssTSE
    Purpose: General survey, breath-hold localizer
    Respiratory: Breath-hold
    Imaging plane: Coronal
    Slice thickness: 8 mm
In-phase and opposed-phase T1: Dual-echo spoiled gradient echo
    Purpose: Characterization of lipid-containing lesions
    Respiratory: Breath-hold
    Imaging plane: Axial
    Slice thickness: 6 to 8 mm
Fat-suppressed T2: FSE/TSE, GraSE, or turboSTIR
    Purpose: Lesion characterization, detection of lymphadenopathy and fluid
    Respiratory: Breath-hold for turboSTIR; triggered for FSE or GraSE
    Imaging plane: Axial
    Slice thickness: 6 to 8 mm
Dynamic gadolinium-enhanced T1: 2D or 3D spoiled gradient echo (fat-suppressed if possible)
    Purpose: Lesion detection and characterization; depiction of vascular anatomy
    Respiratory: Breath-hold (expiration preferred)
    Imaging plane: Axial
    Slice thickness: 6 to 8 mm (2D), <5 mm (3D)
    Injection rate and volume: 2 mL/sec for 20 mL
    Initial scan delay: Based on test bolus and organ of interest
    Number of scans: Precontrast, arterial, venous (45 seconds), equilibrium (90 seconds)
Delayed fat-suppressed T1: 2D or 3D spoiled gradient echo
    Purpose: Lesion characterization (particularly hemangioma and cholangiocarcinoma)
    Respiratory: Breath-hold (expiration preferred)
    Imaging plane: Variable
    Slice thickness: Same as dynamic study

Liver Protocol Modifications

Adjust slice thickness, rectangular FOV, and matrix to cover the entire liver in a single breath-hold for breath-hold sequences. In-phase and opposed-phase imaging and breath-hold T2-weighted imaging may be performed in one or two breath-holds to improve image quality.
    Optional elements:

- Coronal or sagittal imaging for lesions near the liver dome.
- MRCP protocol for assessment of bile ducts.
- Long TE ($\geq$140 msec) T2-weighted images for characterization of cyst or hemangioma (Fig. 1.44).

Pancreas Protocol Modifications

Adjust slice thickness, rectangular FOV, and matrix to cover entire pancreas in a single breath-hold for breath-hold sequences. The use of fat suppression is important for evaluation of the pancreas. If dynamic scans cannot be fat-suppressed, subtraction of the precontrast scan from subsequent contrast-enhanced scans is recommended (as long as misregistration between scans is minimal).
    Optional elements:

- Precontrast fat-suppressed T1-weighted sequence (spin echo or spoiled gradient echo) for assessment of pancreatic parenchyma.
- Coronal or sagittal imaging to determine relationship of pancreatic or peripancreatic masses to adjacent organs (e.g., stomach, spleen).
- MRCP protocol for assessment of biliary and pancreatic ducts.

Renal Protocol Modifications

Adjust slice thickness, rectangular FOV, and matrix to cover both kidneys in a single breath-hold for breath-hold sequences. Include precontrast fat-suppressed T1-weighted sequence for differentiation between fat and blood products. The optimal imaging plane for the dynamic sequence should be based on the location of the lesion. Coronal imaging may show lesions of the renal poles to better advantage than axial imaging. Coronal imaging may also allow for superior vascular anatomic displays in some cases. It may be helpful to acquire the delayed postcontrast scan in an orthogonal plane relative to the dynamic scan.
    Optional elements:

- Noncontrast MRA sequence to evaluate the renal vein and inferior vena cava in the setting of renal cell carcinoma (see Fig. 2.17).
- MR urography sequence to evaluate the collecting system.

Adrenal Protocol Modifications

Adjust slice thickness, rectangular FOV, and matrix to cover both adrenal glands in a single breath-hold. For evaluation of

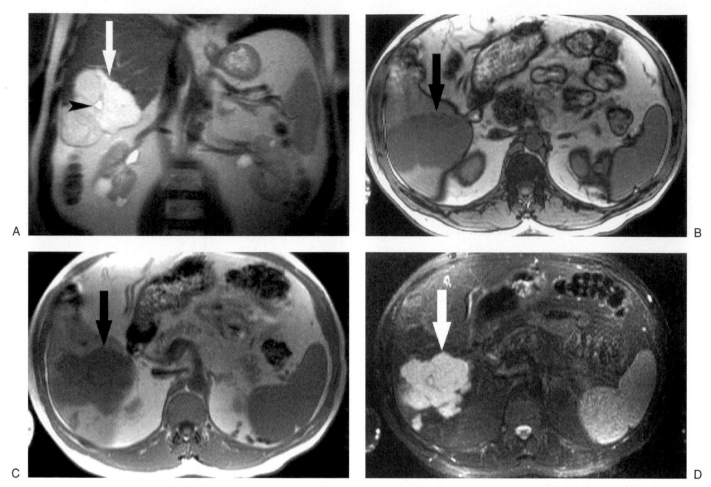

FIG. 1.43. Basic elements of abdominal MRI protocol in a patient with giant hemangioma (*arrows*). Precontrast and equilibrium-phase 3D gradient echo images were also obtained but are not shown. **A:** Coronal HASTE survey/breath-hold localizer. Note high signal intensity central scar (*arrowhead*) within hemangioma (*arrow*). **B:** Breath-hold T1-weighted opposed-phase gradient echo image. Note dark (phase cancellation) lines around organs. **C:** T1-weighted in-phase gradient echo image. This image was obtained during same dual echo sequence as **(B)**. **D:** Fat-suppressed T2-weighted (turboSTIR) image shows hemangioma nearly as bright as cerebrospinal fluid. Note increased signal intensity of spleen relative to liver.

adrenal masses detected with other modalities, intravenous contrast is not indicated in most cases. If the characteristic uniform signal loss of an adrenal mass is demonstrated on opposed-phase imaging, the diagnosis of adrenal adenoma can be made with reasonable certainty, and intravenous contrast is unlikely to further aid in diagnosis.

Optional elements:

- If the characteristic appearance of adrenal adenoma is not present on in-phase and opposed-phase imaging, dynamic contrast-enhanced imaging may be helpful.
- Coronal imaging may show some small adrenal masses to better advantage than axial imaging.
- Thin section (≤3 mm) imaging through the adrenals may be helpful for small adrenal masses.
- Coronal fat-suppressed T2-weighted imaging to include the paraspinal regions and aortic bifurcation may be helpful to evaluate for extraadrenal pheochromocytoma in the absence of an adrenal mass.

MR Cholangiopancreatography Protocol

Because of the high prevalence of hepatic or pancreatic parenchymal abnormalities in patients with disorders of the bile and pancreatic ducts, most MRCP sequences should be performed as part of a complete liver or pancreatic protocol. It may not be necessary to include all of the sequences listed below in all cases. In general, an MRCP protocol should consist of some combination of thin and thick section images. Nonstandard imaging planes may be used to better demonstrate anatomy or abnormalities not well seen with standard views. Most of the sequences listed below are simply variations on a heavily T2-weighted sequence. Selective use of an oral negative contrast agent may be helpful to suppress signal from fluid in bowel.

Multiplanar scout
Thin section multislice images: HASTE/ssFSE/ssTSE
    Respiratory: Breath-hold

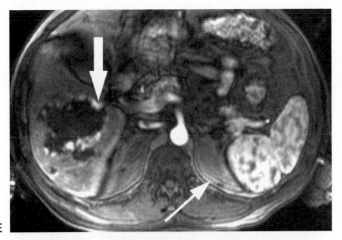

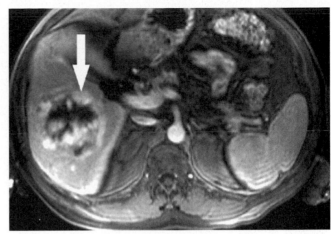

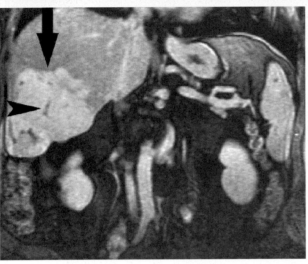

FIG. 1.43. (continued) **E:** Arterial phase image from fat-suppressed 3D dynamic gadolinium-enhanced (VIBE) sequence. Note early peripheral nodular enhancement (*arrow*) of hemangioma and truncation artifact (*thin arrow*). Heterogeneous enhancement of spleen is normal during arterial phase. **F:** Portal venous phase image obtained as part of same dynamic scan as **(E)** shows progressive centripetal filling of hemangioma (*arrow*). Spleen is now homogeneously enhanced. **G:** Coronal delayed fat-suppressed gradient echo image shows complete filling of hemangioma (*arrow*) with exception of central scar (*arrowhead*). Coronal plane was chosen for this sequence to provide alternative display of anatomy.

Imaging plane: Axial and coronal

Slice thickness: 3 mm

Fat suppression: May improve quality of 3D reconstructions

Radial thick slab MRCP: Heavily T2-weighted FSE/TSE

Respiratory: Breath-hold

Imaging plane: Radially oriented around distal common bile duct (minimum of three projections)

Slice thickness: 40 to 80 mm

Optional elements:

- High-resolution, respiratory-triggered thin section MRCP with slice thickness less than 2 mm may be performed, although scans of this type last several minutes and respiratory motion may degrade 3D reconstructions. The use of a fast recovery/driven equilibrium technique (DRIVE), may improve image contrast, reduce flow artifacts, and reduce scan time for respiratory-triggered 3D techniques.

- The above sequences may be repeated in any imaging plane to best display the anatomy of interest.
- A mangafodipir-enhanced MRCP may better demonstrate nondilated bile ducts (Fig. 1.45). Imaging with a 3D spoiled gradient echo sequence beginning approximately 15 to 30 minutes after contrast administration usually yields good results. Results may be suboptimal in the setting of liver failure.

Basic Pelvic Protocol (Fig. 1.46)

General comments: Due to differences in male and female anatomy, there is considerable variability in the protocols used to image the pelvis. In general, T2-weighted images provide the most information on a pelvic MRI examination. The zonal anatomy of the uterus and prostate, presence of fluid collections, and ovarian anatomy are all shown to best

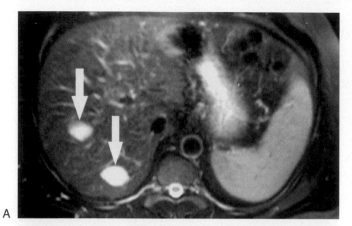

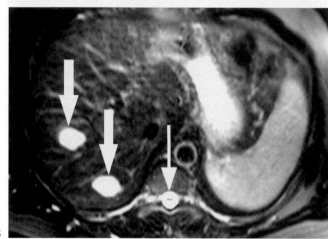

FIG. 1.44. Use of increasing echo time to characterize hepatic lesions. **A:** Fat-suppressed T2-weighted image (echo time [TE] 80 msec) shows two high signal intensity lesions (*arrows*) in right hepatic lobe. **B:** On long TE (160 msec) image, relative signal intensity of liver decreases, but lesions (*arrows*) remain nearly isointense to cerebrospinal fluid (*thin arrow*). Therefore, lesions have very long T2 relaxation times compatible with cysts or hemangiomas (in this case, hemangiomas).

advantage on a T2-weighted scan. T1-weighted images provide little information about the internal structure of the pelvic organs. However, T1-weighted images are useful when performed with and without fat suppression to characterize fat-containing or hemorrhagic abnormalities of the pelvis. When performing MRI of the pelvis, it is often helpful to include the kidneys on the coronal survey to screen for renal anomalies or hydronephrosis. Respiratory motion artifact can be reduced on non–fat-saturated, free-breathing sequences by placement of a saturation band over the anterior abdominal fat.

Multiplanar scout
Coronal T2 survey: HASTE/ssFSE/ssTSE
   Purpose: Overall survey, screening for renal anomalies and
     hydronephrosis
   Respiratory: Breath-hold
   Imaging plane: Coronal
   Slice thickness: 8 mm

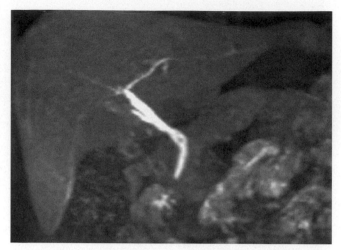

FIG. 1.45. Mangafodipir-enhanced MR cholangiopancreatography. Coronal maximum intensity projection of fat-suppressed 3D gradient echo sequence performed approximately 30 minutes after administration of intravenous mangafodipir.

Axial T1: FSE/TSE
   Purpose: Axial anatomy
   Respiratory: Free-breathing
   Imaging plane: Axial to pelvis
   Slice thickness: 6 to 8 mm
Fat-suppressed axial T1: Spoiled gradient echo
   Purpose: Characterization of fatty or hemorrhagic lesions
   Respiratory: Breath-hold
   Imaging plane: Axial to pelvis
   Slice thickness: 6 to 8 mm
Fat-suppressed axial T2: FSE/TSE
   Purpose: Detection of fluid and cystic structures
   Respiratory: Free-breathing
   Imaging plane: Axial to pelvis
   Slice thickness: 6 to 8 mm
High-resolution sagittal T2 (female only): FSE/TSE
   Purpose: Evaluation of endometrium, junctional zone, and
     cervix
   Respiratory: Free-breathing
   Imaging plane: Sagittal to uterus
   Slice thickness: 6 mm

Congenital Uterus and Adenomyosis Protocol Modifications

Multiplanar (axial and coronal), high-resolution T2-weighted imaging should be performed relative to the plane of the uterus (Fig. 1.47).

Fibroid Protocol Modifications

Dynamic contrast-enhanced imaging using a coronal 3D sequence should be performed before and for follow-up of

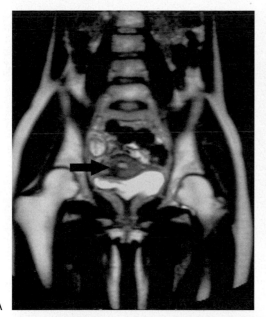

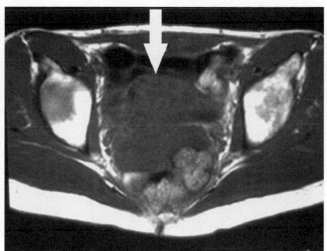

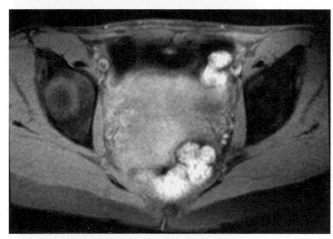

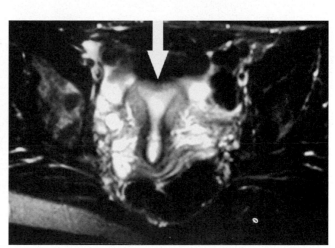

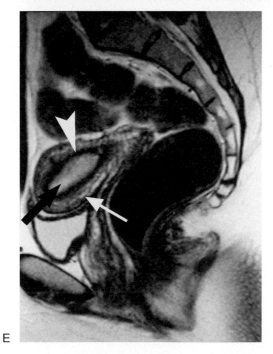

FIG. 1.46. Basic elements of female pelvic protocol. **A:** Coronal HASTE survey shows midline uterus (*arrow*). **B:** Axial T1-weighted fast spin echo sequence demonstrates pelvic fat planes but no internal uterine anatomy (*arrow*). **C:** Axial T1-weighted fat-suppressed gradient echo sequence used to characterize fat-containing or hemorrhagic lesions. Note increased signal intensity of bowel contents, a normal finding. **D:** Axial fat-suppressed T2-weighted fast spin echo sequence shows uterus (*arrow*) to be oriented coronally with respect to scan plane. **E:** Midline sagittal T2-weighted fast spin echo image of different patient shows zonal anatomy of uterus. Arrow denotes bright endometrium, arrowhead denotes dark junctional zone, and thin arrow denotes intermediate signal intensity outer myometrium.

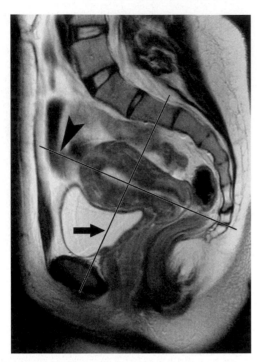

FIG. 1.47. Scan planes for evaluation of uterine anomalies and endometrium. In this case, scan plane (*arrow*) oriented axial to uterus is almost coronal with respect to pelvis on this T2-weighted sagittal image. The scan plane (*arrowhead*) oriented coronal to the uterus is actually almost axial relative to the pelvis.

uterine fibroid embolization. This allows for depiction of fibroid blood supply and enhancement characteristics. Images should be obtained before contrast administration and during the arterial and venous phases of enhancement. The FOV should include the level of the renal arteries to allow for detection of ovarian and lumbar arteries. The venous phase allows for detection of deep vein thrombosis caused by compression of the pelvic veins by the enlarged uterus.

Uterine Malignancy Protocol Modifications

Dynamic contrast-enhanced imaging is helpful for determining the depth of myometrial invasion of endometrial cancer. If myometrial invasion is suspected, orthogonal views should be obtained to confirm. Scans planned relative to the uterus (see Fig. 1.47) are helpful for evaluation of the endometrium.

Optional elements:

- Distention of the vagina with water-soluble lubricant may aid in defining pelvic anatomy or evaluating the cervix and vagina (Fig. 1.48).
- The use of intravenous contrast may be helpful for the evaluation of cervical carcinoma when noncontrast sequences are indeterminate.

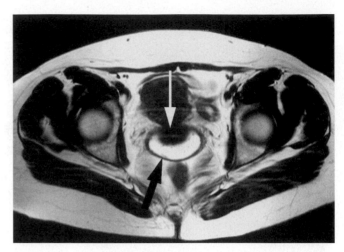

FIG. 1.48. Use of water-soluble lubricant for vaginal distention. T2-weighted image shows vagina (*arrow*) distended with approximately 60 mL of water-soluble lubricant. Note clear demarcation of the cervix (*thin arrow*).

Adnexa Protocol Modifications

Scans performed for the evaluation of the female adnexa can be aligned relative to the pelvis rather than the uterus. T1-weighted images acquired with and without frequency-selective fat suppression should be used to distinguish lipid-containing lesions from hemorrhagic lesions. Contrast administration is useful for the evaluation of cystic ovarian masses, particularly to identify enhancing mural nodules or septations.

Pelvic Floor Relaxation Protocol Modifications (Fig. 1.49)

A single-slice, multiphase, rapid T2-weighted scan (HASTE, ssTSE, ssFSE) can be performed in the midline sagittal plane with the patient at rest and during Valsalva maneuver. Approximately one image per second should be acquired for a total of 20 images. In this manner, approximately five images are sequentially obtained with the patient at rest. Without interrupting acquisition, the command to commence the Valsalva maneuver is then given to the patient while the next 10 images are obtained. The patient is then told to rest during acquisition of the final five images. When performing this type of examination, we advise placing absorbent material beneath the patient in case of urinary incontinence.

Female Urethral Diverticulum Protocol Modifications (Fig. 1.50)

The evaluation of a potential or known urethral diverticulum requires high-resolution imaging, preferably with an endovaginal coil. Small FOV T1- and T2-weighted imaging is primarily performed in the axial plane, although coronal or sagittal imaging may be performed to better define

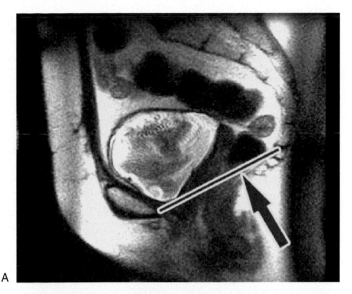

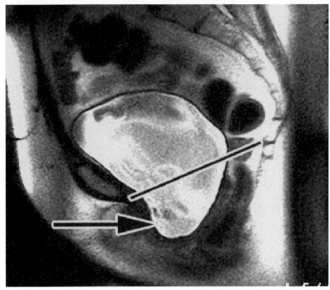

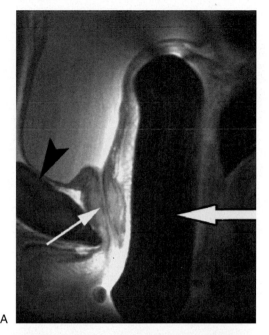

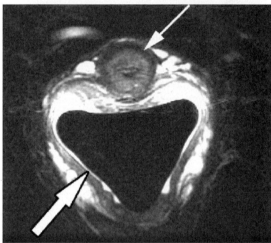

FIG. 1.49. Dynamic imaging of pelvic floor relaxation. **A:** Midline sagittal HASTE image at rest shows bladder base above sacrococcygeal-inferior pubic line (*arrow*). **B:** During Valsalva maneuver, bladder base (*thin arrow*) descends considerably.

FIG. 1.50. Endovaginal imaging of female urethra. **A:** High-resolution sagittal T2-weighted image demonstrates endovaginal coil (*arrow*) and urethra (*thin arrow*). Pubic symphysis is marked by arrowhead. **B:** High-resolution axial image through mid-urethra (*thin arrow*) shows triangular signal void representing coil in vagina (*arrow*).

the anatomy of the diverticulum. Fat-suppressed gadolinium-enhanced axial images are helpful in defining the diverticulum neck.

Bladder Protocol Modifications

The bladder should be moderately full while imaging. The optimal imaging plane differs from patient to patient and should be determined by consulting the initial general survey images. Standard coronal, axial, or sagittal views may assist the urologist in better understanding the anatomic relationships, but a plane perpendicular to the interface between the mass and the bladder wall should be included to ensure the best evaluation for depth of bladder wall invasion. Dynamic

imaging is recommended to help determine the depth of bladder wall invasion, because bladder cancer typically enhances early relative to the bladder wall (Fig. 1.51).

Prostate Protocol Modifications

Adequate evaluation of the prostate at 1.5 T requires imaging with an endorectal coil in addition to the general survey performed with a surface coil (Fig. 1.52). We routinely administer intravenous glucagon to patients undergoing prostate imaging, because use of an endorectal coil may induce rectal spasms that degrade image quality. High-resolution, small

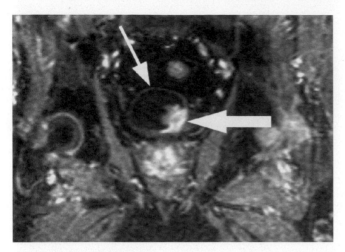

FIG. 1.51. Enhancement of transitional cell carcinoma of the bladder. Arterial phase image from fat-suppressed 3D gadolinium-enhanced dynamic study of bladder demonstrates early enhancement of transitional cell carcinoma (*arrow*) relative to bladder wall (*thin arrow*).

FOV images are usually possible given the relative immobility of the prostate. At a minimum, we acquire T2-weighted images in the axial and coronal planes in addition to an axial T1-weighted sequence. Fat suppression is used selectively. To prevent confusion between prostate carcinoma and postbiopsy hemorrhage, a 3-week waiting period is recommended after biopsy before imaging the prostate.

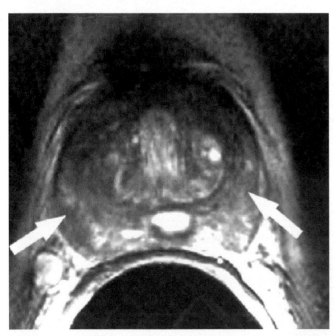

FIG. 1.52. Endorectal prostate MR image. Axial T2-weighted image of prostate performed with endorectal coil shows abnormal low signal intensity within peripheral zone of prostate (*arrows*) in patient with adenocarcinoma.

Optional elements:

- The use of intravenous contrast is usually reserved for problematic cases.
- MR spectroscopy may be beneficial if available.

Scrotum Protocol Modifications

Evaluation of the scrotum requires the use of a surface coil with a limited FOV. Before imaging, the scrotum should be elevated with a towel draped across the patient's upper thighs. The scrotum should then be covered with a sheet or blanket with the surface coil placed directly over it. High-resolution fast spin echo T2-weighted images (FSE, TSE) should be acquired in three planes. The axial and coronal planes have the advantage of including both testes, providing a convenient reference for comparison. The sagittal plane often shows the epididymis to best advantage. Spin echo T1-weighted images are useful for identifying hemorrhage.

Optional elements:

- Contrast enhancement can be valuable for evaluating suspected tumors or vascular lesions.
- Dynamic 3D gradient echo imaging may reveal information about testicular perfusion or vascularity.

Vascular Protocol

A large number of MRA protocol variations exist, although these are mostly variations on four types of MRA techniques: dark blood, time-of-flight, phase-contrast, and 3D gadolinium-enhanced MRA. These techniques are discussed in more detail in Section 2.1. In most situations, 3D gadolinium-enhanced MRA serves as the primary diagnostic sequence, although situations exist when noncontrast MRA is a useful adjunct. Vascular imaging is often combined with soft tissue imaging.

A basic gadolinium-enhanced MR angiogram consists of a 3D gradient echo sequence with a minimum TR and TE and a flip angle of approximately 40 degrees. This flip angle is greater than that used for soft tissue imaging to create more background tissue saturation. Additional time-saving techniques, such as zerofill interpolation, are commonly employed. Slices should be as thin as possible while still allowing coverage of the anatomy of interest during a breathhold. Overlapping or overcontiguous slices allow for excellent quality 3D reconstructions. The scan plane should be aligned along the vessel of interest. Coronal imaging works best for most abdominal and pelvic applications. Fat suppression is optional. A noncontrast data set with identical parameters to the MR angiogram should be acquired to serve as a mask for subtraction.

Renal Artery Stenosis Protocol Modifications

The adrenal glands should be included in the FOV on most sequences to exclude adrenal pathology as a cause of hypertension.

Optional elements:

- On occasion, the addition of a 3D phase-contrast angiogram may salvage a contrast-enhanced study compromised by motion or poor timing.
- Some limited hemodynamic information about the severity of stenosis may be obtained from phase-contrast images (Fig. 1.53).
- The correct velocity-encoding parameter varies by patient, but 50 cm/sec makes a reasonable starting point.

Portal Vein Protocol Modifications

This protocol varies primarily in timing. Because the timing of the portal phase is not as critical as the arterial phase, we typically perform a standard 3D gadolinium-enhanced MR angiogram of the aorta and repeat the sequence twice, stopping briefly to allow the patient to breathe between ac-

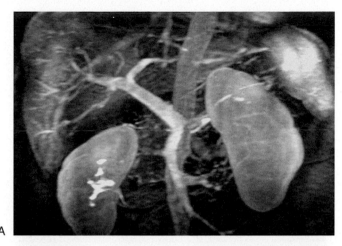

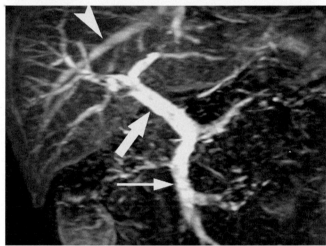

FIG. 1.54. Subtraction technique for displaying venous phase. **A:** Coronal 3D gadolinium-enhanced portal venous phase MRA shows combination of arterial and venous structures. **B:** Pure venous image obtained by subtracting the arterial phase image (not shown) from **(A)**. Portal vein (*arrow*) and hepatic veins (*arrowhead*) are more clearly depicted in **(B)**. Superior mesenteric vein (*thin arrow* **[B]**) is shown without overlapping aorta.

quisitions. If a pure arterial phase image is obtained, it can be subtracted from the venous phase images to provide an image displaying only the venous structures (Fig. 1.54).

Optional elements:

A 3D phase-contrast venogram or a steady-state gradient echo sequence such as trueFISP or balanced FFE may be helpful if intravenous access is difficult. A velocity encoding parameter of 20 to 40 cm/sec usually suffices for phase-contrast imaging.

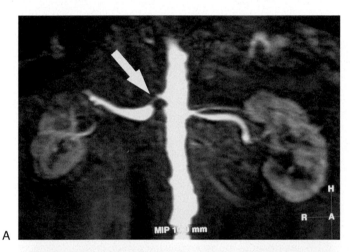

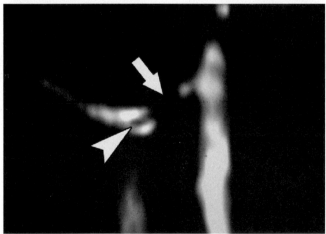

FIG. 1.53. 3D gadolinium-enhanced versus 3D phase-contrast MRA. **A:** Maximum intensity projection image of coronal 3D gadolinium-enhanced renal MRA shows severe stenosis of right renal artery (*arrow*) and poststenotic dilatation. **B:** Coronal reformation of 3D phase-contrast MRA in same patient as **(A)** shows signal void at site of stenosis (*arrow*) and poststenotic jet (*arrowhead*).

Cavagram and Pelvic Venogram Protocol Modifications

Successful demonstration of the inferior vena cava can be a challenge with the standard contrast-enhanced 3D MRA technique (with contrast administered through an upper extremity vein), because the renal vein outflow opacifies the

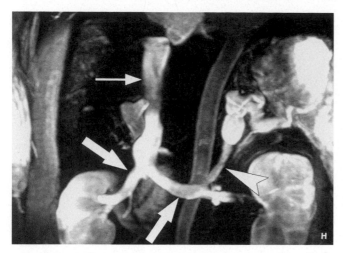

FIG. 1.55. Indirect MR venogram of renal veins and suprarenal inferior vena cava (IVC). Timing run was performed to determine peak opacification of IVC. Coronal 3D gadolinium-enhanced MRA was performed after antecubital intravenous injection of contrast agent. Note excellent depiction of renal veins (*arrows*), suprarenal IVC (*thin arrow*), and splenorenal shunt (*arrowhead*).

upper cava long before the lower cava receives enhanced blood from the lower extremities. In addition, there may be considerable dilution of contrast and surrounding soft tissue enhancement that occurs by the time the cava is fully opacified. When evaluating the upper inferior vena cava with such a technique, we simply perform a timing run to determine peak

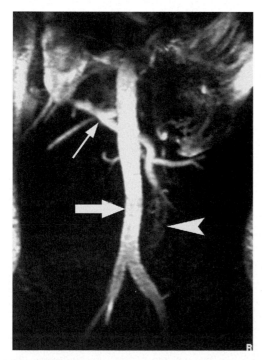

FIG. 1.56. 3D phase-contrast venogram. Inferior vena cava (*arrow*) and portal vein (*thin arrow*) are demonstrated without intravenous contrast. A 30 cm/sec velocity encoding was selected, resulting in little signal from aorta (*arrowhead*).

opacification of the suprarenal segment and adjust the scan delay accordingly (Fig. 1.55). The pelvic veins and inferior vena cava can also be evaluated with either time-of-flight or phase-contrast venography without the need for intravenous contrast (Fig. 1.56).

Uncooperative Patient Protocol

Imaging the uncooperative patient requires rapid sequences that are relatively resistant to patient motion. Two useful sequences for this purpose are HASTE (providing T2-weighted images) and magnetization prepared gradient echo (providing T1-weighted images). Although sensitivity for lesion detection and image quality may be reduced in this setting, sufficient information can often be obtained to make or confirm an important diagnosis. Additional strategies include the use of respiratory triggering or sacrificing in-plane and through-plane resolution to allow shorter breath-holds. Finally, consideration should be given to delaying a nonemergent study until a time when the patient is likely to be more cooperative.

SECTION SUMMARY

1. Most abdominal MRI protocols include the following sequences:
   - Coronal HASTE survey
   - Axial in-phase and opposed-phase T1-weighted gradient echo sequence
   - Axial fat-suppressed T2-weighted sequence (most often fast spin echo)
   - Axial dynamic gadolinium-enhanced T1-weighted gradient echo sequence
2. When imaging the abdomen and pelvis, the scan plane, use of fat suppression, and scan delay following intravenous contrast administration should be individualized based on the specific clinical question.
3. For most abdominal and pelvic indications, imaging should be performed dynamically following the administration of intravenous gadolinium.
4. Breath-hold or respiratory-triggered sequences should be used when possible for the upper abdomen. Free-breathing sequences may routinely be performed in the pelvis (with saturation of the anterior subcutaneous fat).
5. Most MRCP protocols consist of heavily T2-weighted sequences performed in multiple imaging planes with a variety of slice thicknesses.
6. Most MR angiography studies use a gadolinium-enhanced 3D gradient echo sequence. Non–contrast-enhanced sequences may occasionally be helpful.
7. Uncooperative patients may be successfully imaged with rapid sequences such as HASTE or magnetization-prepared gradient echo. However, sensitivity for the detection of some abnormalities is reduced.

Introduction to Specific Abdominal and Pelvic Magnetic Resonance Imaging Techniques

SECTION 2.1

Magnetic Resonance Angiography in the Abdomen and Pelvis

Magnetic resonance angiography (MRA) has become an essential tool in abdominal and pelvic MR imaging (MRI). The utility of MRA has been enhanced by the addition of intravenous contrast agents and the recent proliferation of postprocessing techniques, many of which are largely automated and allow for real-time interaction on commercially available workstations. As a result, MRA examinations account for a significant percentage of the abdominal and pelvic MRI volume at many hospitals. At such centers, the volume of diagnostic catheter angiography performed has decreased proportionately.

MRA TECHNIQUES

Unlike conventional catheter-based angiography, MRA may be performed using a variety of techniques based on entirely different physical principles. Not every MRA technique yields equivalent results in similar situations. Therefore, it is important to understand the advantages and limitations of each technique. MRA techniques may be divided into two basic categories: non–contrast-enhanced and contrast-enhanced.

Non–Contrast-Enhanced Techniques

Dark Blood

The goal of dark blood angiography is to eliminate as much signal as possible from the blood vessels of interest. With most spin echo–based techniques (including fast spin echo and single-shot techniques), flowing blood results in a relative signal void on MR images. However, some signal often remains in the vessel lumen with these techniques if additional steps are not taken. A simple method of reducing intravascular signal on a dark blood sequence is to increase the echo time (TE). This allows more time for intravoxel dephasing and for blood excited by the initial 90-degree pulse to exit before experiencing the subsequent refocusing pulse. Gradient

moment nulling is not used in this setting to allow dephasing caused by the imaging gradients to contribute to the signal loss from flowing blood. Placing a saturation band perpendicular to the vessel of interest upstream from the image slice can also reduce intraluminal signal.

Another technique for eliminating signal from vessels is called *double inversion recovery*. This technique uses slice-selective and non–slice-selective 180-degree inversion prepulses to eliminate signal from flowing blood. Stationary tissues experience both 180-degree pulses and begin the imaging cycle as if no pulses had been applied (the second inversion pulse reverses the effects of the first pulse). Blood flowing into the imaging plane only experiences the second 180-degree pulse and subsequently regrows longitudinal magnetization according to its T1 relaxation time. By beginning the imaging cycle at the null point of blood, the signal from flowing blood can be suppressed.

Dark blood techniques are useful for the depiction of intraluminal abnormalities such as dissection flaps and tumor thrombus (Fig. 2.1).

Time-of-Flight

Time-of-flight MRA is based on the gradient echo pulse sequence and exploits the concept of flow-related enhancement to produce bright intraluminal signal. To minimize the effects of phase shifts experienced by moving protons (these phase shifts contribute to signal loss), flow compensation is used with time-of-flight imaging. Time-of-flight MRA can be performed with either a two-dimensional (2D) or three-dimensional (3D) acquisition. Typically, 2D acquisitions are preferred in the abdomen and pelvis to avoid saturation of blood that occurs when flowing blood remains in the imaging volume too long. In-plane saturation can be reduced for a 2D acquisition by choosing an imaging plane perpendicular to the flow within the vessel of interest. Arteries or veins can be selectively imaged with this technique by applying a

53

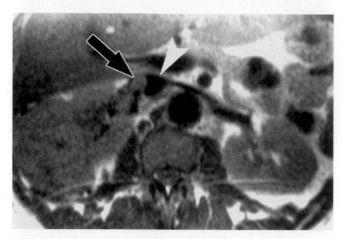

FIG. 2.1. Axial dark blood image performed at level of renal veins with double inversion recovery HASTE technique in patient with right renal cell carcinoma. Tumor thrombus (*arrow*) within inferior vena cava (*arrowhead*) is clearly depicted against signal void of flowing blood.

saturation band above or below the image slice. In this manner, blood flowing through the saturation band before entering the image slice loses signal, allowing display of unidirectional flow. In 2D acquisitions, saturation bands are most effective when traveling with or tracking the imaging slice (as opposed to remaining stationary while the imaging slice moves). Signal from any blood vessel passing through a saturation band is eliminated, regardless of whether it is arterial or venous. This can create a false impression of thrombosis within a target vessel with retrograde flow.

To allow for efficient imaging and better saturation of background tissues with time-of-flight MRA, the repetition time (TR) and TE are minimized, while the flip angle is kept between 30 and 60 degrees. Minimizing the TE also helps reduce the effects of dephasing (and resulting signal loss) due to complex flow. Cardiac gating may dramatically improve image quality for vessels with highly pulsatile flow (e.g., aorta and iliac vessels), but it significantly prolongs acquisition time (Fig. 2.2). Thin overlapping slices allow for more appealing 3D reconstructions. Time-of-flight MRA is seldom used to image the arterial system of the abdomen and pelvis, because it is time consuming and susceptible to artifacts. However, it remains useful for assessing the abdominal and pelvic veins.

Phase-Contrast

Flowing protons develop a net phase accumulation relative to stationary tissues when a bipolar gradient (two gradients of equal strength but opposite polarity) is applied. This phase shift, which can be measured, forms the basis of phase-contrast angiography (the term *contrast* here refers to image contrast created by phase differences, not intravenous contrast material). Faster flowing protons experience a greater phase shift than slower moving protons, allowing for the

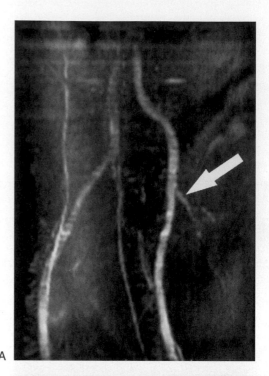

A

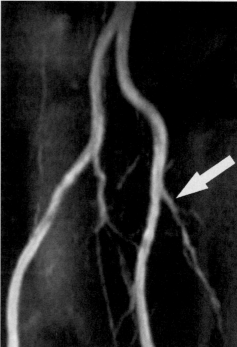

B

FIG. 2.2. Two-dimensional time-of-flight MRA (oblique maximum intensity projection) of pelvis showing benefit of cardiac gating. **A:** Ungated MRA demonstrates variable signal intensity of common and external iliac arteries. Internal iliac arteries (*arrow*) are poorly seen. Signal from veins eliminated by traveling inferior saturation band. **B:** Repeat study with cardiac gating demonstrates even distribution of high signal intensity throughout iliac arteries. Internal iliac arteries are clearly seen (*arrow*). Acquisition time for gated study exceeded 15 minutes, however.

calculation of flow velocity. Therefore, phase-contrast MRA is inherently quantitative, unlike time-of-flight or gadolinium-enhanced MRA. The signal intensity of blood is proportional to its flow velocity in phase-contrast MRA, and the direction of flow can be determined based on the direction of the phase shift. However, flowing blood experiencing a phase shift in excess of 180-degrees is represented as flowing in the opposite direction (a phenomenon referred to as *aliasing*). Therefore, it is necessary to specify in advance the velocity of flow that is to be imaged by selecting the velocity-encoding parameter (frequently referred to as *Venc*). The velocity-encoding parameter determines the bipolar gradient strength, which in turn determines the flow velocity that results in a 180-degree phase shift. It is critical to estimate the velocity of flow in the vessel of interest with reasonable accuracy before the sequence is run (Fig. 2.3).

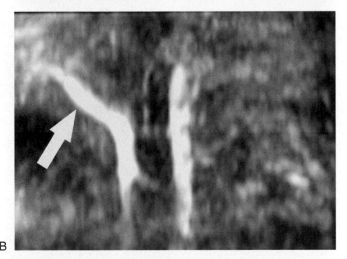

A

B

FIG. 2.3. Importance of proper velocity encoding for phase-contrast MRA. **A:** Three-dimensional phase-contrast MR portogram performed in patient without intravenous access using velocity-encoding of 25 cm/sec. Portal vein was poorly visualized and initially interpreted as thrombosed. Arrow denotes hepatic artery. **B:** Examination repeated later same day with velocity-encoding of 5 cm/sec demonstrates very slow portal flow (*arrow*).

In vessels for which the flow velocity is unknown, a series of 2D images performed while varying the velocity-encoding parameter can provide an estimated value. The velocity value for each axis or direction must be assigned separately, and for each flow direction encoded, the scan time is increased.

As with time-of-flight MRA, the signal from vessels can be selectively eliminated based on flow direction with the use of a saturation band. This may be unnecessary if the velocity-encoding parameter is appropriately selected, because the signal intensity of flowing blood is dependent upon its velocity. Phase-contrast technique is seldom used alone for abdominal and pelvic MRA, but it may be useful to confirm the significance of a stenosis identified using other techniques (see Fig. 1.53).

Additional Non–Contrast-Enhanced MRA Techniques

Newer methods of imaging blood vessels are continually being developed or refined. Balanced steady-state gradient echo sequences (TrueFISP, balanced FFE, FIESTA) have increased in popularity recently, due in part to their utility in cardiac imaging. The contrast mechanisms of these types of sequences are complex, demonstrating both bright blood and bright fluid (Fig. 2.4).

Contrast-Enhanced Techniques

Three-Dimensional Gadolinium-Enhanced MRA (CE-MRA)

The introduction of gadolinium chelates has dramatically expanded the clinical utility of MRA (Fig. 2.5). The basic sequence for contrast-enhanced MRA is 3D gradient echo. A 3D acquisition is preferable, because it allows for relatively thin contiguous image sections to be obtained during a single

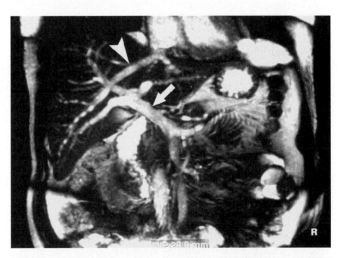

FIG. 2.4. Portal MR venogram performed with balanced-FFE sequence. Portal (*arrow*) and hepatic (*arrowhead*) veins are clearly demonstrated on this coronal maximum intensity projection image. This sequence required 20 seconds and no intravenous contrast.

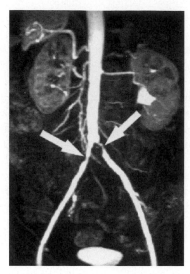

FIG. 2.5. Maximum intensity projection image of three-dimensional gadolinium-enhanced abdominal and pelvic MRA performed with 20 mL of contrast agent injected at 2 mL/sec via antecubital vein. Note bilateral iliac artery stenoses (*arrows*).

breath-hold. Because this sequence relies on the T1 shortening effects of the gadolinium to enhance the target vasculature, saturation effects are not problematic like they are with time-of-flight techniques. In the typical 3D CE-MRA sequence, the TR and TE are minimized to allow for the most efficient imaging, while the flip angle is maintained at 30 to 60 degrees to allow for saturation of stationary tissues. This sequence closely resembles the 3D gradient echo sequence used for dynamic imaging of the liver, although the latter sequence uses a lower flip angle to prevent saturation of stationary tissues.

Critical to CE-MRA is the ability to time the data acquisition to coincide with arrival of the contrast bolus in the vessel of interest. The dose of contrast necessary to perform abdominal and pelvic CE-MRA varies by scanner, target vessel, and operator confidence. We have found that most MRA examinations can be adequately performed with approximately 20 mL of gadolinium chelate. It is important to follow the contrast agent injection with approximately 15 to 20 mL of normal saline flush at the same injection rate to clear residual contrast material from the intravenous tubing and ensure adequate dose delivery.

Blood Pool Contrast Agents

Blood pool contrast agents have a prolonged intravascular phase, which means that a wide window of opportunity exists for imaging the blood vessels after contrast agent administration. However, imaging during the arterial phase is still necessary to avoid interference from venous structures. Blood pool contrast agents are not currently approved for routine clinical use at the time of this writing, and the utility of these agents for imaging the vessels of the abdomen and pelvis remains to be proven in clinical trials.

Methods of Background Suppression

Suppression of signal from nonvascular structures is usually desirable during MRA. Background tissue suppression typically occurs during MRA as the result of repeated radiofrequency (RF) pulses. By using a short TR and a sufficiently large (usually 30 to 60 degrees) flip angle, the longitudinal magnetization of the background tissues does not have sufficient time to recover between RF pulses and, therefore, becomes saturated. This alone often provides sufficient background suppression for diagnostic quality MRA. However, a variety of techniques may be used to further suppress background tissues.

Fat suppression and magnetization transfer are two easily performed techniques that must be selected *before* imaging. Magnetization transfer is used primarily for cerebral MRA, but fat suppression is commonly used in the abdomen and pelvis.

Another method of background suppression for CE-MRA involves image subtraction. With this technique, a precontrast scan (also known as a *mask*) is digitally subtracted from a postcontrast scan (Fig. 2.6). For this method to succeed, the two data sets must spatially match, because any movement between sequences results in spatial misregistration and poor image quality.

Additional background suppression techniques are unnecessary with phase-contrast imaging, because stationary tissues accumulate no phase shift and are automatically subtracted to produce the angiographic images.

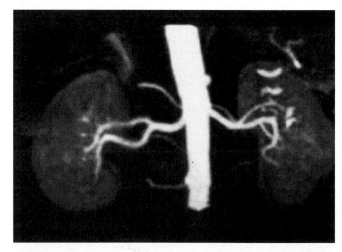

FIG. 2.6. Elimination of background signal. Renal artery MRA shows excellent visualization of renal arteries with minimal background signal. This was accomplished by subtracting precontrast data set from arterial phase data set and limiting thickness of reconstruction volume for this maximum intensity projection.

Timing of Contrast-Enhanced MRA

A properly timed CE-MRA sequence is one in which the portions of the acquisition related to image contrast (the center of k-space) are obtained when the contrast bolus is at peak concentration in the vessel of interest. If the image acquisition begins too soon, the critical image data are acquired before the contrast bolus peaks, causing a characteristic artifact (Fig. 2.7) (1). If the image acquisition begins too late, the vessel of interest is not maximally intense, and venous contamination may prevent optimal visualization of the arteries.

Various methods exist to ensure proper timing of CE-MRA. To properly employ these methods, however, it is essential to know how the MRI system acquires data. In general, there are two widely available types of data acquisition used for CE-MRA. The standard type of acquisition is referred to as *linear* or *sequential*. In this situation, the data most responsible for image contrast (the critical data for CE-MRA) are acquired at the center of the acquisition. If a scanner uses this type of data acquisition, the scan must be timed so that the contrast bolus peaks near the center of the acquisition. In other words, if the acquisition is 20 seconds long, the contrast bolus should peak halfway through the acquisition, around 10 seconds into the scan. Therefore, a scanner acquiring data in a sequential manner should begin collecting data before the signal intensity peaks in the vessel of interest.

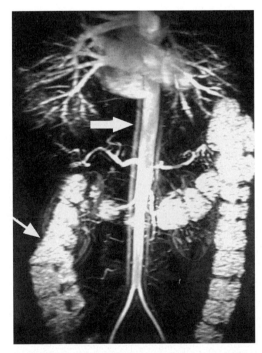

FIG. 2.7. Artifact from premature data acquisition during contrast-enhanced MRA. Centric ordered k-space acquisition initiated before contrast bolus peaked in aorta resulted in "ringing" artifact (*arrow*) on maximum intensity projection image. Note high signal intensity of colon contents (*thin arrow*), a common finding on three-dimensional MRA sequences that can be reduced through use of subtraction.

The other common method of data collection in CE-MRA is centric (also referred to as *low-high*, because the weakly phase-encoded echoes from the center of k-space are acquired first). In this instance, the data most responsible for image contrast are acquired near the beginning of the acquisition. One advantage of this technique is that the most critical data are acquired early, minimizing the effects of respiratory motion in patients who cannot tolerate a prolonged breath-hold. If the CE-MRA sequences of a scanner are centric ordered, the data acquisition should begin slightly later than with a sequential acquisition to ensure that the central lines of k-space are sampled when the contrast bolus is at peak concentration in the vessel of interest.

Timing Bolus/Test Injection

The time between injection of the contrast material and initiation of data acquisition is referred to as the *scan delay*. One method of determining the proper scan delay is with a timing bolus, which involves administering a bolus of 1 to 2 mL of gadolinium chelate while acquiring rapid sequential images of the vessel of interest. (**Note:** Follow the test dose with a bolus of approximately 15 to 20 mL of flush administered at the same injection rate as the test dose.) Imaging after the test injection is typically performed with a low spatial resolution 2D gradient echo sequence acquired at a rate of one image per second. This allows for determination of the time it takes from injection to peak concentration of contrast in the vessel of interest (referred to as the *circulation time, bolus arrival time,* or *time-to-peak*). This can then be entered into the following formula to obtain the scan delay for a *sequential* data acquisition:

$$\text{Scan delay} = \text{bolus arrival time} + [1/2 \text{ (duration of contrast injection)} - 1/2 \text{ (scan acquisition time)}]$$

For example, assume a renal MRA is being done in a patient in whom a bolus arrival time of 15 seconds, an acquisition time of 24 seconds, and injection duration of 10 seconds (2 mL/sec for 20 mL) has been determined. In this scenario, the scan should be initiated 8 seconds after the contrast delivery is started. Because the scan delay is calculated in advance, this technique has the benefit of allowing precise timing of the breath-hold. For most patients, the scan delay will be between 10 and 20 seconds, depending on cardiovascular status and site of injection.

The timing bolus method is best performed using the aorta as the reference vessel, because smaller vessels may not be well visualized with this technique. Flow-related enhancement in the aorta during the timing run may result in a periodic increase in signal intensity in the vessel of interest unrelated to the arrival of the contrast bolus. Therefore, any increased aortic signal intensity should persist for several seconds before being interpreted as the test bolus. Also, it is important to remember that the bolus arrival time refers to the time for the test injection to peak in the aorta, not the time to when it is first visualized. For a centric ordered acquisition, the scan delay corresponds to the bolus arrival time.

Automatic Bolus Detection

Some scanners have software allowing the scan to be triggered automatically when the contrast bolus is detected (2). With this technique, the signal intensity is monitored within a region of interest placed over the abdominal aorta, or vessel of interest, following injection of the full diagnostic dose of contrast material. When the signal intensity exceeds a preset threshold value, data acquisition is triggered automatically. Because the scan delay is not known in advance, the patient must hold his or her breath quickly once the bolus is detected and the scan is triggered. Because the data acquisition begins when the contrast bolus is detected, a centric ordered acquisition should be used.

Real-Time Monitoring

Another method of timing the acquisition for CE-MRA involves real-time monitoring of the vessel of interest during injection of the full diagnostic dose of contrast material. With this technique, the technologist must coordinate monitoring the images for contrast arrival in the vessel of interest, initiation of patient breath-holding, and starting the scan. A delay of several seconds typically occurs between triggering the scan (i.e., pushing the button) and when the scan actually begins. This delay must be taken into account when timing the initiation of the scan.

Time-Resolved MRA

In some situations, it may be preferable to sacrifice spatial resolution for superior temporal resolution during the vascular phases of enhancement. This can be accomplished with a technique known as *time resolved* MRA (3–5). One approach to time-resolved imaging is simply to repeat the MRA sequence several times after the initiation of contrast material injection. The acquisition that best displays the vessels of interest is then used for image interpretation. With parallel imaging techniques (such as SENSE or SMASH), a complete MRA data set can be collected in a matter of seconds, and multiple data sets can be collected during a single breath-hold (Fig. 2.8). Alternatively, a dedicated time-resolved MRA sequence (such as TRICKS or Time-Resolved Imaging of Contrast Kinetics) can be used to collect data continuously after contrast injection during a single breath-hold. By alternating collection of the central and peripheral portions of k-space at several-second intervals, complete data sets can be reconstructed retrospectively with high temporal resolution. Future software and hardware innovations in this area will make time-resolved MRA commonplace, although few centers routinely use this technique currently.

Regardless of the timing technique used, we recommend that most CE-MRA sequences be repeated at least once after a time interval of several seconds, during which the patient may catch his or her breath. This allows for a venous phase to be obtained and serves as a backup in case the initial sequence was not timed adequately. Even experienced MR angiographers occasionally produce poorly timed examinations. When this happens, the MR angiographer should check the quality of the source data and edit the data set on a 3D workstation. Although the study may not look pretty, it may be diagnostic. If the source data are inadequate, it may be possible to repeat the study using an additional contrast injection, a new mask, and subtraction technique (be sure to stay within safe and acceptable contrast material dose limits). Alternatively, using a noncontrast-enhanced technique, such as phase-contrast or time-of-flight MRA, can often salvage a suboptimal study (the previous dose of intravenous contrast improves the quality of some non–contrast-enhanced MRAs).

MRA Reconstruction Techniques

Recent technologic developments in computer hardware and software have increased available image reconstruction options (Table 2.1). A basic understanding of these techniques is essential to the accurate and efficient interpretation of MRA studies. However, reconstructed images are best used to complement the source data. Any abnormalities suspected on the reconstructed images should be reexamined and confirmed on the source images.

Maximum Intensity Projection

Perhaps the most widely used reconstruction technique is the maximum intensity projection (MIP) algorithm (see Figs. 2.2, 2.5, 2.8). A common misconception is that a MIP represents a compression of the full volume of data into a single plane. In fact, most data are discarded when producing a MIP, because only the highest signal intensity voxel within each projection ray becomes a pixel on the final image. Therefore, these images have no depth and must be viewed in multiple projections to detect findings that might otherwise be obscured by overlapping structures with higher signal intensity. A commonly used postprocessing technique to improve image quality is to include only a portion of the source images in the reconstruction volume. This technique, referred to as *targeted* or *partial volume* MIP, reduces interference from overlapping structures and background noise, making the vessels of interest more conspicuous.

Shaded Surface Display

Shaded surface display (SSD) results in dramatic depiction of anatomy and overcomes problems related to depth perception (Fig. 2.9). With this technique, a minimum signal intensity threshold is set, below which the data are discarded. Voxels above the user-defined signal intensity threshold are retained for the next step in image rendering. Subsequently, the surface

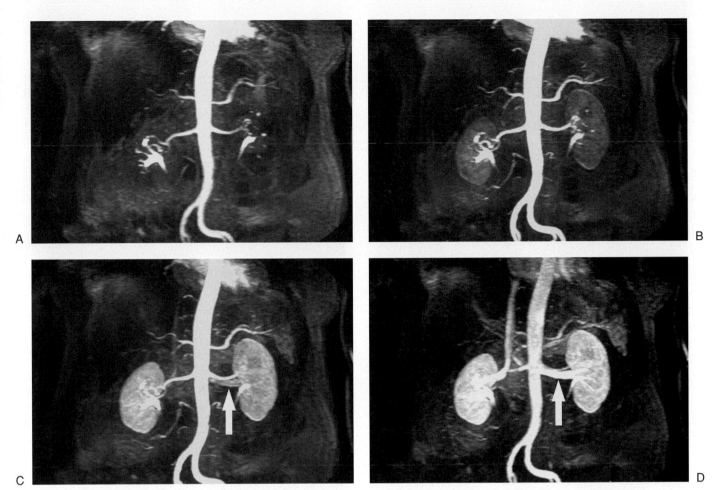

FIG. 2.8. Time-resolved breath-hold contrast-enhanced MRA of renal arteries. Phases A through D were acquired in a total of 19 seconds (<5 seconds per acquisition) using parallel imaging technique (SENSE). Note progressive enhancement of renal veins (*arrow*).

of the vessel of interest is represented, commonly by polygons illuminated with a virtual light source. Shading of the surface allows for depth perception. However, visually pleasing as they may be, these images are best left for impressing clinical colleagues or depicting complex anatomy. In particular, they

TABLE 2.1. *Summary of magnetic resonance angiography reconstruction techniques*

Technique	Application
Multiplanar reformation	Routine part of interpretation
Maximum intensity projection	Overall survey; identify areas for further scrutiny
Targeted maximum intensity projection	Isolate vessel of interest; reduce background signal
Curved re-formation	Obtain vessel measurements
Shaded surface display	Convey depth perception
Volume rendering	Convey anatomic relationships; virtual angioscopy
Subtraction	Eliminate background; produce pure venous images

should never be used to estimate degree of stenosis. The edge voxels of a vessel are typically of lower signal intensity (due to partial volume effects) than the central intraluminal voxels. As a result, the edge voxels may be discarded along with the background in an SSD algorithm, thereby falsely increasing the apparent severity of stenosis.

Multiplanar and Curved Re-formation

One of the most useful techniques for analyzing MRA data is also one of the simplest to apply. Multiplanar re-formation (MPR) allows rapid assessment of MRA data in any plane (Fig. 2.10). By scrolling through the images in multiple planes, one quickly gains a 3D appreciation of the data while avoiding problems with vessel overlap and background projection. Intraluminal vascular abnormalities such as thrombus or dissection flaps are readily depicted. However, because most vessels are curved structures, it is often difficult to display a vessel completely on a single image with MPR. Oblique re-formations allow one to align the image plane along the long axis of a vessel, but images presented in this

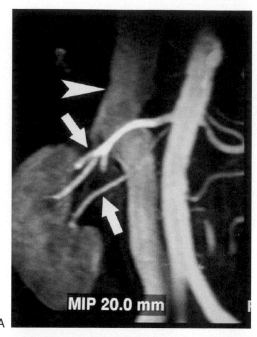

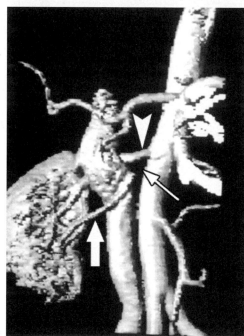

FIG. 2.9. Shaded surface display. **A:** Coronal maximum intensity projection image of three-dimensional gadolinium-enhanced renal MRA shows two right renal arteries (*arrows*) projected over inferior vena cava (IVC) (*arrowhead*). It cannot be determined from this image whether arteries pass anterior or posterior to the IVC. **B:** Shaded surface display of same data set as **(A)** shows inferior artery (*arrow*) to pass anterior to the IVC, while the superior artery (*arrowhead*) passes posterior to the IVC. The apparent gap (*thin arrow*) in the inferior artery was caused by the choice of signal intensity threshold settings used to create this image.

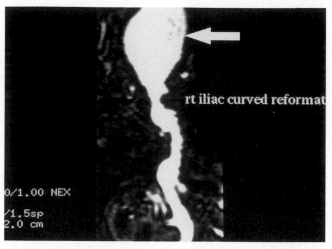

FIG. 2.10. Curved re-formation. Longitudinal view of patient's abdominal aortic aneurysm (*arrow*) and right iliac artery presented on a single image using curved re-formation drawn down the center of the vessel lumen. Such views may be useful for planning interventions such as stent graft placement.

manner may be disorienting. One variation of MPR is curved re-formation. This technique allows the user to project data along a hand-drawn line down the center of a vessel. By using a curved re-formation, one can produce an image of a vessel in its entirety. Such a display allows accurate measurements to be performed for procedures such as stent graft placement. When creating a curved re-formation, one must be careful to follow the exact center of the vessel to avoid generating a pseudostenosis.

Volume Rendering

Volume rendering is the most recent commercially available addition to the 3D reconstruction armamentarium. Despite its growing popularity as a means of data display for computed tomography (CT), volume rendering has not yet been widely used for body MRI applications. Unlike other means of data reconstruction, volume rendering makes use of the entire volume of data (i.e., data are not discarded as they are with MIP or SSD). In addition to allowing window width and level adjustments as with other reconstruction techniques, volume rendering assigns groups of voxels an opacity score from 0% (transparent) to 100% (completely opaque). This function allows one to "see through" selected tissues on the final image. Volume rendering is useful for displaying multiple structures (e.g., tumor, adjacent vessels, and surrounding organs) simultaneously while preserving anatomic relationships. Volume rendering also allows fly-through (e.g., virtual angioscopy) (Fig. 2.11) and fly-around functions.

Subtraction

Subtraction is commonly used before image reconstruction to improve vessel conspicuity by eliminating signal from other

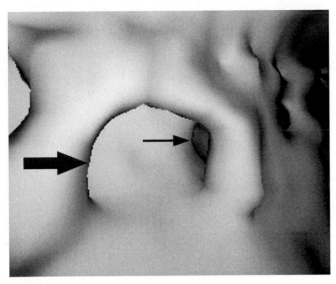

FIG. 2.11. Virtual angioscopy. Virtual angioscopic view through aortic dissection fenestration (*arrow*) showing relationship to left renal artery ostium (*thin arrow*).

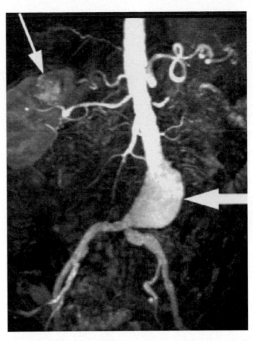

FIG. 2.12. Abdominal aortic aneurysm. Maximum intensity projection image of three-dimensional gadolinium-enhanced MRA of infrarenal abdominal aortic aneurysm (*arrow*) that extends to bifurcation. Note incidentally discovered renal cell carcinoma in right kidney (*thin arrow*).

structures (see Figs. 1.54 and 2.6). The use of subtraction requires a mask, which simply represents a precontrast scan obtained with identical parameters to the subsequent CE-MRA. The mask is then digitally subtracted from the postcontrast scan, resulting in improved image contrast between vessels and background. Subtraction is particularly helpful in eliminating signal from enhancing tissues when two separate contrast injections are used (e.g., when performing a combined study of the chest and abdomen) and for displaying a pure venous phase during indirect MR venography. It is important to have the patient hold his or her breath at the same point in the respiratory cycle for both the mask and the CE-MRA to avoid spatial misregistration artifacts. Requesting the breath-hold at end-expiration can minimize misregistration.

CLINICAL APPLICATIONS OF MRA

Abdominal Aortic Aneurysm

MRA can accurately assess aneurysm extent and the presence of accessory renal arteries (Fig. 2.12) (6,7). The data obtained with MRA can also be used to perform accurate measurements before endoluminal stent graft placement (8). Some aortic stent grafts can be successfully imaged after placement (Fig. 2.13).

It is important to remember that CE-MRA primarily depicts the aortic lumen, particularly when displayed as a MIP. Therefore, the extent of mural thrombus may not be readily apparent on MIP images of an aortic aneurysm, and the true diameter of the aneurysm may be underestimated (Fig. 2.14). In addition, the bulging aortic walls may hide an osteal stenosis or the true aneurysm neck.

Aortic Dissection

The volumetric nature of MRA data provides tremendous benefit over catheter angiography for the evaluation of patients with known or suspected aortic dissection. Through a variety of reconstruction algorithms, the precise origins of the major branch vessels can be determined with respect

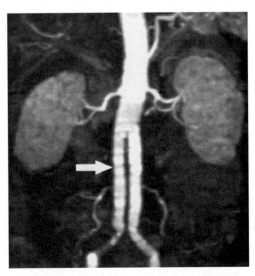

FIG. 2.13. Abdominal aortic aneurysm repair. Maximum intensity projection image of three-dimensional gadolinium-enhanced MRA of infrarenal abdominal aortic aneurysm after endoluminal repair with bifurcated nitinol stent graft (*arrow*).

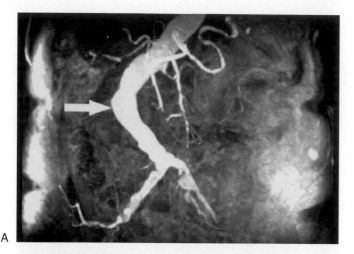

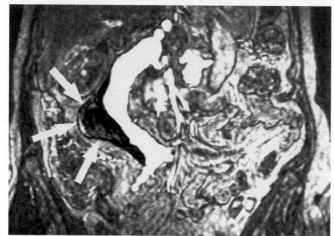

FIG. 2.14. Underestimation of extent of abdominal aortic aneurysm on maximum intensity projection (MIP) image. **A:** MIP image from three-dimensional gadolinium-enhanced aortogram shows mild ectasia of infrarenal aortic lumen (*arrow*). True extent of aneurysm is shown on source image **(B)**, which has been postprocessed to better demonstrate nonenhancing mural thrombus (*arrows*).

to the dissection flap (Fig. 2.15). The dissection flap is typically best demonstrated on MPR images. A thrombosed false lumen may appear as high signal intensity on T1-weighted images performed before injecting contrast material.

Renal MRA

One of the most common indications for abdominal MRA is to evaluate patients with suspected renal artery stenosis (see Fig. 1.53). Several studies have reported sensitivities exceeding 90% for detection of renal artery stenosis with MRA. It is important to detect and assess accessory renal arteries that may arise from the abdominal aorta (or as low as the common iliac arteries). The renal arteries do not always originate from the lateral-most aspect of the aorta. Therefore, an osteal stenosis involving a renal artery with an anterior origin from the aorta may be obscured on a MIP image ori-

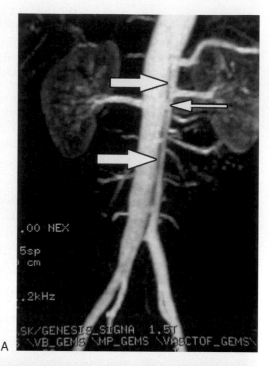

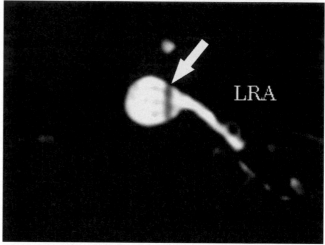

FIG. 2.15. Aortic dissection. **A:** Maximum intensity projection image from three-dimensional gadolinium-enhanced MRA of abdominal aorta shows dissection flap (*arrows*) and fenestrations (*thin arrow* points to same fenestration shown in Figure 2.11). **B:** Flap (*arrow*) is clearly demonstrated on axial re-formation at level of left renal artery.

ented in the anteroposterior (AP) plane. Fibromuscular dysplasia (FMD) may be demonstrated on MRA, although the sensitivity of MRA for the detection of FMD is unknown (Fig. 2.16).

MRA is often used as a component of the preoperative MR evaluation of renal cell carcinoma. Tumor thrombus extending into the renal vein and inferior vena cava (IVC) from renal cell carcinoma may enhance and become inconspicuous on CE-MRA images. Therefore, we recommend that contrast-enhanced images of the renal veins be supplemented with a

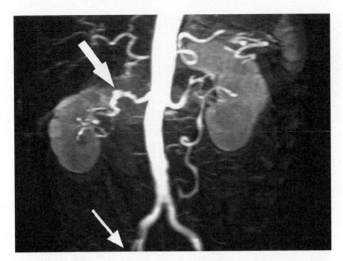

FIG. 2.16. Fibromuscular dysplasia (FMD). Maximum intensity projection image from three-dimensional gadolinium-enhanced MRA shows beading of right renal artery (*arrow*) secondary to FMD. Multiple additional arteries were involved, such as the right external iliac artery (*thin arrow*).

time-of-flight, phase-contrast, or dark blood MRA sequence when tumor thrombus is suspected (Fig. 2.17). Also, peak renal vein enhancement occurs within 5 to 10 seconds of peak renal artery enhancement. Therefore, a biphasic examination designed to optimally depict the renal arteries and veins may be difficult to accomplish with a single contrast injection unless very rapid imaging is performed. Bland renal vein thrombus is clearly depicted on contrast-enhanced studies (Fig. 2.18).

MRA also has utility for the assessment of renal transplant vessels. The most common postoperative arterial anatomy is an end-to-side anastomosis from the transplant renal artery to the recipient external iliac artery. Similarly, the transplant renal vein is attached to the recipient external iliac vein using an end-to-side anastomosis. MRA can assess postoperative vascular complications such as renal artery stenosis, renal arterial or venous thrombosis, and posttransplant pseudoaneurysm or arteriovenous fistula. MRA is also useful for diagnosing pseudo-renal artery stenosis, in which renovascular hypertension or allograft dysfunction occurs secondary to stenosis in the native iliac arteries proximal to the transplant renal artery.

Mesenteric Vessels

MRA of the mesenteric vessels is performed in a similar manner to renal MRA. However, the mesenteric arterial and venous phases are separated by a longer time interval than the arterial and venous phases of the kidney. Therefore, separate evaluation of the mesenteric arteries and veins is easily accomplished by running two consecutive acquisitions after a single injection of contrast material. A coronal imaging plane provides satisfactory images if sufficiently thin partitions are used (≤3 mm) (Fig. 2.19). We do not recommend MRA for the evaluation of small vessel disease or active gastrointestinal bleeding.

Hepatic Vessels

The liver has a dual blood supply via the hepatic artery and portal vein. Contrast-enhanced MRA images of both the hepatic artery and portal vein are obtained simply by performing two separate data acquisitions after contrast injection, allowing approximately 10 seconds for the patient to breathe between acquisitions. A relatively wide window of opportunity exists for imaging the portal vein. Therefore, timing for the portal venous phase is not as critical as for the arterial phase.

Requests to image the hepatic artery are common at centers performing liver transplants or caring for transplant recipients. Most often, patients are referred following an abnormal sonogram. In this situation, MRA frequently identifies the source of the abnormality (Fig. 2.20).

High-quality images of the portal venous system can be obtained with time-of-flight, phase-contrast, or contrast-enhanced MRA. MRA techniques can accurately diagnose acute or chronic thrombosis, tumor invasion, flow reversal, and stenosis of the portal vein. Acute thrombosis is characterized by a nonenhancing portal vein during the venous phase, often associated with a transient hepatic intensity difference related to increased arterial perfusion in the territory supplied by the thrombosed vein. Acute thrombus may occasionally demonstrate increased signal intensity on T1-weighted images and may be confused with flow on noncontrast MRA images (Fig. 2.21). When using noncontrast techniques to image the portal vein, one must also be careful not to confuse flow artifact with thrombus (see Fig. 1.18). Chronic portal vein thrombosis, often referred to as *cavernous transformation*, manifests as absence of a clearly defined main portal vein associated with numerous tortuous collateral veins in the region of the porta hepatis (Fig. 2.22). Tumor thrombus within the portal vein may enhance following contrast material administration and is typically contiguous with a hepatic parenchymal mass (most often hepatocellular carcinoma).

Flow direction within the portal vein can be determined using a 2D gradient echo image with and without a saturation band placed across the proximal aspect of the portal vein. A second saturation band should be placed perpendicular to the aorta above the hepatic dome to eliminate signal from within the hepatic artery. If the distal (closer to the liver) portion of the portal vein loses signal beyond the portal saturation band, the flow is in the normal hepatopetal direction (toward the liver) (Figs. 2.23, 2.24). Similar information can be obtained with phase-contrast MRA, although a saturation band is not necessary in this case, because phase-contrast images are directionally encoded.

Varices associated with portal hypertension are a common finding when performing MRI for evaluation of cirrhosis. There are many potential collateral venous pathways, and it is important to be familiar with the more common patterns visible with MRA.

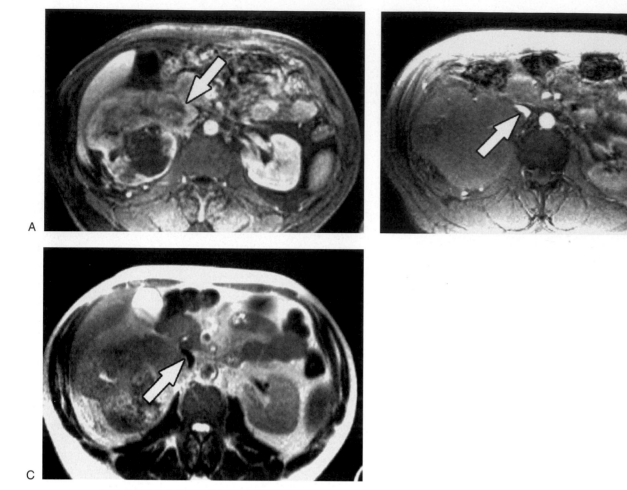

FIG. 2.17. Inferior vena cava (IVC) invasion of renal cell carcinoma demonstrated with three techniques. **A:** Venous phase gadolinium-enhanced three-dimensional interpolated MRI shows large renal mass invading IVC (*arrow*). Due to heterogeneous enhancement of tumor, the precise tumor margins are indeterminate. Two-dimensional time-of-flight **(B)** and dark blood **(C)** techniques more clearly show interface between tumor (*arrow*) and blood. Because artifacts occur with all methods of MRA, we recommend assessment of tumor invasion be confirmed with more than one technique.

The hepatic veins are often well visualized on hepatic MRA examinations, although they are seldom specifically targeted. Important exceptions include hepatic vein thrombosis (Budd-Chiari syndrome). Hepatic vein thrombosis manifests as nonvisualization of the hepatic veins on a flow-sensitive MR sequence or nonenhancement of the hepatic veins on a venous phase contrast-enhanced examination. Often, small curvilinear intrahepatic collateral vessels are present, and the peripheral hepatic parenchyma enhances heterogeneously.

Deep Venous Thrombosis

MRA is not a first line examination for patients with suspected lower extremity deep venous thrombosis (DVT), in that sonography is highly sensitive, specific, and easy to perform. However, MRA is helpful for the evaluation of abdominal and pelvic DVT, because sonography and conventional pedal venography often fail to adequately demonstrate the iliac veins and IVC. Time-of-flight MRA works well for venography, because venous flow is less pulsatile than arterial flow and the major veins are relatively large structures (Fig. 2.25). However, one must be aware of the following common pitfalls when studying the pelvic veins with time-of-flight venography: (1) complex flow patterns may result in signal loss due to intravoxel dephasing, (2) the left common iliac vein crosses under the right iliac artery, resulting in compression of the vein at this location, (3) extrinsic compression of the veins by a mass may simulate DVT (Fig. 2.26). These phenomena may be inadvertently interpreted as thrombus. When performing time-of-flight venography, a 5-mm slice thickness and axial scan plane usually suffice for evaluation of the pelvic veins and IVC.

Contrast-enhanced MRA may also be used to evaluate the pelvic veins using one of two methods. The traditional contrast-enhanced method of pelvic vein evaluation involves

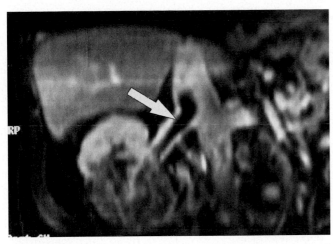

FIG. 2.18. Renal vein thrombus in patient with renal cell carcinoma. Coronal reformation of axial three-dimensional gadolinium-enhanced MRI of patient with renal cell carcinoma. Note nonenhancing bland thrombus (*arrow*) extending from renal vein into inferior vena cava. The patient also had enhancing tumor thrombus (not shown).

a standard antecubital injection of contrast material followed by a sufficient imaging delay to allow for the contrast agent to reach the pelvic veins (a technique referred to as *indirect venography*). When this technique is used, however, peak signal intensity in the veins may be suboptimal due to dilution of the contrast agent. In addition, both arteries and veins are visualized with indirect venography, resulting in overlapping vessels. This latter problem can be resolved by obtaining an initial pure arterial phase acquisition, which can be subtracted from the subsequent venous phase images. The problem of contrast agent dilution can be overcome through a technique referred to as *direct venography* (Fig. 2.27), which is analogous to conventional contrast venography using a pedal injection of contrast material. This technique can produce clear images of systemic venous structures without interference from arteries or enhancing background tissues. When using this technique, however, it is necessary to dilute the contrast agent before injection to reduce the T2-shortening effects of concentrated gadolinium chelate. An appropriate concentration of contrast material can be obtained by mixing 15 mL of gadolinium chelate into a 250-mL bag of normal saline. Direct venography requires bilateral foot vein injections to visualize the entire pelvis and cannot be used to evaluate the internal iliac veins.

PITFALLS OF MRA

Successful MRA interpretation requires familiarity with the many potential pitfalls of the technique. Many pitfalls can be avoided by careful review of the source data. Some common pitfalls afflict both MRA and catheter angiography. For example, some 3D reconstruction techniques such as MIP only depict the opacified vessel lumen. Therefore, mural thrombus

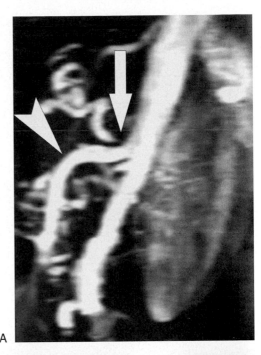

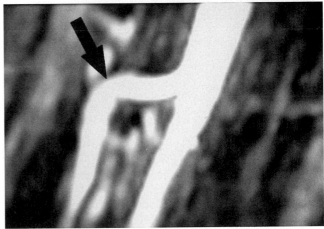

FIG. 2.19. Mesenteric MRA. **A:** Sagittal maximum intensity projection of data from three-dimensional gadolinium-enhanced MRA obtained in coronal plane clearly shows severe celiac artery stenosis (*arrow*) and widely patent superior mesenteric artery (SMA) (*arrowhead*). **B:** No signal is present in proximal celiac artery on phase contrast MRA due to severity of stenosis (*arrow* denotes SMA).

contained within an aneurysm may not be depicted, resulting in underestimation of the aneurysm size (Figs. 2.14 and 2.28). Furthermore, the origins of major branch vessels may be obscured by the adjacent aorta if not viewed in the optimal imaging plane.

Proper positioning of the imaging volume is essential to the success of MRA. One must be careful to ensure that the vessel of interest is included within the imaging volume in its entirety. If the vessel of interest courses partially or completely out of the imaging volume, a stenosis or occlusion may be incorrectly diagnosed. This is particularly true of the renal

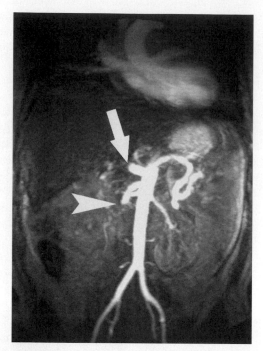

FIG. 2.20. Hepatic artery thrombosis after liver transplantation. Partial volume coronal maximum intensity projection image from three-dimensional gadolinium-enhanced MRA shows abrupt termination of hepatic artery (*arrow*). Acute thrombosis of hepatic artery was found at surgery, and biliary necrosis eventually developed in the patient. Superior mesenteric artery (*arrowhead*) travels out of reconstruction volume, resulting in pseudo-occlusion.

and iliac vessels, which appear to follow a straight course on a frontal projection while possibly being quite tortuous in the axial or sagittal plane.

Endovascular stents and metallic clips adjacent to vessels are common in patients with peripheral vascular disease. Although most stents and metallic clips produce artifact limited to the immediate vicinity of the offending object, susceptibility artifact can simulate an occlusion or stenosis if sufficiently close to or within a vessel (see Fig. 2.28). Some types of embolization coils may produce sufficient artifact to render an MRA examination nondiagnostic. Devices made of nitinol produce relatively little susceptibility artifact and allow imaging of the stent lumen in larger vessels.

Some MRA pitfalls are unique to non–contrast-enhanced techniques. For example, a major limitation of time-of-flight imaging involves the saturation band used to selectively suppress signal from the arteries or veins. Because suppression of flow-related enhancement is based on flow direction, flow-related signal may be suppressed in retrograde-flowing segments of a highly tortuous vessel. This elimination of signal from a retrograde-flowing segment mimics the appearance of occlusion. Other causes of signal loss within a patent vessel include RF saturation of in-plane flow (see Fig. 1.16) and complex flow resulting in intravoxel dephasing. This latter phenomenon is common at major venous confluences

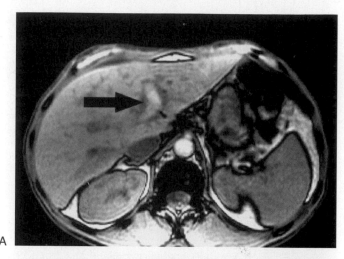

A

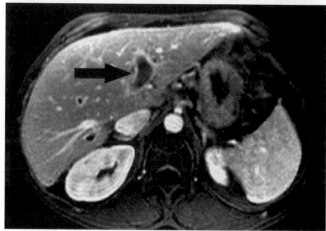

B

FIG. 2.21. Acute portal vein thrombosis. **A:** Noncontrast T1-weighted spoiled gradient echo image shows high signal intensity within left portal vein (*arrow*). **B:** Following administration of intravenous gadolinium, nonenhancing thrombus (*arrow*) is clearly demonstrated.

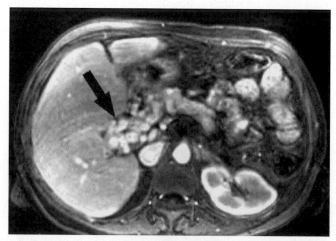

FIG. 2.22. Chronic portal vein thrombosis. Numerous periportal collateral vessels are present in porta hepatis (*arrow*) without clearly defined main portal vein.

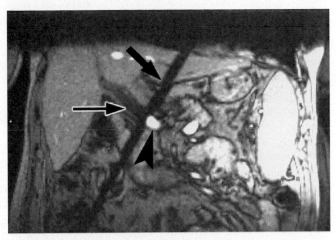

FIG. 2.23. Antegrade portal flow. Coronal gradient echo image performed with narrow saturation band (*arrow*) over portal vein shows high signal intensity portal flow proximal to saturation band (*arrowhead*) and low signal intensity portal flow on hepatic side of saturation band (*thin arrow*) consistent with hepatopetal flow.

(e.g., at the portal confluence [see Fig. 1.18] or where the renal veins enter the IVC).

Although most MRA pitfalls and artifacts involve signal loss within a patent vessel, a thrombosed vessel may occasionally appear patent because methemoglobin contained within the thrombus appears bright on MRA images (many MRA sequences are somewhat T1-weighted) (see Fig. 2.21A).

Abnormalities may also be created or exacerbated through the use of postprocessing. Both MIPs and SSDs may obscure an intraluminal abnormality such as thrombus if the thrombus

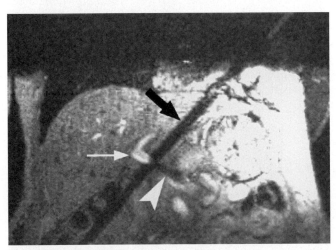

FIG. 2.24. Retrograde portal flow. Coronal gradient echo image performed with narrow saturation band (*arrow*) over portal vein shows low signal intensity portal flow proximal to saturation band (*arrowhead*) and high signal intensity portal flow on hepatic side of saturation band (*thin arrow*) consistent with hepatofugal flow.

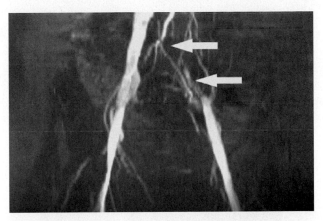

FIG. 2.25. Time-of-flight (TOF) MR venogram of pelvis. Thrombosis of left common iliac vein (*arrows*) is demonstrated on coronal maximum intensity projection image from TOF MR venogram obtained in axial plane. Superior saturation band was used to eliminate signal from arteries.

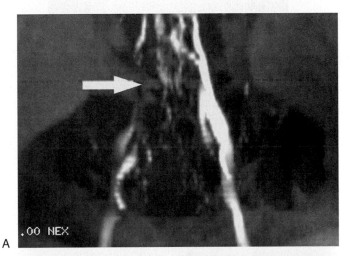

A

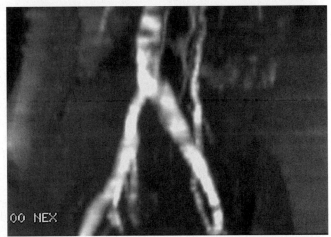

B

FIG. 2.26. Time-of-flight MR venogram of pelvis in patient with large fibroid uterus. **A:** Examination performed with patient supine demonstrates absence of signal in right common iliac vein (*arrow*), which could be confused with thrombus. **B:** Examination performed with patient on her left side demonstrates veins to be patent. Source images (not shown) confirmed venous compression by enlarged uterus.

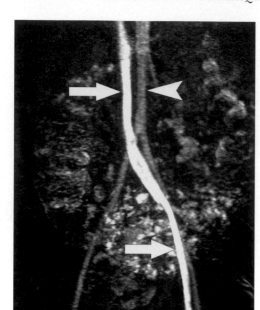

FIG. 2.27. Direct MR venography. Dilute gadolinium chelate (1:15) injected via left foot vein clearly demonstrates patent left iliac veins and inferior vena cava (*arrows*) on maximum intensity projection image from three-dimensional gradient echo acquisition. Note that this technique fails to visualize right pelvic and internal iliac veins. Faint aortoiliac arterial enhancement (*arrowhead*) is present from recirculation of contrast medium.

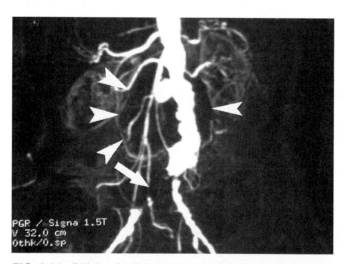

FIG. 2.28. Pitfalls of MRA. Maximum intensity projection image of three-dimensional gadolinium-enhanced MRA of patient with aortic pseudoaneurysm underestimates true size of pseudoaneurysm (*arrowheads* mark extent of largely thrombosed pseudoaneurysm sac found at surgery). Metallic susceptibility artifact from right common iliac artery stainless steel endovascular stent (*arrow*) could be mistaken for occlusion.

is surrounded by high signal intensity blood. Full-thickness MIP displays are also limited by high signal intensity background noise projected onto the reconstructed image (background projection). It is more likely that a projection ray will encounter a voxel of high signal intensity noise if the reconstruction volume is relatively thick. The resulting background projection may obscure low signal intensity, but clinically relevant, structures. In addition, lower signal intensity voxels at the edge of a vessel may be obscured by projected noise, contributing to the apparent severity of a stenosis. Inappropriate threshold settings for an SSD reconstruction may further worsen this effect, making this technique inaccurate for estimating stenosis severity.

SECTION SUMMARY

1. A variety of MRA techniques can be performed without intravenous contrast agents. These include dark blood, time-of-flight, phase-contrast, and steady-state gradient echo techniques.
2. Most contrast-enhanced MRA techniques involve performing a 3D gradient echo sequence following intravenous bolus administration of gadolinium.
3. Accurate timing is critical to the successful performance of 3D gadolinium-enhanced MRA. This can be accomplished through the use of a low-dose timing injection, automated bolus detection technique, or real-time monitoring.
4. A variety of reconstruction techniques can be used to display MRA data. Multiplanar re-formations are most useful for interpretation, whereas maximum intensity projection is the most commonly used display algorithm. Most reconstruction techniques result in loss of data. Volume rendering uses entire data sets and will likely increase in popularity for this reason.
5. MRA has utility for a wide range of clinical indications in the abdomen and pelvis. The arterial, systemic venous, and portal venous systems can all be successfully imaged with MRA techniques.
6. Accurate interpretation of MRA examinations requires familiarity with the potential pitfalls and artifacts that may result from data acquisition and reconstruction.

REFERENCES

1. Svensson J, Petersson JS, Stahlberg F, et al. Image artifacts due to a time-varying contrast medium concentration in 3D contrast-enhanced MRA. *J Magn Reson Imaging* 1999;10:919–928.
2. Foo TK, Saranathan M, Prince MR, et al. Automated detection of bolus arrival and initiation of data acquisition in fast, three-dimensional, gadolinium-enhanced MR angiography. *Radiology* 1997;203:275–280.
3. Korosec FR, Frayne R, Grist TM, et al. Time-resolved contrast-enhanced 3D MR angiography. *Magn Reson Med* 1996;36:345–351.
4. Masunaga H, Takehara Y, Isoda H, et al. Assessment of gadolinium-enhanced time-resolved three-dimensional MR angiography for evaluating renal artery stenosis. *AJR* 2001;176:1213–1219.

5. Schoenberg SO, Bock M, Knopp MV, et al. Renal arteries: optimization of three-dimensional gadolinium-enhanced MR angiography with bolus-timing-independent fast multiphase acquisition in a single breath hold. *Radiology* 1999;211:667–679.

6. Prince MR, Narasimham DL, Stanley JC, et al. Gadolinium-enhanced magnetic resonance angiography of abdominal aortic aneurysms. *J Vasc Surg* 1995;21:656–669.

7. Petersen MJ, Cambria RP, Kaufman JA, et al. Magnetic resonance angiography in the preoperative evaluation of abdominal aortic aneurysms. *J Vasc Surg* 1995;21:891–898.

8. Nasim A, Thompson MM, Sayers RD, et al. Role of magnetic resonance angiography for assessment of abdominal aortic aneurysm before endoluminal repair. *Br J Surg* 1998;85:641–644.

SUGGESTED READINGS

Earls JP, Rofsky NM, DeCorato DR, et al. Breath-hold single-dose gadolinium-enhanced MR aortography: usefulness of a timing examination and a power injector. *Radiology* 1996;201:705–710.

Erden A, Erden I, Karayalcin S, et al. Budd-Chiari syndrome: evaluation with multiphase contrast-enhanced three-dimensional MR angiography. *AJR* 2002;179:1287–1292.

Glockner JF. Three-dimensional gadolinium-enhanced MR angiography: applications for abdominal imaging. *Radiographics* 2001;21:357–370.

Hany TF, McKinnon GC, Leung DA, et al. Optimization of contrast timing for breath-hold three-dimensional MR angiography. *J Magn Reson Imaging* 1997;7:551–556.

Jara H, Barish MA. Black-blood MR angiography. Techniques and clinical applications. *Magn Reson Imaging Clin N Am* 1999;7:303–317.

Kaufman JA, McCarter D, Geller SC, et al. Two-dimensional time-of-flight MR angiography of the lower extremities: artifacts and pitfalls. *AJR* 1998;171:129–135.

Korosec FR, Mistretta CA. MR angiography: basic principals and theory. *Magn Reson Imaging Clin N Am* 1998;6:223–256.

Maki JH, Chenevert TL, Prince MR. Contrast-enhanced MR angiography. *Abdom Imaging* 1998:23;469–484.

Okumura A, Watanabe Y, Dohke M, et al. Contrast-enhanced three-dimensional MR portography. *Radiographics* 1999;19:973–987.

Pavone P, Luccichenti G, Cademartiri F. From maximum intensity projection to volume rendering. *Semin Ultrasound CT MRI* 2001;22:413–419.

Ruehm SG, Zimny K, Debatin JF. Direct contrast-enhanced 3D MR venography. *Eur Radiol* 2001;11:102–112.

Saeed M, Wendland MF, Higgins CB. Blood pool MR contrast agents for cardiovascular imaging. *J Magn Reson Imaging* 2000;12:890–898.

Watanabe Y, Dohke M, Okumura A, et al. Dynamic subtraction contrast-enhanced MR angiography: technique, clinical applications, and pitfalls. *Radiographics* 2000;20:135–152.

SECTION 2.2

Magnetic Resonance Cholangiopancreatography

The refinement and dissemination of magnetic resonance cholangiopancreatography (MRCP) techniques have revolutionized evaluation of the biliary tree and pancreatic duct. MRCP has proven particularly useful in patients for whom endoscopic retrograde cholangiopancreatography (ERCP) is contraindicated, technically difficult, or incomplete. When combined with standard abdominal imaging sequences, MRCP provides a complete assessment of the abdomen not possible with endoscopic techniques.

TECHNIQUE

Most MRCP techniques use heavily T2-weighted sequences, which exploit the long T2 relaxation time of fluid. Background suppression results from the T2 decay of non–fluid-containing structures, which have shorter T2 relaxation times than fluid. The additional application of fat suppression further suppresses background signal, improving the conspicuity of ductal structures. MRCP images may be acquired as a single thick slab using a single-shot fast spin echo sequence or as a series of thin slices that can be reconstructed via the maximum intensity projection (MIP) algorithm (Fig. 2.29). Data acquired as a thick slab cannot be manipulated to create multiple views. Therefore, thick-slab MRCP techniques require the acquisition of multiple separate projections. Even though thin slice techniques overcome this limitation by allowing multiplanar three-dimensional (3D) reconstructions of acquired data, such reconstructions are potentially limited by respiratory motion-induced slice misregistration. Because most MRCP sequences can be performed in less than 30 seconds on newer scanners, both techniques can be routinely used to capitalize on the advantages of each method.

A thick-slab, single-shot fast spin echo sequence with a very long effective echo time (TE) provides a useful overview of the ducts. At a minimum, coronal and bilateral oblique projections should be performed with thick-slab techniques. A slab thickness of 4 to 8 cm generally provides adequate coverage and minimizes overlap from other fluid-containing structures. Thin section images (2 to 4 mm) can be easily obtained with a HASTE sequence in the coronal (or oblique coronal) and axial planes. With this sequence, the entire biliary and pancreatic ductal systems can be covered in one or two breath-holds. Some magnetic resonance imaging (MRI) scanners can perform a 3D respiratory-triggered fast spin echo sequence with extremely thin partitions or slices. When successful, such acquisitions enable very fine 3D reconstructions (Fig. 2.30). However, these sequences are relatively time consuming and easily degraded by inconsistent breathing. Therefore, we do not perform a respiratory-triggered sequence when the breath-hold images are diagnostic.

A successful MR practitioner takes advantage of the infinite multiplanar capability of MRI. For thick-slab imaging, an oblique axial view of the pancreatic or intrahepatic bile ducts is often helpful in delineating anatomy obscured in other planes. Thin slices obtained parallel or perpendicular to a duct of interest may be helpful to confirm the presence of an intraductal stone or demonstrate a communication between the duct and a cystic structure. MRCP sequences take relatively little time to perform, and creativity in choosing imaging planes is often rewarded with informative data (Fig. 2.31).

Negative oral contrast agents may be helpful to suppress the signal from the stomach, duodenum, or other fluid-filled loops of bowel that overlap the biliary or pancreatic ducts. However, the use of negative oral contrast agents is usually unnecessary for diagnostic purposes. Furthermore, visualization of the duodenum is often desirable, because it allows one to localize the position of the ampulla and accurately determine the presence and length of a biliary or pancreatic duct obstruction or stricture.

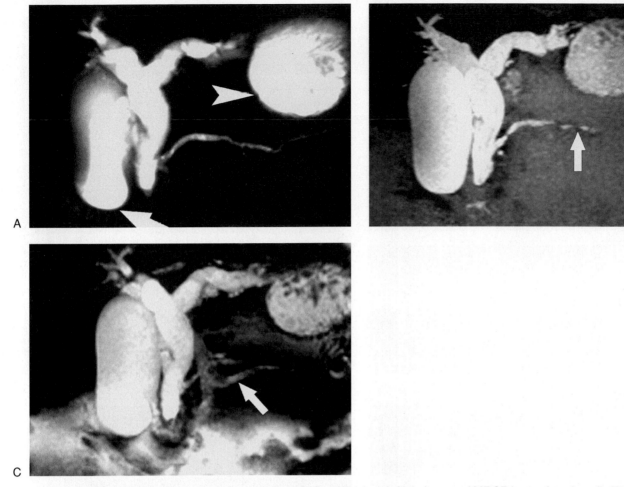

FIG. 2.29. Breath-hold techniques for MRCP. **A:** Thick slab (8 cm) coronal MRCP image from heavily T2-weighted fast spin echo (RARE) sequence in patient with biliary obstruction. Note that fluid in gallbladder (*arrow*) and stomach (*arrowhead*) also appear bright. **B:** Maximum intensity projection (MIP) image of same patient as **(A)** created from 3-mm coronal HASTE images. Note that lack of fat-suppression interferes with visualization of pancreatic duct (*arrow*). **C:** MIP image of same patient as **(A)** created from 3-mm coronal steady-state gradient echo images (balanced FFE). Note that vessels (*arrow*) appear bright on this sequence, potentially complicating interpretation. Data sets for **(B)** and **(C)** can be viewed in any projection.

The use of secretin has been studied for use with MRCP of the pancreatic duct (1–4). Secretin is a hormone produced by the duodenum that stimulates pancreatic secretion in response to acidic contents from the stomach. When administered as part of an MRCP examination, secretin enhances visualization of the pancreatic duct and has been successfully used in the assessment of exocrine reserve in chronic pancreatitis. A synthetic form of secretin has recently been approved for clinical use in the United States.

Hepatobiliary contrast agents, such as mangafodipir (Teslascan), offer an alternative technique for visualizing the bile ducts (Fig. 2.32). These agents are taken up by hepatocytes and are partially excreted in the bile. The time from intravenous administration to appearance of the contrast agent in the bile varies with hepatic function. However, timing of the acquisition is not critical, in that contrast may be excreted in bile for several hours after injection. For mangafodipir-enhanced MR cholangiography, we typically begin imaging the bile ducts with a high-resolution 3D gradient echo sequence approximately 15 to 30 minutes after injection. Currently, mangafodipir remains the only approved hepatobiliary agent for clinical use in the United States.

Kinematic MRCP may be useful in distinguishing biliary dilatation caused by an obstructing ampullary or periampullary lesion from nonobstructive causes of biliary dilatation. This assessment can be performed by repeatedly imaging through the sphincteric segment of the distal common bile duct in the oblique coronal plane using a heavily T2-weighted thick-slab (2 to 3 cm), single-shot fast spin echo or HASTE sequence (5,6).

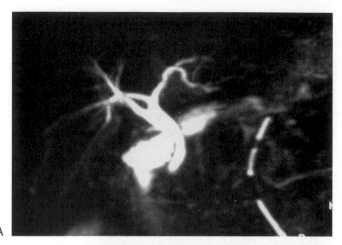

A

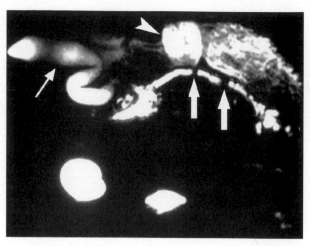

FIG. 2.31. Use of noncoronal imaging plane for MRCP. Pancreatic duct was partially obscured on coronal MRCP (not shown) by gastric fluid in patient with chronic pancreatitis. Thick slab MRCP in oblique axial plane aligned along pancreatic duct clearly demonstrates full length of duct containing two stones (*arrows*) without interference from gallbladder (*thin arrow*) or stomach (*arrowhead*). Bright circle at lower left of image is renal cyst.

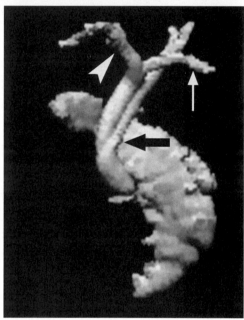

B

FIG. 2.30. Respiratory triggered MRCP. **A:** Coronal maximum intensity projection MRCP image from three-dimensional, respiratory triggered, heavily T2-weighted fast spin echo sequence in patient with aberrant biliary anatomy. Partition thickness was approximately 1.5 mm. **B:** Shaded surface display created from same data set as **(A)** viewed from posterior projection shows low confluence (*arrow*) of right anterior segment duct and duct draining left hepatic (*arrowhead*) and right posterior segment (*thin arrow*) ducts.

CLINICAL APPLICATIONS

Biliary Applications

Preoperative Imaging

MRCP clearly demonstrates biliary anatomy in most patients. Therefore, MRCP has become a useful adjunct to standard MRI of the liver performed as part of the preoperative assessment of patients with liver tumors and for evaluation of potential living-related hemiliver donors (7,8). In the assessment of living-related donors, complete visualization of the

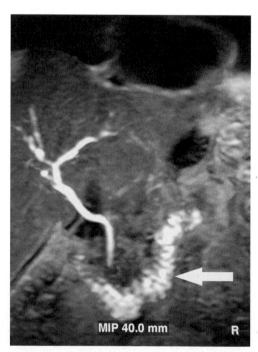

FIG. 2.32. Mangafodipir-enhanced MR cholangiography. Coronal maximum intensity projection of T1-weighted, three-dimensional, interpolated gradient echo sequence performed 1 hour after intravenous administration of mangafodipir clearly demonstrates bile ducts. Note excretion of contrast into duodenum (*arrow*).

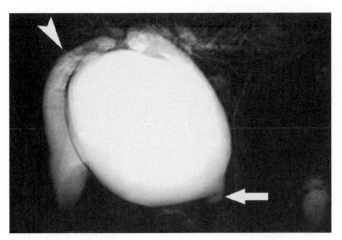

FIG. 2.33. Choledochal cyst. Thick slab coronal MRCP image demonstrates large choledochal cyst arising from common bile duct (*arrow*). Gallbladder and cystic duct are draped over cyst (*arrowhead*).

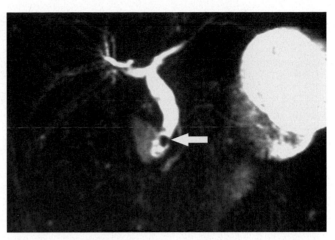

FIG. 2.34. Choledocholithiasis. Coronal thick slab MRCP demonstrates distal common bile duct stone (*arrow*).

relevant intrahepatic bile ducts can be achieved in approximately 90% of individuals. However, smaller or more peripheral branches may elude detection in some individuals. Hepatobiliary agents such as mangafodipir may alleviate this problem by better demonstrating small intrahepatic radicles (9,10).

Congenital Biliary Anomalies

Choledochal cysts (Fig. 2.33) are congenital biliary dilatations thought to result from anomalous union of the common bile and pancreatic ducts, allowing reflux of pancreatic enzymes into the bilary tree. MRCP may be useful for establishing the diagnosis of choledochal cyst and for demonstrating anomalous pancreaticobiliary ductal union, although the latter finding may prove more difficult to demonstrate (11–13).

Choledocholithiasis

Choledocholithiasis (Fig. 2.34) remains one of the most common indications for MRCP of the biliary system. The sensitivity and specificity of MRCP for the diagnosis of choledocholithiasis are approximately 91% to 98% and 89% to 98%, respectively (14–17). Because MRCP does not rely on retrograde injections of contrast material to visualize ducts, it may be more sensitive than ERCP for the diagnosis of intrahepatic bile duct stones (18).

Trauma

Traumatic injury of the biliary system may result from blunt or penetrating abdominal trauma or surgical intervention. Conventional MRCP may demonstrate disruption of a bile duct, although T2-weighted images alone cannot reliably distinguish between a biloma and other fluid collections. Preliminary evidence suggests that hepatobiliary agents such as

mangafodipir may be useful in the diagnosis and characterization of bile leaks and bilomas (Fig. 2.35) (19).

Sclerosing Cholangitis

Sclerosing cholangitis (Fig. 2.36) may occur in isolation or in association with other conditions such as inflammatory bowel disease (most commonly ulcerative colitis), retroperitoneal fibrosis, retroorbital pseudotumor, cirrhosis, and pancreatitis. MRCP compares favorably with ERCP for the diagnosis, depiction, and localization of sclerosing cholangitis. In some patients, MRCP may be superior to ERCP for intrahepatic bile duct visualization in the setting of sclerosing cholangitis (20–22). This is not surprising in that opacification of some ducts peripheral to areas of stricture may not be possible with ERCP.

Neoplastic Involvement of the Bile Ducts

Neoplastic biliary obstruction may result from tumors of biliary or nonbiliary origin. MRCP excels at defining the level of biliary obstruction, thereby helping to build an appropriate differential diagnosis in patients with presumed malignant biliary obstruction.

Most primary biliary tumors are cholangiocarcinomas (Fig. 2.37). Accurate staging is critical to the management of patients with cholangiocarcinoma, because surgical resection offers the best hope of long-term survival. MRCP may play an important role in determining the location and extent of tumor, thereby precluding unnecessary intervention in some patients with malignant hilar strictures (23,24).

Pancreatic Applications

Congenital Anomalies

Congenital anomalies and variants of the pancreatic duct are well demonstrated with MRCP (25–27). Pancreas divisum is

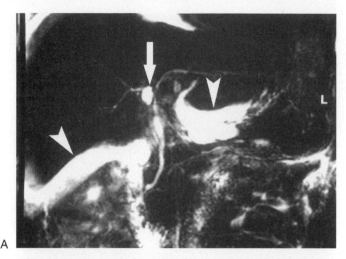

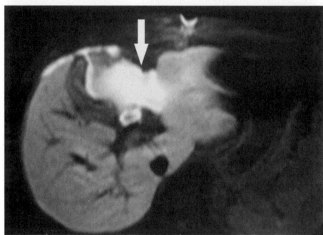

FIG. 2.35. Bile duct laceration. **A:** Conventional coronal thick slab MRCP in patient with stab wound to liver demonstrates focal fluid collection (*arrow*) near right hepatic duct and perihepatic fluid (*arrowheads*). **B:** Fat-suppressed T1-weighted image acquired through liver approximately 1 hour after intravenous administration of mangafodipir demonstrates enhancement of perihepatic fluid (*arrow*) consistent with bile leak. Based on these findings, the patient underwent successful percutaneous drainage of bile ducts.

commonly diagnosed in patients with a history of pancreatitis. However, there is no definitive proof that divisum causes pancreatitis; it is also commonly encountered on MRCP examinations performed for other reasons (Fig. 2.38). Annular pancreas is considerably less common but equally well demonstrated with MRCP techniques (Fig. 2.39).

Pancreatitis

In patients with acute pancreatitis, MRCP compares favorably with ERCP and may assist in identifying underlying structural abnormalities or obstruction of the pancreaticobiliary tract (28,29). Imaging of the pancreatic duct may be difficult during the acute phase due to the presence of edema

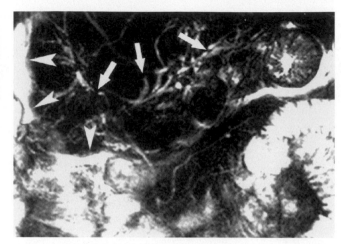

FIG. 2.36. Sclerosing cholangitis. Coronal thick slab MRCP image in patient with sclerosing cholangitis demonstrates multiple intrahepatic biliary strictures (*arrows*). Note lobular liver contour typical of sclerosing cholangitis (*arrowheads*).

and peripancreatic fluid. During acute pancreatitis, MRCP may demonstrate duodenal fold thickening with widening of the c-loop that resembles similar findings on barium studies (Fig. 2.40).

Irreversible pancreatic parenchymal damage characterizes chronic pancreatitis. MRCP accurately depicts the pancreatic ductal abnormalities associated with chronic pancreatitis such as strictures, dilatations of the main duct and side branches, and intraductal calculi (Fig. 2.41) (30). Pancreatic pseudocysts and fistulae can also be demonstrated with MRCP, although communication with the pancreatic duct cannot be established in all cases of pseudocyst. Some of the manifestations of chronic pancreatitis on MRCP

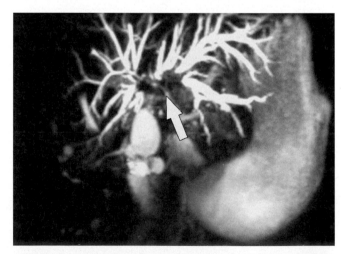

FIG. 2.37. Cholangiocarcinoma. Coronal maximum intensity projection from a respiratory-triggered MRCP demonstrates central obstruction of left and right bile ducts resulting from unresectable hilar cholangiocarcinoma (*arrow*).

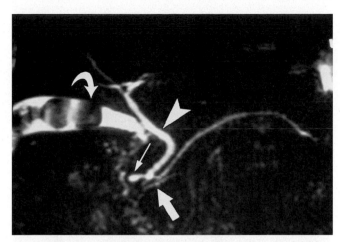

FIG. 2.38. Pancreas divisum. Coronal thick slab MRCP demonstrates small ventral pancreatic duct (*arrow*) draining with common bile duct (*arrowhead*) into ampulla. The majority of pancreatic drainage is via dorsal duct through minor papilla (*thin arrow*). Note focal dilatation of dorsal duct at minor papilla (sometimes referred to as *santorinicele*). Gallstones (curved *arrow*) are present within gallbladder.

overlap with imaging findings of adenocarcinoma or intraductal mucinous tumors. Dilatation of the common bile duct and main pancreatic duct (double duct sign), a finding typically associated with adenocarcinoma, may be seen with chronic inflammation and may be associated with an inflammatory mass, mimicking a neoplasm. Penetration of a mass by a nonobstructed pancreatic duct favors an inflammatory etiology (duct-penetrating sign) (31).

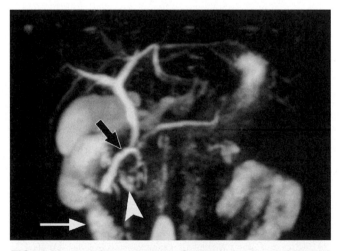

FIG. 2.39. Annular pancreas. Coronal maximum intensity projection of respiratory-triggered MRCP in patient with recurrent episodes of pancreatitis shows dilated annular pancreatic duct (*arrow*) encircling duodenum (*arrowhead*). Patient had intestinal bypass (*thin arrow*) surgery at early age. (From Leyendecker JR, Elsayes KM, Gratz BI, et al. MR cholangiopancreatography: spectrum of pancreatic duct abnormalities. *AJR* 2002;179:1465–1471, with permission.)

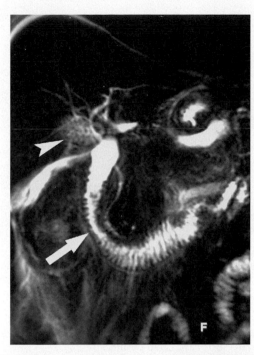

FIG. 2.40. Acute pancreatitis. Coronal thick slab MRCP in patient with acute pancreatitis shows abnormal duodenal c-loop (*arrow*) due to pancreatic inflammation. Note pancreatic duct is poorly visualized. *Arrowhead* denotes gallstones.

Trauma

Documenting main pancreatic duct injury in the setting of abdominal trauma has important prognostic significance. MRCP can be useful in establishing the site of disruption or in confirming ductal integrity in the setting of trauma (Fig. 2.42)(32,33). Because it does not rely on the

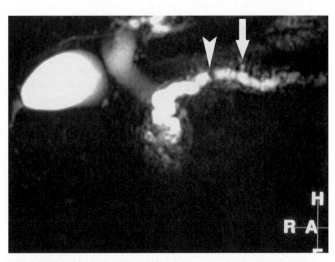

FIG. 2.41. Chronic pancreatitis. Coronal thick slab MRCP in patient with chronic pancreatitis shows dilated main pancreatic duct associated with branch duct ectasia (*arrow*) and intraductal stone (*arrowhead*).

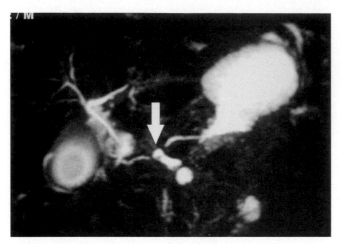

FIG. 2.42. Traumatic disruption of pancreatic duct. Coronal maximum intensity projection from thin section respiratory triggered MRCP demonstrates interruption of pancreatic duct and associated fluid collection (*arrow*) caused by blunt abdominal trauma 2 weeks earlier. (From Leyendecker JR, Elsayes KM, Gratz BI, et al. MR cholangiopancreatography: spectrum of pancreatic duct abnormalities. *AJR* 2002;179:1465–1471, with permission.)

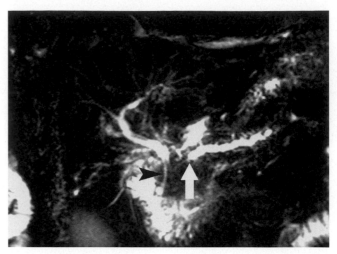

FIG. 2.43. Pancreatic adenocarcinoma. Coronal thick slab MRCP demonstrates abrupt cutoff of pancreatic duct (*arrow*) with upstream dilatation due to adenocarcinoma of pancreatic head. A biliary stent (*arrowhead*) is in place for coexistent biliary obstruction.

retrograde injection of contrast material, MRCP has the advantage over ERCP of reliably demonstrating the pancreatic duct beyond a site of disruption. Because most MR scanners are not optimized for the evaluation of acutely traumatized patients, MRCP may be most practical in the subacute setting, once a trauma patient's condition is stabilized. Pancreatic duct injury should be suspected on MRCP when discontinuity of the duct is documented. An associated fluid collection may be present in the region of the pancreatic duct injury.

Neoplastic Involvement of the Pancreatic Duct

Most malignant pancreatic tumors are adenocarcinomas of ductal origin, with the majority occurring in the pancreatic head. Therefore, most patients with ductal adenocarcinoma have dilatation of the bile duct, pancreatic duct, or both. Abrupt obstruction of the pancreatic duct associated with atrophy of the pancreatic body and tail should raise concern for pancreatic carcinoma (Fig. 2.43). Occasionally, duct dilatation may be the only direct imaging sign of pancreatic cancer. MRCP can be combined with standard parenchymal MRI and MR angiography to provide a comprehensive evaluation of pancreatic adenocarcinoma, particularly with respect to resectability (34).

Intraductal papillary mucinous tumor (IPMT) of the pancreas originates from duct epithelium and produces mucin, resulting in duct dilatation or cyst formation. Therefore, the location and extent of these tumors are readily demonstrated with MRCP (35,36). A simple classification system for IPMT divides this entity into a main duct type and a branch duct type, although features of both types may coexist in a sin-

gle patient. Main duct IPMT is associated with diffuse or segmental dilatation of the main pancreatic duct (Fig. 2.44). Because mucin resembles fluid on heavily T2-weighted sequences, main duct IPMT may be confused with chronic pancreatitis on MRCP images. Chronic pancreatitis may coexist with IPMT, a fact that may further confound the diagnosis. The branch duct type of IPMT can appear unilocular or multilocular, and communication with the main pancreatic duct may be visible with MRCP (Fig. 2.45). The presence of soft tissue filling defects in IPMT suggests malignancy, as does

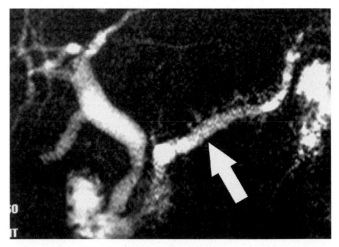

FIG. 2.44. Main duct intraductal papillary mucinous tumor. Coronal thick slab MRCP demonstrates diffuse dilatation of pancreatic duct (*arrow*) with branch duct ectasia. At endoscopy, pancreatic duct was filled with mucin. (From Leyendecker JR, Elsayes KM, Gratz BI, et al. MR cholangiopancreatography: spectrum of pancreatic duct abnormalities. *AJR* 2002;179:1465–1471, with permission.)

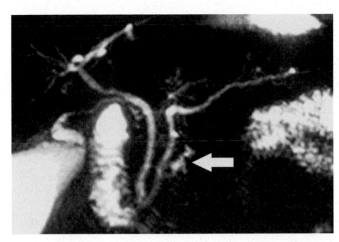

FIG. 2.45. Branch duct intraductal papillary mucinous tumor (IPMT). Coronal thick slab MRCP demonstrates lobulated cystic mass (*arrow*) arising from main pancreatic duct. Benign IPMT was found at surgery. (From Leyendecker JR, Elsayes KM, Gratz BI, et al. MR cholangiopancreatography: spectrum of pancreatic duct abnormalities. *AJR* 2002;179:1465–1471, with permission.)

main pancreatic duct enlargement associated with a branch duct type (37).

PITFALLS OF MRCP

As with all MRI techniques, one must be constantly vigilant about the possibility of artifacts masquerading as abnormalities on MRCP images. One must also be aware of some of the common pitfalls that may lead to an errant interpretation.

A number of entities may lead to a false-positive diagnosis of choledocholithiasis on MRCP images. Air within the bile duct from recent instrumentation or a biliary-enteric anastomosis is a common cause of filling defects within the bile duct. This pitfall can usually be recognized by noting that air rises to the nondependent part of the duct and exhibits susceptibility artifact on gradient echo images. Surgical clips are another cause of susceptibility artifact that may create a pseudostenosis within the bile duct or simulate a filling defect. Susceptibility artifact worsens as the TE increases with gradient echo images, so consulting in-phase and opposed-phase images may be helpful when air bubbles or surgical clips are suspected.

A crossing right hepatic artery may compress the bile duct, creating an impression indistinguishable from a stone on thick-slab images or maximum intensity projection reconstructions (Fig. 2.46). The nature of this extrinsic compression should be evident on thin section images obtained through the duct.

On axial thin section HASTE images, it is common to see a small signal void centered in the common bile duct, simulating a stone. Bile is a dynamic fluid, and HASTE images are particularly sensitive to flow artifact. By repeating the axial images with a sequence that is less susceptible to flow

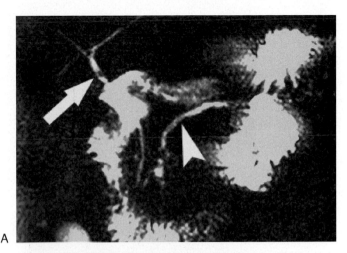

A

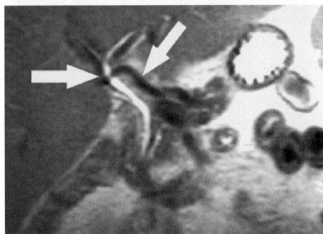

B

FIG. 2.46. Hepatic artery impression on bile duct. **A:** Coronal thick slab MRCP in patient with history of recurrent pancreatitis shows apparent filling defect (*arrow*) in common hepatic duct originally interpreted as stone by inexperienced observer. Note dilated pancreatic duct (*arrowhead*). **B:** Coronal HASTE image shows defect to be caused by crossing right hepatic artery (*arrows*).

artifact, such as TrueFISP or balanced FFE, the true nature of the artifact may be revealed (Fig. 2.47).

False-negative interpretations for stones may also occur, most commonly when a stone is impacted at the ampulla and not surrounded by high signal intensity bile. Thick-slab acquisitions or MIP reconstructions may also obscure stones that are of lower signal intensity than bile. Because all fluid-containing structures appear bright on MRCP images, a fluid-filled stomach, duodenum, or gallbladder may obscure abnormalities of the biliary or pancreatic ducts. Acquiring thinner slabs or performing partial volume reconstructions of the data can minimize this latter problem. However, a duct that courses partially or completely outside of a limited reconstruction volume may falsely appear stenosed or occluded.

Elimination of signal from bowel may also alleviate the problem of overlapping structures, although the duodenum

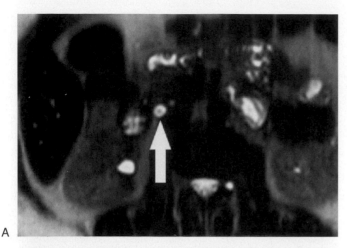

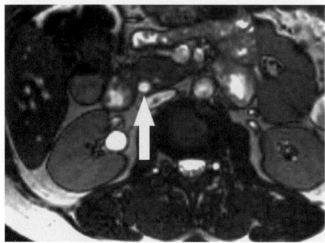

FIG. 2.47. Flow artifact in common bile duct. **A:** Thin section axial HASTE image demonstrates low signal focus in center of distal common bile duct (*arrow*). **B:** Steady-state gradient echo (TrueFISP) image shows no stone in distal duct (*arrow*).

serves as a useful landmark for the position of the ampulla. The use of negative oral contrast agents with MRCP may cause one to misjudge the distance from the visualized portion of the bile or pancreatic duct to the ampulla. As a result, a stricture or tumor involving one or both of these ducts may be missed on MRCP images. Therefore, if the duodenum is not visualized on an MRCP image, it is important to refer to soft tissue images to ensure that the ducts are visualized to the level of the ampulla.

SECTION SUMMARY

1. Most MRCP techniques are based on heavily T2-weighted sequences optimized for the display of fluid-filled structures.
2. MRCP data can be acquired as a thick slab that cannot be manipulated or as multiple thin sections that can be reconstructed and viewed in any projection.
3. Mangafodipir is a hepatobiliary MR contrast agent that shows promise for imaging of the bile ducts.

4. MRCP is useful for evaluation of a variety of congenital, inflammatory, traumatic, and neoplastic processes involving the biliary and pancreatic ducts.
5. Accurate interpretation of MRCP examinations requires familiarity with the potential pitfalls and artifacts that may result from data acquisition and reconstruction.

REFERENCES

1. Cappeliez O, Delhaye M, Deviere J, et al. Chronic pancreatitis: evaluation of pancreatic exocrine function with MR pancreatography after secretin stimulation. *Radiology* 2000;215:358–364.
2. Fukukura Y, Fujiyoshi F, Sasaki M, et al. Pancreatic duct: morphologic evaluation with MR cholangiopancreatography after secretin stimulation. *Radiology* 2002;222:674–680.
3. Manfredi R, Costamagna G, Brizi MG, et al. Severe chronic pancreatitis versus suspected pancreatic disease: dynamic MR cholangiopancreatography after secretin stimulation. *Radiology* 2000;214:849–855.
4. Hellerhoff KJ, Helmberger H 3rd, Rosch T, et al. Dynamic MR pancreatography after secretin administration: image quality and diagnostic accuracy. *AJR* 2002;179:121–129.
5. Kim JH, Kim MJ, Park SI, et al. Using kinematic MR cholangiopancreatography to evaluate biliary dilatation. *AJR* 2002;178:909–914.
6. Van Hoe L, Gryspeerdt S, Vanbeckevoort D, et al. Normal Vaterian sphincter complex: evaluation of morphology and contractility with dynamic single-shot MR cholangiopancreatography. *AJR* 1998;170:1497–1500.
7. Fulcher AS, Szucs RA, Bassignani MJ, et al. Right lobe living donor liver transplantation: preoperative evaluation of the donor with MR imaging. *AJR* 2001;176:1483–1491.
8. Lee VS, Morgan GR, Teperman LW, et al. MR imaging as the sole preoperative imaging modality for right hepatectomy: a prospective study of living adult-to-adult liver donor candidates. *AJR* 2001;176:1475–1482.
9. Lee VS, Rofsky NM, Morgan GR, et al. Volumetric mangafodipir trisodium-enhanced cholangiography to define intrahepatic biliary anatomy. *AJR* 2001;176:906–908.
10. Kapoor V, Peterson MS, Baron RL, et al. Intrahepatic biliary anatomy of living adult liver donors: correlation of mangafodipir trisodium-enhanced MR cholangiography and intraoperative cholangiography. *AJR* 2002;179:1281–1286.
11. Irie H, Honda H, Jimi M, et al. Value of MR cholangiopancreatography in evaluating choledochal cysts. *AJR* 1998;171:1381–1385.
12. Matos C, Nicaise N, Deviere J, et al. Choledochal cysts: comparison of findings at MR cholangiopancreatography and endoscopic retrograde cholangiopancreatography in eight patients. *Radiology* 1998;209:443–448.
13. Kim MJ, Han SJ, Yoon CS, et al. Using MR cholangiopancreatography to reveal anomalous pancreaticobiliary ductal union in infants and children with choledochal cysts. *AJR* 2002;179:209–214.
14. Hochwalk SN, Dobryansky M, Rofsky NM, et al. Magnetic resonance cholangiopancreatography accurately predicts the presence or absence of choledocholithiasis. *J Gastrointest Surg* 1998;2:573–579.
15. Boraschi P, Neri E, Braccini G, et al. Choledocholithiasis: diagnostic accuracy of MR cholangiopancreatography. Three-year experience. *Magn Reson Imaging* 1999;17:1245–1253.
16. Taylor AC, Little AF, Hennessy OF, et al. Prospective assessment of magnetic resonance cholangiopancreatography for noninvasive imaging of the biliary tree. *Gastrointest Endosc* 2002;55:17–22.
17. Calvo MM, Bujanda L, Calderon A, et al. Role of magnetic resonance cholangiopancreatography in patients with suspected choledocholithiasis. *Mayo Clin Proc* 2002;77:422–428.
18. Kim TK, Kim BS, Kim JH, et al. Diagnosis of intrahepatic stones: superiority of MR cholangiopancreatography over endoscopic retrograde cholangiopancreatography. *AJR* 2002;179:429–434.
19. Vitellas KM, El-Dieb A, Vaswani KK, et al. Using contrast-enhanced MR cholangiography with IV mangafodipir trisodium (Teslascan) to evaluate bile leaks after cholecystectomy: a prospective study of 11 patients. *AJR* 2002;179:409–416.
20. Fulcher AS, Turner MA, Franklin KJ, et al. Primary sclerosing

cholangitis: evaluation with MR cholangiography—a case-control study. *Radiology* 2000;215:71–80.

21. Vitellas KM, El-Dieb A, Vaswani KK, et al. MR cholangiopancreatography in patients with primary sclerosing cholangitis: interobserver variability and comparison with endoscopic retrograde cholangiopancreatography. *AJR* 2002;179:399–407.

22. Vitellas KM, Enns RA, Keogan MT, et al. Comparison of MR cholangiopancreatographic techniques with contrast-enhanced cholangiography in the evaluation of sclerosing cholangitis. *AJR* 2002;178:327–334.

23. Zidi SH, Prat F, Le Guen O, et al. Performance characteristics of magnetic resonance cholangiography in the staging of malignant hilar strictures. *Gut* 2000;46:103–106.

24. Lee SS, Kim MH, Lee SK, et al. MR cholangiography versus cholangioscopy for the evaluation of longitudinal extension of hilar cholangiocarcinoma. *Gastrointest Endosc* 2002;56:25–32.

25. Bret PM, Reinhold C, Taourel P, et al. Pancreas divisum: evaluation with MR cholangiopancreatography. *Radiology* 1996;199:99–103.

26. Ueno E, Takada Y, Yoshida I, et al. Pancreatic diseases: evaluation with MR cholangiopancreatography. *Pancreas* 1998;16:418–426.

27. Manfredi R, Costamagna G, Brizi MG, et al. Pancreas divisum and "santorinicele": diagnosis with dynamic MR cholangiopancreatography with secretin stimulation. *Radiology* 2000;217:403–408.

28. Sica GT, Braver J, Cooney MJ, et al. Comparison of endoscopic retrograde cholangiopancreatography with MR cholangiopancreatography in patients with pancreatitis. *Radiology* 1999;210:605–610.

29. Shimizu T, Suzuki R, Yamashiro Y, et al. Magnetic resonance cholangiopancreatography in assessing the cause of acute pancreatitis in children. *Pancreas* 2001;22:196–199.

30. Takehara Y, Ichijo K, Tooyama N, et al. Breath-hold MR cholangiopancreatography with a long-echo-train fast spin echo sequence and a surface coil in chronic pancreatitis. *Radiology* 1994;192:73–78.

31. Ichikawa T, Sou H, Araki T, et al. Duct-penetrating sign at MRCP: usefulness for differentiating inflammatory pancreatic mass from pancreatic carcinomas. *Radiology* 2001;221:107–116.

32. Fulcher AS, Turner MA, Yelon JA, et al. Magnetic resonance cholangiopancreatography (MRCP) in the assessment of pancreatic duct trauma and its sequelae: preliminary findings. *J Trauma* 2000;48:1001–1007.

33. Soto JA, Alvarez O, Múnera F, et al. Traumatic disruption of the pancreatic duct: diagnosis with MR pancreatography. *AJR* 2001;176:175–178.

34. Catalano C, Pavone P, Laghi A, et al. Pancreatic adenocarcinoma: combination of MR imaging, MR angiography and MR cholangiopancreatography for the diagnosis and assessment of resectability. *Eur Radiol* 1998;8:428–434.

35. Sugiyama M, Atomi Y, Hachiya J. Intraductal papillary tumors of the pancreas: evaluation with magnetic resonance cholangiopancreatography. *Am J Gastroenterol* 1998;93:156–159.

36. Usuki N, Okabe Y, Miyamoto T. Intraductal mucin-producing tumor of the pancreas: diagnosis by MR cholangiopancreatography. *J Comput Assist Tomogr* 1998;22:875–879.

37. Irie H, Honda H, Aibe H, et al. MR cholangiopancreatographic differentiation of benign and malignant intraductal mucin-producing tumors of the pancreas. *AJR* 2000;174:1403–1408.

SUGGESTED READINGS

Fayad LM, Kowalski T, Mitchell DG. MR cholangiopancreatography: evaluation of common pancreatic diseases. *Radiol Clin North Am* 2003;41:97–114.

Fulcher AS, Turner MA. Pitfalls of MR cholangiopancreatography (MRCP). *J Comput Assist Tomogr* 1998;22:845–850.

Fulcher AS, Turner MA. MR pancreatography: a useful tool for evaluating pancreatic disorders. *Radiographics* 1999;19:5–24.

Irie H, Honda H, Kuroiwa T, et al. Pitfalls in MR cholangiopancreatographic interpretation. *Radiographics* 2001;21:23–37.

Leyendecker JR, Elsayes KM, Gratz BI, et al. MR cholangiopancreatography: spectrum of pancreatic duct abnormalities. *AJR* 2002;179:1465–1471.

Motohara T, Semelka RC, Bader TR. MR cholangiopancreatography. *Radiol Clin North Am* 2003;41:89–96.

SECTION 2.3

Magnetic Resonance Urography

Magnetic resonance (MR) urography refers to MR imaging (MRI) of the urinary collecting systems in a way that provides information roughly analogous to conventional intravenous urography (IVU). Magnetic resonance imaging is well suited to evaluation of the urinary collecting systems for several reasons. First, the collecting systems are fluid-filled structures that can be imaged using techniques described for magnetic resonance cholangiopancreatography (MRCP). Second, the multiplanar capability of MRI allows optimization of scan planes for evaluation of the ureters and bladder. Third, the extracellular gadolinium chelates are excreted by glomerular filtration. In addition to providing excellent anatomic depiction of the kidneys and renal collecting systems, gadolinium chelates allow functional studies of the collecting systems to be performed without aggravating or inducing renal insufficiency. Despite these theoretical advantages, MR urography is rarely performed as a standalone procedure, because conventional IVU, computed tomography (CT), or ultrasound suffices for diagnosis of the majority of urologic abnormalities. However, MR urography remains a useful adjunct technique when combined with renal parenchymal imaging, particularly in patients with compromised renal function.

TECHNIQUE

The simplest method of performing MR urography involves the use of long echo train, heavily T2-weighted sequences identical to those employed for MRCP. This method is often referred to as static MR urography, and long echo train T2-weighted sequences are sometimes referred to as *RARE* (rapid acquisition with relaxation enhancement) sequences. The use of a relatively long effective echo time (TE) (>140 msec) results in greater conspicuity of fluid-containing structures. The use of fat suppression further increases conspicuity of the collecting systems by eliminating signal from retroperitoneal and intraabdominal fat. As with MRCP, these sequences may be performed as multiple thin slices that can be postprocessed or as a thick slab performed in multiple projections (Fig. 2.48). Breath-hold sequences are preferable to free-breathing sequences. However, for patients unable to hold their breath, respiratory triggering is helpful to reduce motion artifact. Images should be obtained in the coronal plane with a large field of view that includes the entire collecting system. As with conventional IVU, oblique imaging of the intrarenal collecting systems may be helpful to better define anatomy. Although static MR urography is effective in depicting obstructed urinary tracts, nondistended collecting systems may be difficult to portray. If necessary, this problem can be mitigated by hydrating the patient before the examination and administering a low dose of furosemide. An advantage of static MR urography over contrast-enhanced techniques is that it is independent of renal function and eliminates the need for delayed imaging to define the level of ureteral obstruction. Therefore, static MR urography may be more time efficient than excretory urography in this setting.

Excretory MR urography using an intravenous gadolinium chelate is an alternative strategy for imaging the renal collecting systems (Fig. 2.49). This is most often performed as an adjunct to a contrast-enhanced MRI performed for other reasons. However, specific indications for performing contrast-enhanced MR urography include preoperative localization of nondistended ureters or demonstration of a communication between the renal collecting system and a cystic structure or fluid collection (Fig. 2.50). The feasibility of MR renography, in which renal function is quantified with gadolinium-enhanced dynamic MRI, has been demonstrated (1). However, this technique is not widely used.

MR urographic techniques are still evolving. The optimal intravenous contrast dose, method of administration, sequence parameters, and timing of image acquisition for excretory MR urography have yet to be determined. A simple test dose of 1 to 2 mL of contrast material often provides a useful MR urogram on subsequent coronal T1-weighted three-dimensional (3D) gradient echo sequences, as long as sufficient time has elapsed to allow the contrast material to enter the collecting systems (Fig. 2.51). However, this *low-dose* method may be limited by incomplete ureteral visualization due to inadequate patient hydration (2).

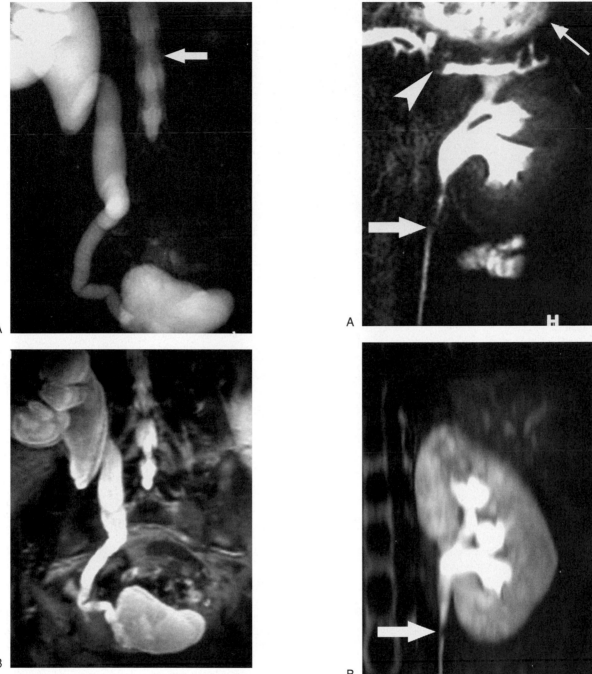

FIG. 2.48. A: Coronal thick-slab static MR urogram in patient with obstructing transitional cell carcinoma. Note incidental MR myelogram (*arrow*). **B:** Maximum intensity projection MR urogram created from multiple coronal thin section HASTE images in same patient as **(A)**.

FIG. 2.49. Static versus excretory MR urography. **A:** Coronal static MR urogram in patient with tiny proximal left ureter stone (*arrow*) demonstrates multiple overlapping fluid-filled structures such as stomach (*thin arrow*) and pancreatic duct (with intraductal stone) (*arrowhead*). **B:** Excretory urogram performed with 20 mL intravenous gadolinium is not limited by overlying fluid and demonstrates nonobstructing nature of ureteral stone (*arrow*).

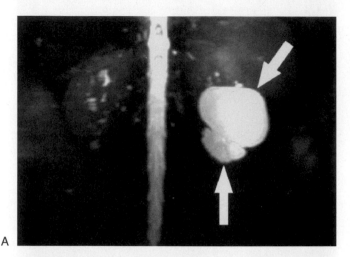

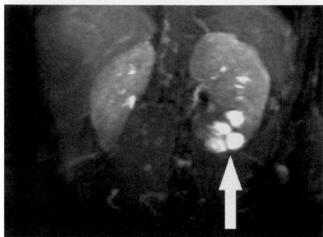

FIG. 2.50. Excretory urography to evaluate cystic renal mass. **A:** Coronal static MR urogram demonstrates large complex cystic mass (*arrows*) involving lower left kidney. **B:** Excretory urogram performed with intravenous gadolinium chelate shows lower part of mass to represent collecting system (*arrow*) obstructed by larger simple cyst (not filled with contrast).

The use of a standard 0.1-mmol/kg dose of gadolinium chelate often results in signal loss within the renal collecting systems due to the T2 shortening effect of gadolinium at high concentrations (Fig. 1.32). This T2 shortening effect of gadolinium is one reason that MR urograms using T2-weighted techniques are commonly performed *before* gadolinium administration (Fig. 1.35). Hydrating the patient and administering a low dose of diuretic such as furosemide (typically 5 to 10 mg) prevents excessive concentration of the contrast material within the collecting systems while improving ureteral distention and contrast distribution in patients without obstruction (3). Gadolinium-based contrast agents have a higher specific gravity than urine and layer dependently within the renal collecting systems and bladder if undisturbed. Turning a supine patient prone or rolling the patient from side to side may alleviate this problem. The infusion of normal saline may augment the effects of furosemide or serve as a standalone

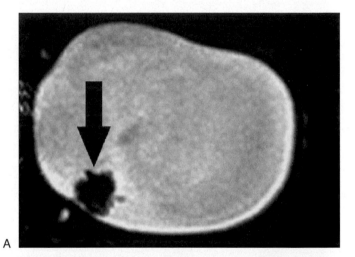

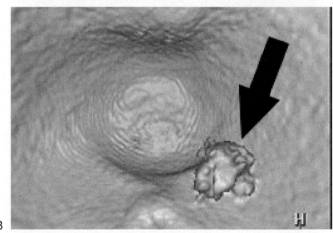

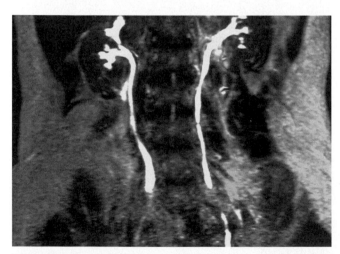

FIG. 2.51. Low-dose MR urogram. Coronal maximum intensity projection image created from three-dimensional gradient echo sequence performed 5 minutes after 2-mL dose of intravenous gadolinium.

FIG. 2.52. Virtual cystoscopy. **A:** Source image from a three-dimensional fast spin echo acquisition of the urinary bladder demonstrates a small polypoid transitional cell carcinoma (*arrow*) arising from the left lateral bladder wall. **B:** Virtual cystoscopic view demonstrates carcinoma (*arrow*) from different perspective. (Images courtesy of Markus Lämmle, M.D.)

TABLE 2.2. *Comparison of static versus excretory magnetic resonance urography*

	Static	Excretory
Can be used in setting of severe renal insufficiency	Yes	No
Imaging delay necessary	No	Yes
Intravenous contrast necessary	No	Yes
Visualization of nondistended ureters	Poor	Good
Problems with overlapping fluid	Yes	No

method of improving gadolinium dilution and distribution. However, neither the optimal gadolinium dosage nor the role of saline infusion in MR urography has been thoroughly established. Excretory MR urography is unlikely to succeed in patients with severely compromised renal function, and saline infusion is not recommended for fluid-restricted patients.

3D gradient echo sequences, preferably combined with fat suppression, provide high-resolution MR urographic images following gadolinium administration that can be used to create maximum intensity projections in multiple views. The coronal plane provides the greatest anatomic coverage in the shortest time, although additional planes may occasionally be useful. If coronal images are of sufficiently high resolution with nearly isotropic voxel dimensions, multiplanar re-formations may substitute for additional acquisitions in other planes. High-performance imaging gradients are necessary to allow complete image acquisition within a single breath-hold.

Although maximum intensity projection and multiplanar re-formation are the most common display methods for MR urography, occasionally other novel reconstruction techniques may be beneficial. For example, virtual cystoscopy or ureteroscopy may be performed using high-resolution, 3D fast spin echo data sets (Fig. 2.52). As with static MR urography, virtual cystoscopy using T2-weighted images must be performed before administration of intravenous gadolinium.

Table 2.2 compares static with excretory MR urography.

CLINICAL APPLICATIONS

Urinary Tract Obstruction

In an obstructed urinary tract, MR urography demonstrates the level of obstruction with an accuracy approaching 100% (4). When T2-weighted (static) MR urography is combined with gadolinium-enhanced 3D gradient echo (excretory) MR urography, the sensitivity for detection of ureteral stones may exceed 90% (see Fig. 2.49) (5,6). Gadolinium-enhanced 3D MR urographic techniques probably have a higher sensitivity for the detection of stones than T2-weighted techniques. Despite the feasibility of MR urography for the evaluation of patients with acute flank pain, it is likely that MR urography will remain a rarely performed adjunct pro-

cedure in this population given the continued use of conventional excretory urography and widespread adoption of CT. However, MR urography will likely assume greater importance in the pediatric and obstetric populations, in whom there is a greater need to avoid ionizing radiation exposure.

Neoplastic obstruction of the collecting system can result from intrinsic urothelial tumors or extrinsic masses that have invaded, encased, or compressed the ureter. Obstructing transitional cell carcinoma involving the ureter is well demonstrated with static techniques in the absence of hemorrhage (Figs. 2.53, 2.54). Primary transitional cell carcinoma of the ureter is much less common than

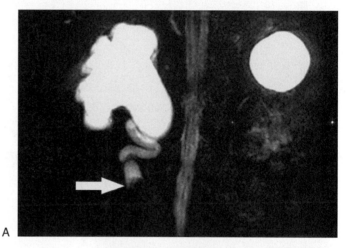

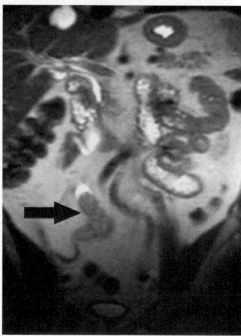

FIG. 2.53. Transitional cell carcinoma of ureter. **A:** Coronal thick-slab static MR urogram demonstrates obstructing tumor of right ureter with inverted "goblet sign." **B:** Coronal HASTE image shows extent of tumor (*arrow*) in right ureter.

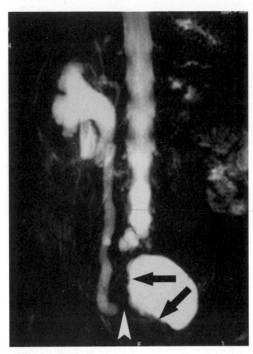

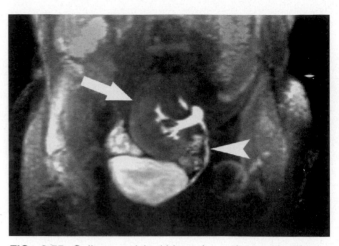

FIG. 2.55. Solitary pelvic kidney in patient with Mayer-Rokitansky-Küster-Hauser syndrome. Ultrasound evaluation (not shown) of patient's pelvic kidney questioned ureteral dilatation. Low-dose excretory urography of pelvic kidney (*arrow*) demonstrates nondilated collecting system (*arrowhead*).

FIG. 2.54. Transitional cell carcinoma of bladder. Coronal thick-slab static MR urogram demonstrates transitional cell carcinoma of bladder (*arrows*) obstructing distal right ureter (*arrowhead*).

secondary involvement of the ureter from bladder cancer. Because urothelial tumors grow slowly, resulting in ureteral dilatation, the administration of gadolinium is unnecessary to visualize the site of obstruction. However, intravenous gadolinium is beneficial in demonstrating the extent of the tumor, which enhances after contrast administration. Likewise, fat-suppressed gadolinium-enhanced sequences are useful for demonstrating extrinsic processes that involve the ureter, such as cervical carcinoma or retroperitoneal fibrosis.

Congenital Abnormalities

Congenital urinary tract abnormalities can be accurately assessed with MR urography (Figs. 2.55, 2.56) (7,8). MR urography combined with MRI provides detailed anatomic information in patients with duplex kidneys and a variety of other congenital renal anomalies. In children with congenital urinary tract anomalies, MR urography and MRI can be combined to provide functional and anatomic information needed for treatment planning and monitoring.

Surgical Evaluation

MR urography may be combined with MR angiography (MRA) and parenchymal sequences to provide a comprehensive preoperative imaging examination. In addition to

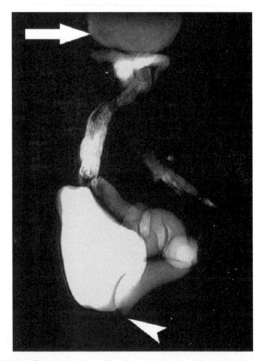

FIG. 2.56. Duplicated collecting system with ectopic ureteral insertion. Oblique sagittal thick-slab static MR urogram in young female with urinary incontinence shows obstructed upper pole moiety (*arrow*) due to ectopic insertion of ureter (*arrowhead*) below bladder (actual insertion site was proximal urethra).

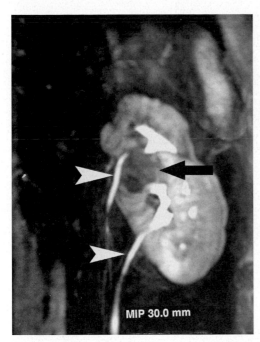

FIG. 2.57. Excretory MR urogram in patient with renal mass considered for partial nephrectomy. Maximum intensity projection image clearly shows relationship of left renal mass (low signal intensity) (*arrow*) to duplicated ureters (*arrowheads*). This portion of the examination was combined with evaluation of the renal artery, vein, and upper abdomen during the same imaging session (not shown).

delineating the size, number, and location of renal masses, the relationship of masses to renal vessels and the collecting systems can be accurately determined (Fig. 2.57). A comprehensive evaluation of potential living renal donors may be performed without concern for nephrotoxicity (9,10). The combination of MR urography, contrast-enhanced renal parenchymal imaging, and MRA may also be beneficial in the evaluation of complications such as abscess, ureteral injury, and vascular compromise in patients after renal transplantation (11,12).

PITFALLS OF MR UROGRAPHY

Because MR urograms are often displayed as maximum intensity projections, many of the same pitfalls afflicting the interpretation of MR angiograms apply to MR urograms. For example, a low signal intensity ureteral stone surrounded by high signal intensity urine may be obscured on maximum intensity projection images. Likewise, improper choice of projection angle or reconstruction volume may create false-positive findings or obscure true abnormalities as a result of overlapping structures or increased background signal intensity. Superimposition of overlapping structures is particularly problematic for static MR urography, in that any fluid-filled structure (e.g., bowel loops, gallbladder and

bile ducts, the spinal canal, or perinephric fluid collections) may have the same signal intensity as urine on the images.

Nondistended ureters may escape detection on static MR urograms, resulting in the incorrect diagnosis of complete ureteral obstruction in the setting of a high-grade partial obstruction. If the distinction between complete and partial obstruction is clinically relevant, excretory MR urography should also be performed.

Parapelvic cysts may masquerade as hydronephrosis, and calyceal diverticula may simulate simple renal cysts on static MR urograms. Once again, gadolinium administration quickly clarifies this issue. However, gadolinium may create different problems when it becomes too concentrated within the collecting system. Sufficiently concentrated gadolinium shortens T2-relaxation times to the point that signal loss from T2 relaxation exceeds the T1-shortening effects of the contrast agent. This may result in poor visualization of all or a portion of the collecting system on T1-weighted images. Concentrated gadolinium in the renal collecting system also causes signal loss on T2-weighted images, particularly when long echo times are used (see Fig. 1.35).

Blood products resulting from hemorrhage within the collecting system may create several problems confounding the interpretation of MR urograms (Fig. 2.58). Methemoglobin from subacute hemorrhage can produce bright signal within the urine, potentially obscuring enhancing intraluminal tumors on early postcontrast T1-weighted images. Subtraction imaging may be helpful in this regard. Hemosiderin or intracellular deoxyhemoglobin can cause T2 shortening that limits the utility of heavily T2-weighted static MR urograms.

Susceptibility effects from metallic objects such as surgical clips can cause apparent ureteral narrowing or obstruction. Also, HASTE sequences may demonstrate flow artifacts resulting from urine in motion. These artifacts are particularly common in the bladder as a result of the ureteral jets and may simulate a bladder abnormality. If a flow artifact is suspected, we recommend repeating the sequence, because flow artifacts often change in appearance on subsequent images. Alternatively, a flow-insensitive steady-state gradient echo sequence (trueFISP, balanced FFE, FIESTA) can be performed.

When interpreting MR urograms (as with all MR techniques), it is important not to rely entirely on reconstructed images for interpretation. A careful review of source images often eliminates potential pitfalls. Proper window and level settings must be used to avoid missing subtle findings of lower signal intensity such as thin septations and walls, small tumors, or stones that may be obscured by the bright surrounding urine. One must also remember that dilatation of the collecting system is not synonymous with obstruction. Vesicoureteral reflux and residual postobstructive dilatation are managed differently from ureteral

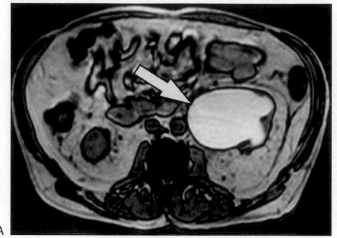

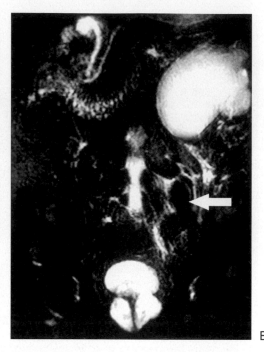

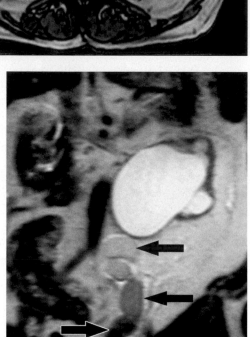

FIG. 2.58. Patient with transitional cell carcinoma of left distal ureter and hematuria. **A:** Blood products within obstructed collecting system have resulted in high signal intensity urine (*arrow*) on T1-weighted gradient echo image. **B:** Coronal static MR urogram performed with a heavily T2-weighted sequence shows ureter as signal void (*arrow*) outlined by fluid due to presence of more concentrated blood products in ureter. **C:** Less heavily T2-weighted coronal HASTE image demonstrates gradual loss of urine signal intensity (*arrows*) due to increasing concentration of blood products as ureter approaches distal tumor.

obstruction, and an effort should be made to distinguish these entities.

SECTION SUMMARY

1. MR urography may be performed using heavily T2-weighted sequences similar to those used for MRCP (static MR urography). As with MRCP, either a thick slab or thin section acquisition can be performed.

2. MR urography may also be performed by imaging after administration of intravenous gadolinium chelate using a 3D gradient echo sequence similar to that used for MRA (excretory MR urography). Excretory MR urography may be performed using either a low dose or conventional dose of intravenous contrast material.

3. Static MR urography works best for dilated collecting sys-

tems and can be successfully employed independent of renal function.

4. Excretory MR urography is preferred over static techniques for demonstration of nondistended ureters. However, excretory MR urography cannot be used in the setting of severely impaired renal function.

5. Patient hydration and diuretic administration may improve ureteral distention and contrast agent distribution during MR urography. These additional modifications may also reduce the T2-shortening effects of excreted gadolinium chelate following administration of a conventional dose of the contrast agent.

6. Clinical applications of MR urography include the evaluation of ureteral obstruction and congenital urinary tract abnormalities.

7. Accurate interpretation of MR urography examinations

requires familiarity with the potential pitfalls and artifacts that may result from data acquisition and reconstruction.

REFERENCES

1. Katzberg RW, Buonocore MH, Ivanovic M, et al. Functional, dynamic, and anatomic MR urography: feasibility and preliminary findings. *Acad Radiol* 2001;8:1083–1099.
2. Szopinski K, Szopinska M, Borówka A, et al. Magnetic resonance urography: initial experience of a low-dose Gd-DTPA-enhanced technique. *Eur Radiol* 2000;10:1158–1164.
3. Nolte-Ernsting CC, Bucker A, Adam GB, et al. Gadolinium-enhanced excretory MR urography after low-dose diuretic injection: comparison with conventional excretory urography. *Radiology* 1998;209:147–157.
4. Blandino A, Gaeta M, Minutoli F, et al. MR pyelography in 115 patients with a dilated renal collecting system. *Acta Radiol* 2001;42:532–536.
5. Sudah M, Vanninen R, Partanen K, et al. MR urography in evaluation of acute flank pain: T2-weighted sequences and gadolinium-enhanced three-dimensional FLASH compared with urography. *AJR* 2001;176:105–112.
6. Sudah M, Vanninen RL, Partanen K, et al. Patients with acute flank pain: comparison of MR urography with unenhanced helical CT. *Radiology* 2002;223:98–105.
7. Avni FE, Nicaise N, Hall M, et al. The role of MR imaging for the assessment of complicated duplex kidneys in children: preliminary report. *Pediatr Radiol* 2001;31:215–223.
8. Rohrschneider WK, Haufe S, Wiesel M, et al. Functional and morphologic evaluation of congenital urinary tract dilatation by using combined static-dynamic MR urography: findings in kidneys with a single collection system. *Radiology* 2002;224:683–694.
9. Low RN, Martinez AG, Steinberg SM, et al. Potential renal transplant donors: evaluation with gadolinium-enhanced MR angiography and MR urography. *Radiology* 1998;207:165–172.
10. Israel GM, Lee VS, Edye M, et al. Comprehensive MR imaging in the preoperative evaluation of living donor candidates for laparoscopic nephrectomy: initial experience. *Radiology* 2002;225:427–432.
11. Schubert RA, Gockeritz S, Mentzel HJ, et al. Imaging in ureteral complications of renal transplantation: value of static fluid MR urography. *Eur Radiol* 2000;10:1152–1157.
12. Cohnen M, Brause M, May P, et al. Contrast-enhanced MR urography in the evaluation of renal transplants with urological complications. *Clin Nephrol* 2002;58:111–117.

SUGGESTED READINGS

Blandino A, Gaeta M, Minutoli F, et al. MR urography of the ureter. *AJR* 2002;179:1307–1314.

Gaeta M, Blandino A, Scribano E, et al. Diagnostic pitfalls of breath-hold MR urography in obstructive uropathy. *J Comput Tomogr* 1999;23:891–897.

Nolte-Ernsting CC, Staatz G, Tacke J, et al. MR urography today. *Abdom Imaging* 2003;28:191–209.

SECTION 2.4

Magnetic Resonance Imaging of the Gastrointestinal Tract

Multiplanar capability, lack of ionizing radiation, and potential for superior tissue characterization represent distinct advantages of magnetic resonance imaging (MRI) over other imaging modalities for evaluation of the gastrointestinal tract. However, respiratory motion, peristalsis, susceptibility artifact from air, and the presence of stool have impeded progress in the development of gastrointestinal MRI applications. With the advent of newer imaging sequences and an increasing array of intravenous and enteric contrast agents, a renewed interest in gastrointestinal applications of MRI has emerged in recent years, although many of the MRI techniques discussed herein are still undergoing clinical testing and optimization.

TECHNIQUE

The two most commonly used sequences for imaging the gastrointestinal tract are HASTE and gadolinium-enhanced, fat-suppressed, T1-weighted gradient echo. Both of these sequences are relatively rapid, allowing imaging of the entire region of interest during a single breath-hold. Half-Fourier single-shot techniques are highly sensitive for intraluminal fluid and are resistant to the susceptibility effects of intraluminal air, although signal-to-noise issues limit the spatial resolution attainable with HASTE sequences (Fig. 2.59). Fat-suppressed, contrast-enhanced techniques allow visualization of enhancing gastrointestinal mucosa and inflammatory tissues but are plagued by the susceptibility artifact created by intraluminal air. This latter limitation is becoming less problematic as sequences with shorter echo times become available. Alternative rapid steady-state sequences such as trueFISP or balanced FFE are being used by some MR practitioners to image fluid-filled bowel. These sequences provide sharp, motion-free images of the bowel during a single breath-hold.

Various oral contrast agents have been investigated for bowel imaging, including man-made and naturally occurring (e.g., blueberry juice) paramagnetic substances, barium, perfluorocarbon, polyethylene glycol, methylcellulose, and particulate iron oxides. Aside from obvious safety and patient acceptance issues, desirable attributes of an oral contrast agent include lack of significant intestinal absorption, uniform distribution, and a dilution-resistant effect on intraluminal signal intensity. A substance that improves bowel distention is also desirable in certain clinical settings. Agents that are bright on T2-weighted images and dark on T1-weighted images may be preferable, because they act as positive intraluminal contrast agents on T2-weighted images while improving conspicuity of the bowel wall and inflammatory processes on fat-suppressed gadolinium-enhanced T1-weighted images.

Despite the wide variety of MRI techniques and contrast agents reported in the literature, gastrointestinal MRI can be relatively simple. Water makes an excellent contrast agent for evaluation of the stomach and proximal small bowel, especially when combined with the motion-resistant HASTE sequence (Fig. 2.60). Water can also be administered rectally for colonic distension before imaging. Oral 2% barium sulfate makes a readily available, inexpensive small bowel contrast medium that is particularly effective when combined with intravenous gadolinium and fat-suppressed T1-weighted gradient echo imaging (1). For the evaluation of inflammatory and neoplastic processes, we prefer the combination of fat-suppressed T2-weighted images and gadolinium-enhanced, fat-suppressed T1-weighted images. Fat-suppressed T2-weighted images are superior for the detection of abnormal fluid collections and edema, whereas the latter images provide the best evaluation of the bowel wall. Fat-suppressed T1-weighted imaging may be performed serially after the administration of intravenous contrast using either a two-dimensional (2D) or three-dimensional (3D) spoiled gradient echo sequence (SPGR, FFE, FLASH) during breath-holding. Delayed imaging performed 3 to 5 minutes after contrast administration using a high spatial

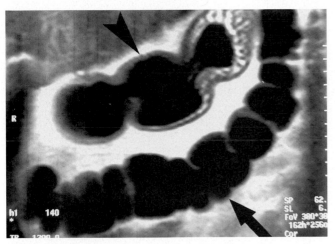

FIG. 2.59. HASTE image of normal bowel. Air-distended transverse colon (*arrow*) and stomach (*arrowhead*) are clearly demonstrated on this coronal HASTE image.

resolution T1-weighted sequence is also suggested. Intravenous glucagon can be used to minimize bowel motion during image acquisition. We suggest injecting 1 mg in a split dose of 0.5 mg per injection just before HASTE and gadolinium-enhanced imaging.

CLINICAL APPLICATIONS

Inflammatory Bowel Diseases

Inflammatory processes of the bowel (Figs. 2.61, 2.62) are characterized by wall edema, thickening, and enhancement, features that are easily demonstrated with available MRI techniques. Despite the potential of MRI for imaging a wide variety of inflammatory bowel processes, much interest has centered on the assessment of Crohn disease.

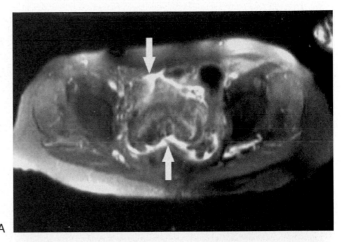

A

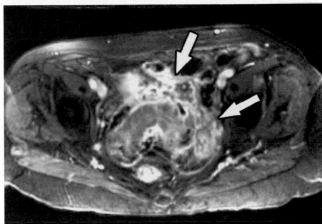

B

FIG. 2.61. Sigmoid diverticulitis. **A:** Axial fat-suppressed T2-weighted image through the pelvis in a patient with acute diverticulitis shows marked colon thickening with high signal intensity pericolonic fluid and edema (*arrows*). **B:** Fat-suppressed T1-weighted gradient echo image at same level as (**A**) shows enhancement of inflamed tissues (*arrows*).

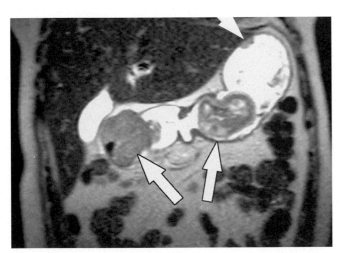

FIG. 2.60. Water as oral contrast agent. Multiple gastric masses (gastrointestinal stromal tumors) (*arrows*) are demonstrated in stomach on coronal HASTE image obtained after ingestion of water.

In patients with Crohn disease, transmural inflammation of the bowel wall develops, resulting in wall thickening, surrounding inflammation, and, in some cases, fistula and abscess formation. Contrast-enhanced, fat-suppressed gradient echo images performed after ingestion of dilute oral barium can accurately depict the site and degree of bowel wall thickening. The intensity of bowel wall enhancement provides a qualitative measure of the activity of inflammation, which can help guide therapy (2,3). T2-weighted and contrast-enhanced T1-weighted images are used together to assess extraluminal inflammation, fistulae, and abscesses. The presence of intestinal strictures (which require adequate bowel distention to demonstrate) and fibrofatty proliferation do not, by themselves, imply active inflammation.

Several other techniques have been investigated for the evaluation of patients with Crohn disease. These include MR enteroclysis with a nasojejunal tube using a variety of intraluminal contrast agents. The sensitivity and specificity of

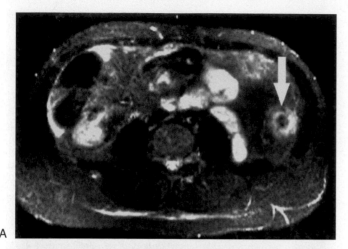

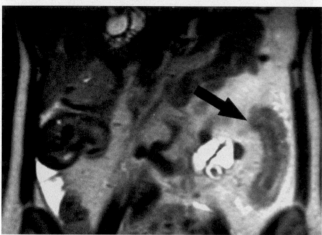

FIG. 2.62. Crohn disease. A: Fat-suppressed T2-weighted image of lower abdomen demonstrates thickening and increased signal intensity of left colon (*arrow*) in patient with active Crohn disease. **B:** Non–fat-suppressed coronal HASTE image of same patient as **(A)** demonstrates colon wall thickening (*arrow*), but lack of fat suppression limits assessment of edema and fluid.

MR enteroclysis for diagnosing inflammatory bowel disease and demonstrating fistulae and abscesses may exceed that of conventional enteroclysis (4).

Bowel Obstruction

MRI is sensitive for detecting bowel obstruction and is accurate in determining its cause (Figs. 2.63, 2.64) (5–7). Fluid-sensitive fast MR techniques such as half-Fourier single-shot echo train spin echo (HASTE, ssFSE, ssTSE) are particularly useful for imaging of small bowel obstruction. The multiplanar capability of MRI should be exploited in determining the precise location of obstruction. In some cases, the ability of MRI to determine the location and cause of bowel obstruction may exceed that of helical computed tomography (CT).

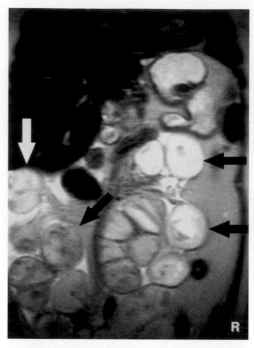

FIG. 2.63. Small bowel obstruction. Coronal HASTE image of abdomen demonstrates multiple dilated loops of small bowel (*arrows*) in patient with small bowel obstruction secondary to adhesions.

Tumor Staging

Accurate staging of gastrointestinal tumors is critical to ensure that patients receive appropriate treatment. The role of MRI in staging gastrointestinal malignancies has not yet been firmly established. In recent years, however, data have accumulated supporting the use of MRI in the staging of gastrointestinal malignancies.

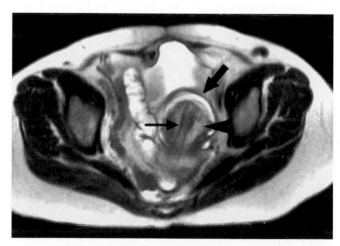

FIG. 2.64. Colonic intussusception. Axial T2-weighted image demonstrates layers of sigmoid colonic intussusception with outer colon wall (*arrow*), pericolonic fat (*arrowhead*), and inner colon wall (*thin arrow*).

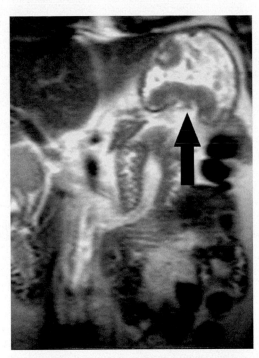

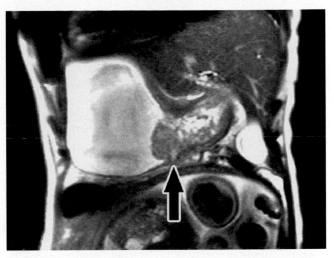

FIG. 2.67. Adenocarcinoma of the stomach in pregnant patient. Oblique coronal HASTE image demonstrates large gastric mass outlined by water. Serosal involvement (*arrow*) was found at surgery.

FIG. 2.65. Malignant gastrointestinal stromal tumor. Coronal HASTE image of same patient as in Figure 2.60 demonstrates transserosal extension of tumor in fundus of stomach as indicated by disruption of low signal intensity gastric wall (*arrow*). Tumor was invading into perigastric fat at surgery.

Gastric cancer is well demonstrated with MRI (Figs. 2.65, 2.66, 2.67). Gastric cancer staging is based on the TNM classification. Staging of the primary tumor (T) is based on depth of invasion into the gastric wall and MRI accurately predicts the T stage of gastric cancer in approximately 73% to 88% of patients (9–12). T1 disease invades the lamina propria or submucosa, T2 disease invades the muscularis propria or subserosa, T3 disease penetrates the serosa without

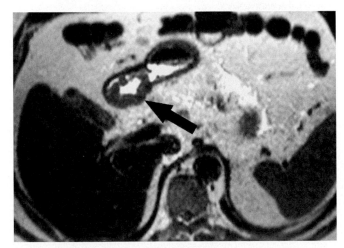

FIG. 2.66. Adenocarcinoma of the stomach. Axial HASTE image demonstrates ulcerated mass in gastric antrum (*arrow*) outlined by fluid.

invading adjacent organs, and T4 disease invades adjacent structures. Wall invasion is probably best appreciated on fat-suppressed, gadolinium enhanced, breath-hold T1-weighted gradient echo images. Dynamic and delayed (approximately 2 minutes) imaging typically reveals focal thickening of the stomach wall or a mass that enhances differently (greater or less) than the normal gastric wall. In general, increased enhancement of the tumor relative to the normal gastric wall is more common. Extraserosal invasion is suggested by disruption of the low signal intensity band normally present around the outer gastric wall (8). Extraserosal invasion is easier to detect when the gastric wall is surrounded by fat. Fat-suppressed, contrast-enhanced gradient echo images may demonstrate enhancing tumor extending into the perigastric fat. The sensitivity of MR for detecting extraserosal tumor invasion may be as high as 93% using dynamic contrast-enhanced techniques (13).

The N stage of gastric cancer is determined by the presence and number of regional or distant lymph node metastases. Because microscopic lymph node metastases cannot be reliably detected with any current cross-sectional imaging modality, nodal disease tends to be understaged. Sensitivity for detection of lymph node metastases depends on the pulse sequence used, and MR generally suffers from the same limitation as CT in that nodal size is not a reliable indicator of malignancy (14).

The imaging protocol for gastric cancer evaluation should include a breath-hold HASTE sequence performed in multiple planes, a fat-suppressed fast spin echo sequence, and dynamic and delayed gadolinium-enhanced spoiled gradient echo images. Fat suppression is recommended for postcontrast imaging when possible. Recently, steady-state free precession images (true-FISP, balanced FFE, FIESTA) have shown utility in imaging gastric cancer and may be beneficial if available. Water administered orally immediately before imaging makes an excellent contrast agent, and more expensive alternatives are probably unnecessary (15).

As with gastric cancer, the accurate staging of rectal carcinoma has important prognostic and therapeutic implications. However, studies have reported a wide range of tumor staging accuracies for MRI. In part, this is because techniques for MRI of rectal cancer continue to evolve and vary considerably from one clinical setting to another.

At present, MRI is capable of achieving similar accuracy to endorectal sonography for T-staging of rectal cancer (16–18). MRI tends to overstage early disease and cannot reliably distinguish between T1 (limited to the submucosa) and T2 (limited to the muscularis propria) tumors. In addition, interobserver variation is considerable for T1 and T2 tumors, even with the use of an endorectal coil (19). The accuracy of MRI improves with more advanced disease, but tends to understage T3 disease. The accuracy rate for determining metastatic lymphadenopathy remains relatively poor, because size criteria remain the sole basis for distinguishing benign from malignant lymph nodes with MRI (20).

The appropriate imaging protocol for staging rectal carcinoma is controversial, although high-resolution imaging and the use of intravenous gadolinium are beneficial (21–24). The use of an endorectal coil may improve one's ability to visualize the layers of the bowel wall, although satisfactory results for detecting T3 and T4 disease can be achieved with the use of an external phased-array coil when an endorectal coil is unavailable or contraindicated (25). Endorectal coils have several disadvantages. Insertion of an endorectal coil in patients with circumferential, stenosing tumors may be difficult and painful. Endorectal coils allow only a limited field of view and may not completely visualize proximal tumor, perirectal structures, or lymph nodes. Although endorectal coil MRI can be combined with a phased-array body coil examination, this adds considerably to the examination time. Ultimately, higher field strength scanners (e.g., 3 T) may completely eliminate the need for endorectal coil imaging, although this remains speculative. The need for rectal distention with an endoluminal contrast agent is similarly controversial, and further studies are needed before the routine use of rectal distention with contrast agents can be completely endorsed.

High-resolution T2-weighted images of the rectum using a phased-array body coil demonstrate three layers of the rectal wall (26). The high signal intensity innermost layer consists of mucosa and submucosa. This layer is bordered by the low signal intensity muscularis propria. The outermost layer consists of relatively hyperintense perirectal fat. Following contrast administration, the muscularis propria remains relatively low signal intensity compared with the enhancing mucosa. Complete interruption of the low signal intensity muscularis propria or invasion of the perirectal fat on T2-weighted or contrast-enhanced T1-weighted images indicates at least stage T3 disease (Fig. 2.68).

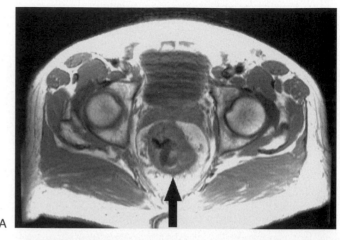
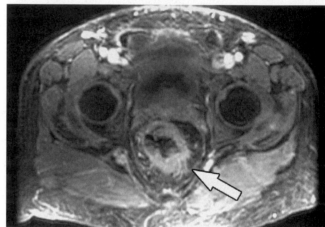

FIG. 2.68. T3 Rectal carcinoma. **A:** Axial T1-weighted fast spin echo image of pelvis demonstrates marked rectal thickening in patient with rectal carcinoma (*arrow*). **B:** Fat-suppressed, gadolinium-enhanced T1-weighted gradient echo image shows infiltration of the perirectal fat (*arrow*) by tumor.

MR Colonography

Current guidelines for colon cancer screening involve testing for occult blood in the stool and periodic endoscopy or barium enema examinations after the age of 50 years. Due to poor compliance with current screening guidelines, CT and MR colonography (MRC) have been proposed as less invasive alternatives to colonoscopy. Although CT colonography has received more attention to date, the use of MRC would avoid exposure of a large segment of the population to ionizing radiation. Currently, there is no consensus as to the optimal technique for MRC. The challenges faced by investigators involve the usual tradeoffs between signal-to-noise, scan time, spatial resolution, and artifact suppression.

A variety of endoluminal contrast agents have been proposed for MRC, including gas, water, gadolinium, and barium. In general, MRC techniques can be divided into bright lumen and dark lumen techniques. The most thoroughly

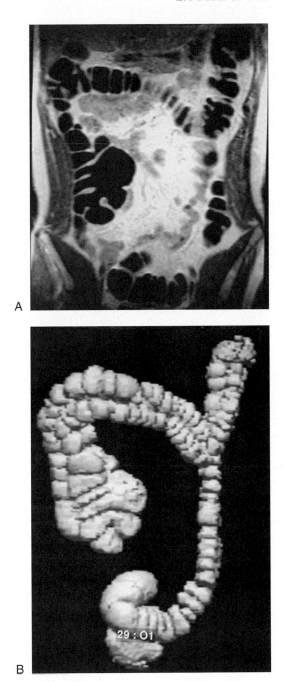

FIG. 2.69. Dark lumen MR colonography. **A:** Coronal source image from air-contrast examination of the colon using T1-weighted fast-spin echo technique optimized for breath-hold imaging. **B:** Surface rendering from same data set as **(A)** demonstrates anatomy of colon.

studied bright lumen technique involves administration of a dilute gadolinium enema and imaging with a T1-weighted 3D gradient echo sequence (27,28). Dark lumen techniques use a negative intraluminal contrast agent such as barium or air and may be combined with intravenous gadolinium to improve conspicuity of the colon wall and polyps (Fig. 2.69). Fecal tagging using an orally administered contrast agent may reduce or eliminate the need for colon

catharsis (29). As with MR enteroclysis, however, much work remains to be done before MRC can be considered mainstream.

SECTION SUMMARY

1. Protocols designed to evaluate abnormalities of the bowel typically include fat-suppressed T2-weighted and

fat-suppressed, gadolinium-enhanced T1-weighted sequences.

2. Half-Fourier single-shot spin echo (HASTE, ssFSE, ssTSE) and steady-state gradient echo (trueFISP, balanced FFE, FIESTA) sequences can rapidly provide motion-free images of the bowel.

3. A variety of substances have been tested as oral MR contrast agents. Two inexpensive, readily available oral contrast agents for gastrointestinal imaging are barium suspension and water.

4. Inflammatory and obstructive processes of the small bowel and colon are well evaluated with currently available MRI techniques.

5. MRI may be useful for staging of gastric and rectal cancer.

6. Initial results with MR colonography and MR enteroclysis are promising, although further development is required before widespread clinical acceptance of these relatively new techniques is gained.

REFERENCES

1. Low RN, Francis IR. MR imaging of the gastrointestinal tract with I.V. gadolinium and diluted barium oral contrast media compared with unenhanced MR imaging and CT. *AJR* 1997;169:1051–1059.
2. Maccioni F, Viscido A, Broglia L, et al. Evaluation of Crohn disease activity with magnetic resonance imaging. *Abdom Imaging* 2000;25:219–228.
3. Koh DM, Miao Y, Chinn RJ, et al. MR imaging evaluation of the activity of Crohn's disease. *AJR* 2001;177:1325–1332.
4. Rieber A, Wruk D, Potthast S, et al. Diagnostic imaging in Crohn's disease: comparison of magnetic resonance imaging and conventional imaging methods. *Int J Colorectal Dis* 2000;15:176–181.
5. Regan F, Beall DP, Bohlman ME, et al. Fast MR imaging and the detection of small-bowel obstruction. *AJR* 1998;170:1465–1469.
6. Beall DP, Fortman BJ, Lawler BC, et al. Imaging bowel obstruction: a comparison between fast magnetic resonance imaging and helical computed tomography. *Clin Radiol* 2002;57:719–724.
7. Matsuoka H, Takahara T, Masaki T, et al. Preoperative evaluation by magnetic resonance imaging in patients with bowel obstruction. *Am J Surg* 2002;183:614–617.
8. Kang BC, Kim JH, Kim KW, et al. Value of the dynamic and delayed MR sequence with Gd-DTPA in the T-staging of stomach cancer: correlation with the histopathology. *Abdom Imaging* 2000;25:14–24.
9. Matsushita M, Oi H, Murakami T, et al. Extraserosal invasion in advanced gastric cancer: evaluation with MR imaging. *Radiology* 1994;192:87–91.
10. Sohn KM, Lee JM, Lee SY, et al. Comparing MR imaging and CT in the staging of gastric carcinoma. *AJR* 2000;174:1551–1557.
11. Kim AY, Han JK, Seong CK, et al. MRI in staging advanced gastric cancer: is it useful compared with spiral CT? *J Comput Assist Tomogr* 2000;24:389–394.
12. Wang CK, Kuo YT, Liu GC, et al. Dynamic contrast-enhanced subtraction and delayed MRI of gastric tumors: radiologic-pathologic correlation. *J Comput Assist Tomogr* 2000;24:872–877.
13. Oi H, Matsushita M, Murakami T, et al. Dynamic MR imaging for extraserosal invasion of advanced gastric cancer. *Abdom Imaging* 1997;22:35–40.
14. Kato M, Saji S, Kanematsu M, et al. Detection of lymph-node metastases in patients with gastric carcinoma: comparison of three MR imaging pulse sequences. *Abdom Imaging* 2000;25:25–29.
15. Kim AY, Han JK, Kim TK, et al. MR imaging of advanced gastric cancer: comparison of various MR pulse sequences using water and gadopentetate dimeglumine as oral contrast agents. *Abdom Imaging* 2000;25:7–13.
16. Blomqvist L, Machado M, Rubio C, et al. Rectal tumour staging: MR imaging using pelvic phased array and endorectal coils vs endoscopic ultrasonography. *Eur Radiol* 2000;10:653–660.
17. Gualdi GF, Casciani E, Guadalaxara A, et al. Local staging of rectal cancer with transrectal ultrasound and endorectal magnetic resonance imaging: comparison with histologic findings. *Dis Colon Rectum* 2000;43:338–345.
18. Hunerbein M, Pegios W, Rau B, et al. Prospective comparison of endorectal ultrasound, three-dimensional endorectal ultrasound, and endorectal MRI in the preoperative evaluation of rectal tumors. *Surg Endosc* 2000;14:1005–1009.
19. Drew PJ, Farouk R, Turnbull LW, et al. Preoperative magnetic resonance staging of rectal cancer with an endorectal coil and dynamic gadolinium enhancement. *Br J Surg* 1999;86:250–254.
20. Kim NK, Kim MJ, Park JK, et al. Preoperative staging of rectal cancer with MRI: accuracy and clinical usefulness. *Ann Surg Oncol* 2000;7:732–737.
21. Brown G, Richards CJ, Newcombe RG, et al. Rectal carcinoma: thin-section MR imaging for staging in 28 patients. *Radiology* 1999;211:215–222.
22. Maier AG, Kersting-Sommerhoff B, Reeders JW, et al. Staging of rectal cancer by double-contrast MR imaging using the rectally administered superparamagnetic iron oxide contrast agent ferristene and IV gadodiamide injection: results of a multicenter phase II trial. *J Magn Reson Imaging* 2000;12:651–660.
23. Wallengren NO, Holtas S, Andren-Sandberg A, et al. Rectal carcinoma: double-contrast MR imaging for preoperative staging. *Radiology* 2000;215:108–114.
24. Torricelli P, Pecchi A, Luppi G, et al. Gadolinium-enhanced MRI with dynamic evaluation in diagnosing the local recurrence of rectal cancer. *Abdom Imaging* 2003;28:19–27.
25. Gagliardi G, Bayar S, Smith R, et al. Preoperative staging of rectal cancer using magnetic resonance imaging with external phase arrayed coils. *Arch Surg* 2002;137:447–451.
26. Laghi A, Ferri M, Catalano C, et al. Local staging of rectal cancer with MRI using a phased array body coil. *Abdom Imaging* 2002;27:425–431.
27. Luboldt W, Bauerfeind P, Wildermuth S, et al. Colonic masses: detection with MR colonography. *Radiology* 2000;216:383–388.
28. Pappalardo G, Polettini E, Frattaroli FM, et al. Magnetic resonance colonography versus conventional colonoscopy for the detection of colonic endoluminal lesions. *Gastroenterology* 2000;119:300–304.
29. Lauenstein TC, Holtmann G, Schoenfelder D, et al. MR colonography without colonic cleansing: a new strategy to improve patient acceptance. *AJR* 2001;177:823–827.

SUGGESTED READINGS

Bartram C, Brown G. Endorectal ultrasound and magnetic resonance imaging in rectal cancer staging. *Gastroenterol Clin North Am* 2002;31:827–839.

Giovagnoni A, Fabbri A, Maccioni F. Oral contrast agents in MRI of the gastrointestinal tract. *Abdom Imaging* 2002;27:367–375.

Lee JK, Marcos HB, Semelka RC. MR imaging of the small bowel using the HASTE sequence. *AJR* 1998;170:1457–1463.

Lomas DJ. Technical developments in bowel MRI. *Eur Radiol* 2003;13:1058–1071.

Low RN, Sebrechts CP, Politoske DA, et al. Crohn disease with endoscopic correlation: single-shot fast spin-echo and gadolinium-enhanced fat-suppressed spoiled gradient-echo MR imaging. *Radiology* 2002;222:652–660.

Luboldt W, Morrin MM. MR colonography: status and perspective. *Abdom Imaging* 2002;27:400–409.

Maccioni F, Viscido A, Marini M, et al. MRI evaluation of Crohn's disease of the small and large bowel with the use of negative superparamagnetic oral contrast agents. *Abdom Imaging* 2002;27:384–393.

Motohara T, Semelka RC. MRI in staging of gastric cancer. *Abdom Imaging* 2002;27:376–383.

Prassopoulos P, Papanikolaou N, Grammatikakis J, et al. MR enteroclysis imaging of Crohn disease. *Radiographics* 2001;21:S161–S172.

Rieber A, Nussle K, Reinshagen M, et al. MRI of the abdomen with positive oral contrast agents for the diagnosis of inflammatory small bowel diseases. *Abdom Imaging* 2002;27:394–399.

Umschaden HW, Gasser J. MR enteroclysis. *Radiol Clin North Am* 2003;41:231–248.

SECTION 2.5

Obstetric Magnetic Resonance Imaging

There has been growing interest in the use of magnetic resonance (MR) for maternal-fetal imaging. The great attraction of MR imaging (MRI) in this setting is the ability to produce high-quality images without the use of ionizing radiation. MRI also provides a global view of pertinent anatomy unencumbered by the restrictions of a sonographic window, and rapid MRI sequences allow the production of detailed, motion-free images. Even though there have been no documented adverse fetal effects of MRI, we believe it is usually prudent to avoid imaging in the first trimester of pregnancy (the period of organogenesis).

TECHNIQUE

Fetal motion limits the choice of pulse sequences. Sequences must be fast enough to be resistant to motion while providing adequate signal-to-noise and tissue contrast. In addition, sequences must be kept within acceptable SAR limits. Currently, the most commonly performed sequence for fetal imaging is HASTE (or ssFSE, ssTSE) (1).

A typical fetal protocol includes a spoiled gradient echo scout sequence to locate the fetus and a series of HASTE images in the axial, sagittal, and coronal planes relative to the fetus. Because of fetal motion, each scan must be planned using the immediate preceding scan as a localizer. To reduce maternal motion, which also contributes to image degradation, images are acquired during maternal breath-holding. The HASTE images provide most of the necessary anatomic information (Fig. 2.70) (2). T1-weighted images may be acquired using a spoiled gradient echo or fast spin echo sequence. Relatively sharp, motion-free images may also be obtained using a steady-state gradient echo sequence (trueFISP, balanced FFE, FIESTA), although the tissue contrast mechanisms are more complex (Fig. 2.71) (3). Steady-state gradient echo sequences produce exceptionally sharp images and have the benefit of relatively low energy deposition in the mother and fetus. Therefore, it is likely that these sequences will eventually become standard for fetal imaging. Gadolinium chelates cross the placental barrier and are not recommended for fetal imaging.

Some additional considerations should be taken into account when imaging pregnant women. Prolonged periods in the supine position may be poorly tolerated, particularly during the last trimester. Therefore, sequences should be as short as possible. Placing the patient in an oblique or decubitus position may be necessary to complete the examination. A phased-array body coil improves signal-to-noise ratio but may limit field of view. Maternal abdominal circumference and position may mandate use of the main body coil. Even though no long-term adverse effects of RF exposure from diagnostic MRI on human fetuses have been documented, our collective experience with fetal MRI is still limited. Therefore, one should make an attempt to limit the SAR to the extent possible.

CLINICAL APPLICATIONS

Fetal Imaging

Ultrasonography remains the screening procedure of choice for fetal anomalies. However, MRI is useful for evaluating potential abnormalities initially detected with ultrasonography. MRI has several advantages over ultrasonography including decreased operator dependence, superior tissue contrast, independence from the need for a sonographic window, and a larger field of view. Imaging of fetal anomalies may be performed as early as the second trimester.

Suspected brain anomalies are particularly well demonstrated with MRI because of the high image contrast achievable between the brain and CSF, regardless of the fetal head position or degree of calvarial ossification (Fig. 2.72, 2.73). Likewise, detailed normal fetal anatomy is well represented on MR images (4). Early in the second trimester, fetal brain gyration may not be apparent, giving the brain a smooth appearance resembling lissencephaly (Fig. 2.74). At some variable point during the second trimester, fetal brain gyri begin to develop and a layered appearance of the cerebrum can be appreciated. As with ultrasonography, the axial diameter of

95

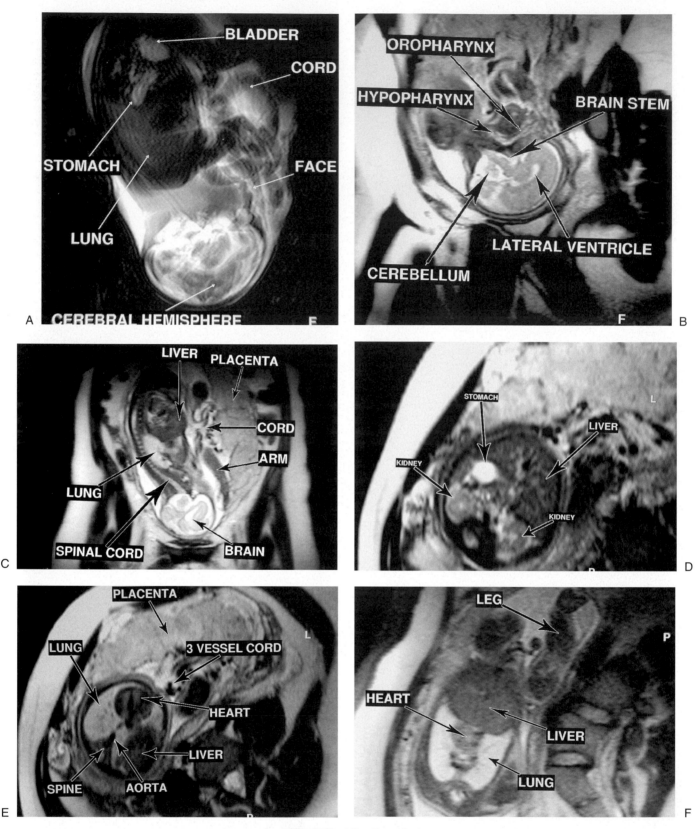

FIG. 2.70. (*Continued*)

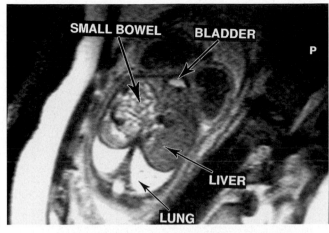
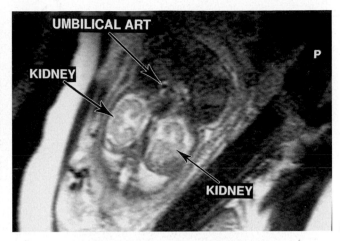

FIG. 2.70. Normal third trimester fetal anatomy (cephalic presentation) demonstrated on **(A)** thick-slab, heavily T2-weighted fast spin echo image, **(B)** sagittal HASTE image through fetal head, **(C)** sagittal HASTE image through fetal spine and body, **(D)** axial HASTE image through fetal abdomen, **(E)** axial HASTE image the through fetal thorax, **(F)** coronal HASTE image through fetal thorax, **(G)** coronal HASTE image through fetal abdomen, and **(H)** coronal HASTE image through fetal kidneys. (Images courtesy of Dacia Napier, M.D.)

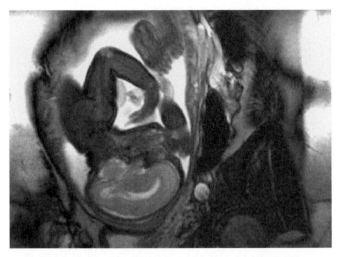

FIG. 2.71. Steady-state gradient echo (trueFISP) sequence for fetal imaging. Anatomy of 32-week fetus is clearly demonstrated.

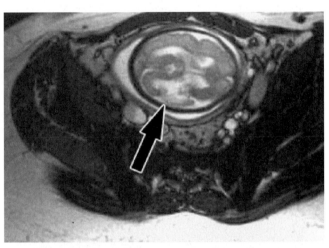

FIG. 2.73. Porencephaly. TrueFISP sequence performed axial with respect to fetal brain demonstrates focal area of porencephaly (*arrow*).

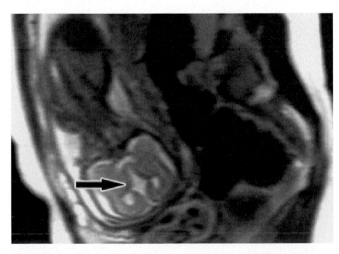

FIG. 2.72. Agenesis of corpus callosum. HASTE sequence performed coronal with respect to fetal brain demonstrates dilated, high-riding third ventricle with absence of corpus callosum (*arrow*).

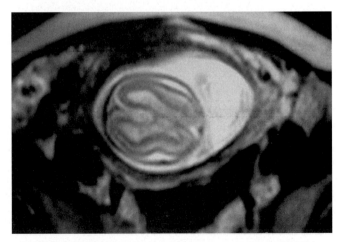

FIG. 2.74. Fetal brain, second trimester. Axial HASTE sequence performed through normal fetal brain early in second trimester demonstrates smooth appearance of cerebral hemispheres.

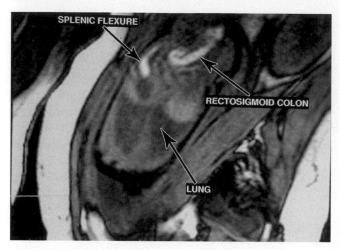

FIG. 2.75. Normal colon during third trimester. Note high signal intensity of colonic contents on this T1-weighted gradient echo sequence.

the lateral ventricle should not exceed 10 mm beyond 25 weeks of gestation. Fetal spine anomalies, such as meningomyelocele, can also be demonstrated with fetal MRI.

Abnormalities elsewhere such as neck masses, diaphragmatic hernias, cystic adenomatoid malformations, pulmonary sequestrations, abdominal wall defects, intestinal and renal abnormalities, and sacrococcygeal teratomas can also be diagnosed or confirmed (5). Fetal contours are clearly outlined by high signal intensity amnionic fluid, which also outlines the oropharynx and proximal gastrointestinal tract. The distal small bowel and colon may appear as high signal intensity on T1-weighted images and low signal intensity on HASTE

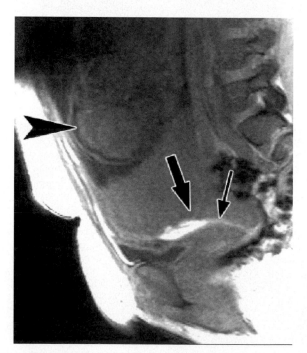

FIG. 2.76. Central placenta previa. Sagittal T1-weighted gradient echo image shows placenta completely covering internal cervical os (*arrow*) in patient with vaginal bleeding. Fetal head notated by (*arrowhead*). High signal intensity within cervical canal (*thin arrow*) represents hemorrhage.

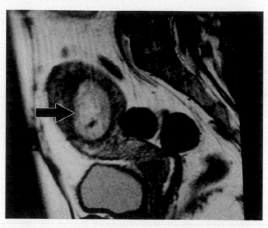

FIG. 2.77. Gestational trophoblastic disease. Sagittal T2-weighted fast spin echo image through uterus in patient with abnormally elevated human chorionic gonadotropin level and abnormal transvaginal ultrasound. Nonspecific thickening of the endometrium is seen (*arrow*) without evidence of fetal development or gestational sac. Dilatation and curettage revealed complete molar pregnancy.

images (Fig. 2.75) (6). The fetal airways, urinary tract, and gallbladder are also fluid-filled and, therefore, of high signal intensity on the T2-weighted sequences routinely used for fetal imaging. The fetal lung parenchyma is not as bright as amniotic fluid but is still relatively high in signal intensity compared to other organs such as the fetal liver. The umbilical cord and its insertion sites are easily identified. Rarely, fetal cardiac abnormalities may be demonstrated with MRI, although MRI is limited in this capacity due to the small size and rapid motion of the fetal heart.

Maternal Imaging

Maternal pathology can also be evaluated with MRI without the concern of exposing the fetus or mother to ionizing radiation (7). Both pregnancy-related and non–pregnancy-related abnormalities can be successfully imaged. Adnexal masses,

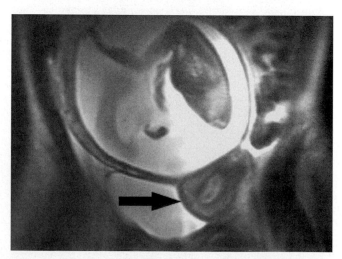

FIG. 2.78. Gravid bicornuate uterus. Coronal HASTE image demonstrates second uterine horn (*arrow*) in pregnant patient with bicornuate uterus.

gestational trophoblastic disease, uterine fibroids, and placental abnormalities can be evaluated with MRI (Fig. 2.76, 2.77, 2.78). Attempts to diagnose placenta accreta (placenta attachment onto myometrium), increta (placental invasion into myometrium), and percreta (invasion through serosa) with MRI have met with mixed success (8–10). Risk factors for placental implantation abnormalities include previous cesarean section and endometrial cavity instrumentation. On MR images, the diagnosis of a placental implantation abnormality can be suggested by focal thinning or disruption of the myometrium subjacent to the placenta. In the case of placenta percreta, high signal intensity placental tissue may be seen extending through the disrupted lower signal intensity myometrium on T2-weighted images. The diagnosis of a placental implantation abnormality is difficult to make prospectively with any imaging modality.

The use of intravenous contrast agents to diagnose maternal disease should only be considered if noncontrast techniques are inadequate for diagnosis, no suitable alternative imaging is possible, and the benefits of contrast administration outweigh the potential risk to the fetus.

Pelvimetry

Pelvimetry may also be performed without exposing the fetus to ionizing radiation by using MRI (Fig. 2.79) (11,12). To

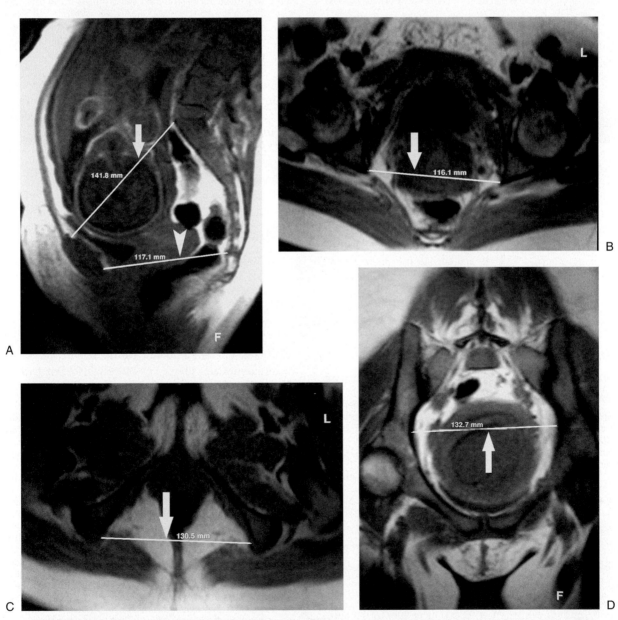

FIG. 2.79. MR pelvimetry. **A:** Midsagittal T1-weighted image demonstrates obstetric conjugate (*arrow*) and outlet sagittal diameter (*arrowhead*). **B:** Axial T1-weighted image demonstrates interspinous distance (*arrow*). **C:** Axial T1-weighted image demonstrates intertuberous diameter (*arrow*). **D:** Oblique T1-weighted image in plane of obstetric conjugate demonstrates transverse diameter of pelvic inlet (*arrow*).

perform MR pelvimetry, axial, mid-sagittal, and oblique images of the maternal pelvis are performed (typically with a gradient echo T1-weighted sequence). The following measurements are made: obstetric conjugate (from sacral promontory to top of pubic symphysis on mid-sagittal image), outlet sagittal diameter (from bottom of sacrum to bottom of pubic symphysis inner cortex on midsagittal image), interspinous distance (between ischial spines on axial image), intertuberous diameter (between ischial tuberosities on axial image), and transverse diameter of the pelvic inlet (obtained from an oblique image performed in the plane of the obstetric conjugate). The measurements associated with the highest error are the intertuberous distance and sagittal outlet (13). A variety of different calculations may be performed with the measurements obtained from MR pelvimetry, none of which has been shown to be clearly superior to others for predicting labor outcome. We recommend consultation with referring obstetricians to determine the best use of pelvimetry data in a particular practice setting.

Postpartum Imaging

On occasion, one may be asked to image the pelvis shortly after delivery to evaluate puerperal fever or other postpartum complication. Uterine or extrauterine fluid collections, uterine dehiscence, and ovarian vein thrombosis are well demonstrated with MRI (Fig. 2.80). During the immediate postpartum period, the uterus is normally enlarged (up to 16 cm in length excluding the cervix). The largest percentage decrease in uterine size occurs during the first week after delivery. Prominent myometrial vessels are commonly present during the postpartum period (14). The normal zonal anatomy of the uterus is not usually visualized on T2-weighted images during the first 2 weeks after delivery and may not return for as long as 6 months after delivery in some patients.

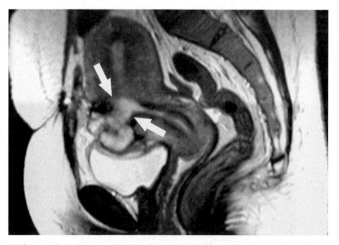

FIG. 2.80. Uterine dehiscence following cesarean section. Sagittal T2-weighted image of uterus in patient with pain and bleeding after cesarean section. Note disruption of myometrium at the incision site (*arrows*).

Although the cervix may demonstrate increased signal intensity immediately after vaginal delivery on T2-weighted images, the cervical fibrous stroma tends to maintain its low signal intensity in the postpartum period. Endometrial fluid is common in the first week and may appear bright on T1-weighted images, reflecting the presence of subacute blood products. The anteroposterior thickness of the endometrial fluid typically measures only a few centimeters. In patients who have undergone cesarean section, evidence of blood products may also be present in the uterine incision and bladder flap. The myometrial incision site has increased signal intensity on T2-weighted images in the postpartum period, which reflects edema. However, there should be no myometrial gap at this site. Increased peri-incisional signal on T2-weighted images should resolve by 3 months after delivery (15,16).

SECTION SUMMARY

1. Motion-free images of fetal anatomy and abnormalities are best obtained using half-Fourier single-shot spin echo (HASTE, ssFSE, ssTSE) or steady-state gradient echo (trueFISP, balanced FFE, FIESTA) sequences.
2. Due to fetal motion, each imaging sequence should be planned using the immediately preceding sequence as a localizer.
3. Fetal anatomy and abnormalities can be clearly demonstrated with MRI as early as the second trimester of pregnancy.
4. MRI during the first trimester of pregnancy and the use of intravenous gadolinium chelates at any time during pregnancy should be avoided unless the potential benefits of such actions clearly outweigh the potential risks to the fetus.
5. When imaging during pregnancy, attempts should be made to limit the specific absorption rate (SAR).
6. MRI is safe and effective for the evaluation of maternal diseases during pregnancy as well as for postpartum complications.
7. MR pelvimetry can assess maternal pelvic dimensions without exposing the fetus to ionizing radiation.

REFERENCES

1. Yamashita Y, Namimoto T, Abe Y, et al. MR imaging of the fetus by a HASTE sequence. *AJR* 1997;168:513–519.
2. Huppert BJ, Brandt KR, Ramin KD, et al. Single-shot fast spin echo MR imaging of the fetus: a pictorial essay. *Radiographics* 1999;19:S215–S227.
3. Ertl-Wagner B, Lienemann A, Strauss A, et al. Fetal magnetic resonance imaging: indications, technique, anatomical considerations and a review of fetal abnormalities. *Eur Radiol* 2002;12:1931–1940.
4. Amin RS, Nikolaidis P, Kawashima A, et al. Normal anatomy of the fetus at MR imaging. *Radiographics* 1999;19:S201–S214.
5. Shinmoto H, Kashima K, Yuasa Y, et al. MR Imaging of non-CNS fetal abnormalities: a pictorial essay. *Radiographics* 2000;20:1227–1243.
6. Saguintaah M, Couture A, Veyrac C, et al. MRI of the fetal gastrointestinal tract. *Pediatr Radiol* 2002;32:395–404.

7. Jung SE, Byun JY, Lee JM, et al. MR imaging of maternal diseases in pregnancy. *AJR* 2001;177:1293–1300.
8. Lam G, Kuller J, McMahon M, et al. Use of magnetic resonance imaging and ultrasound in the antenatal diagnosis of placenta accreta. *J Soc Gynecol Invest* 2002;9:37–40.
9. Levine D, Hulka CA, Ludmir J, et al. Placenta accreta: evaluation with color Doppler US, power Doppler US, and MR imaging. *Radiology* 1997;205:773–776.
10. Maldjian C, Adam R, Pelosi M 3rd, et al. MRI appearance of placenta percreta and placenta accreta. *Magn Reson Imaging* 1999;17:965–971.
11. Van Loon AJ, Mantingh A, Serlier EK, et al. Randomised controlled trial of magnetic resonance pelvimetry in breech presentation at term. *Lancet* 1997;350:1799–1804.
12. Spörri S, Thoeny HC, Raio L, et al. MR imaging pelvimetry: a useful adjunct in the treatment of women at risk for dystocia? *AJR* 2002;179:137–144.
13. Keller TM, Rake A, Michel SC, et al. Obstetric MR pelvimetry: reference values and evaluation of inter- and intraobserver error and intraindividual variability. *Radiology* 2003;227:37–43.
14. Willms AB, Brown ED, Kettritz UI, et al. Anatomic changes in the pelvis after uncomplicated vaginal delivery: evaluation with serial MR imaging. *Radiology* 1995;195:91–94.
15. Woo GM, Twickler DM, Stettler RW, et al. The pelvis after cesarean section and vaginal delivery: normal MR findings. *AJR* 1993;161:1249–1252.
16. Dicle O, Küçükler C, Pirnar T, et al. Magnetic resonance imaging evaluation of incision healing after cesarean sections. *Eur Radiol* 1997;7:31–34.

SUGGESTED READINGS

Hubbard AM, Simon EM. Fetal imaging. *Magn Reson Imaging Clin N Am* 2002;10:389–408.
Huisman TA, Martin E, Kubik-Huch R, et al. Fetal magnetic resonance imaging of the brain: technical considerations and normal brain development. *Eur Radiol* 2002;12:1941–1951.
Huisman TA, Wisser J, Martin E, et al. Fetal magnetic resonance imaging of the central nervous system: a pictorial essay. *Eur Radiol* 2002;12:1952–1961.
Ismail KM, Ashworth JR, Martin WL, et al. Fetal magnetic resonance imaging in prenatal diagnosis of central nervous system abnormalities: 3-year experience. *J Matern Fetal Neonatal Med* 2002;12:185–190.
Levine D, Barnes PD, Edelman RR. Obstetric MR imaging. *Radiology* 1999;211:609–617.
Levine D, Zuo C, Faro CB, et al. Potential heating effect in the gravid uterus during MR HASTE imaging. *J Magn Reson Imaging* 2001;13:856–861.

Interpretation of Abdominal and Pelvic Magnetic Resonance Imaging

SECTION 3.1

Approach to Interpreting Abdominal and Pelvic Magnetic Resonance Imaging Examinations

Many radiologists and radiology trainees are intimidated by the prospect of interpreting abdominal and pelvic magnetic resonance imaging (MRI) studies, but such fear is unfounded. We remind our residents and fellows of two reassuring facts. First, the anatomy of the human body does not change with changes in imaging modality or scan plane. Second, the diseases of the human body remain the same, no matter how they are imaged. The pancreas is in the same location on a coronal MRI scan as it is on an axial computed tomography (CT) scan, although it is displayed differently. Likewise, there is a limited differential diagnosis for a cystic pancreatic mass, regardless of the modality used to image it.

Individuals new to abdominal and pelvic MRI should adopt a systematic approach. When faced with an abdominal or pelvic MR image, we recommend going through the following checklist:

1. Is the image T1- or T2-weighted? A T2-weighted image is easily identified by the presence of high signal intensity fluid within the spinal canal, bile ducts, or urinary tract. Using the signal intensity of fat to distinguish a T1- from a T2-weighted image is not recommended.
2. If the image is T1-weighted, is it in-phase or out-of-phase? This applies to gradient echo images. An out-of-phase image demonstrates phase cancellation at fat-water interfaces, resulting in a characteristic dark rim around the solid organs.
3. Is the image fat-suppressed or non–fat-suppressed?
4. Which direction is phase-encoded and which is frequency-encoded? This is important because one needs to be able to distinguish phase ghosts and other artifacts from actual lesions within the abdomen.
5. Are any artifacts present? Initially looking for artifacts such as phase ghosting, wraparound, and susceptibility artifact may prevent misinterpreting such artifacts later in the interpretive process.

6. Has intravenous contrast been administered? A fat-suppressed, T1-weighted, contrast-enhanced image may look similar to a fat-suppressed T2-weighted image (Fig. 3.1).
7. For contrast-enhanced images, what is the phase of enhancement (e.g., arterial, venous, equilibrium, delayed)?

When an abnormality is seen, we recommend the following considerations:

1. In what organ or anatomic compartment is the abnormality located?
   a. In which direction are adjacent organs or structures displaced?
   b. Between what structures does the abnormality occur?
   c. What is the blood supply (if any) of the abnormality?
   d. Are fat planes visible between the abnormality and adjacent structures?
   e. Are all organs in the region accounted for? (e.g., If normal adrenal glands or ovaries are identified, it is unlikely that a mass arises from these structures. However, failure to identify a normal structure increases the likelihood that it is the source of the abnormality.)
2. Are there any MR artifacts that could explain the abnormality?
3. Are there any associated findings that could improve specificity (e.g., metastatic lesions, findings suggestive of a particular syndrome)?
4. What are the signal characteristics of the abnormality on T1- and T2-weighted images, and how does the lesion enhance?

Once an abdominal or pelvic abnormality is detected, its probable organ of origin identified, and its signal characteristics delineated, it is helpful to characterize its basic tissue components. By identifying the basic components (e.g., fluid, fat, blood) of an abnormality, one can significantly narrow the differential diagnosis. The following is a guide to the basic

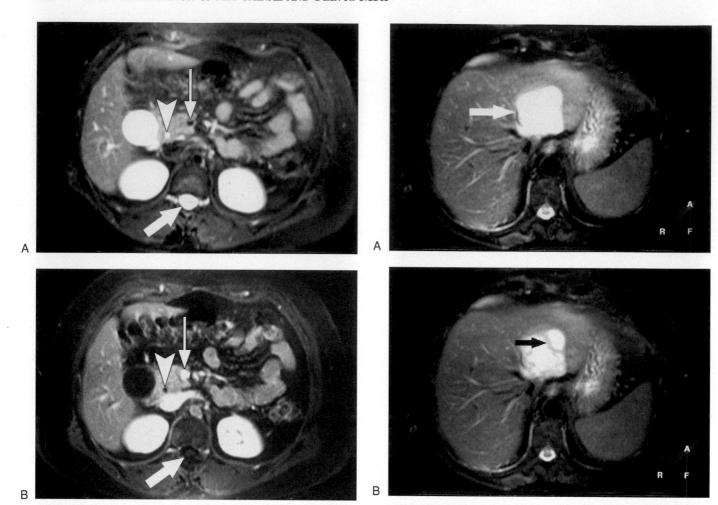

FIG. 3.1. Fat-suppressed T2-weighted images **(A)** may look similar to fat-suppressed, gadolinium-enhanced T1-weighted images **(B)**. The bright cerebrospinal fluid (*arrow*) in **(A)** is clue that the image is T2-weighted. Note that common bile duct (*arrowhead*) is bright and superior mesenteric vein (*thin arrow*) is dark on T2-weighted image **(A)**. Note that common bile duct (*arrowhead*) is dark and superior mesenteric vein (*thin arrow*) is bright on fat-suppressed, gadolinium-enhanced T1-weighted image **(B)**.

FIG. 3.2. Importance of appropriate window and level settings. **A:** Fat-suppressed T2-weighted image of liver demonstrates what appears to be a simple cystic lesion (*arrow*) in left hepatic lobe. **B:** After adjustment of the window and level settings, septations (*arrow*) and debris are detected in hepatic abscess.

substances and tissues likely to be encountered during interpretation of abdominal and pelvic MRI examinations.

Fluid: Simple fluid is very bright on T2-weighted images and dark on T1-weighted images. When evaluating a lesion with very high signal intensity on T2-weighted images, proper window and level settings are critical to evaluate the internal architecture of the lesion (Fig. 3.2). Mobile fluid, such as ascites, may appear heterogeneous on HASTE sequences because of flow artifacts. Fluid containing blood products or protein usually has intermediate or high signal intensity on T1-weighted images.

Fat: Fat appears very bright on T1-weighted images and on fast spin echo T2-weighted images (Fig. 3.3). The use of fat suppression greatly reduces signal from fat. Fat shows little or no enhancement after contrast administration. Lesions containing intracytoplasmic lipid lose signal on opposed-phase gradient echo images (relative to in-phase images).

Fibrous tissue: Mature fibrosis demonstrates low signal intensity on T1-weighted and T2-weighted images. Fibrous tissue with some component of active inflammation may demonstrate high signal intensity on fat-suppressed T2-weighted images. Delayed enhancement is typical of fibrosis and of lesions containing fibrous tissue. Early enhancement is rare in the absence of acute inflammation.

Hematoma/hemorrhage: Extravascular blood products have a highly variable appearance on MR images (see Fig. 3.3). Hemorrhage may appear homogeneous or heterogeneous with areas of variable high signal intensity on T1-weighted images due to the presence of methemoglobin. Hemorrhage does not lose signal with frequency-selective fat saturation techniques. In fact, it may appear brighter on fat-suppressed images because background signal is eliminated from surrounding fat. The signal intensity of hemorrhage on T2-weighted images varies from very dark to very bright depending on the concentration of intracellular deoxyhemoglobin and hemosiderin, both of which can reduce

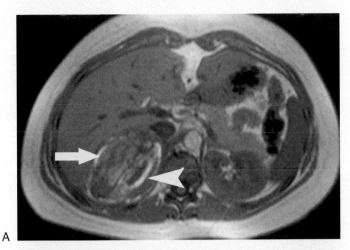

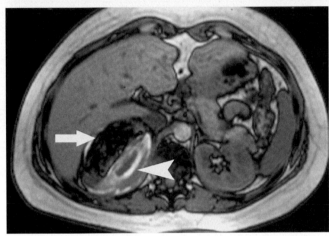

FIG. 3.3. Fat and hemorrhage (hemorrhaging angiomyolipoma). **A:** T1-weighted in-phase gradient echo image through right renal mass demonstrates a lesion with lateral (*arrow*) and medial (*arrowhead*) components having increased signal intensity. **B:** Opposed-phase image acquired as part of same sequence shows signal loss in lateral component (*arrow*) signifying the presence of fat but persistent high signal intensity without chemical shift artifact in medial component signifying hemorrhage.

signal as a result of T2 or T2* shortening. Hematomas may demonstrate fluid-fluid or fluid-debris levels. Hematomas do not enhance, which helps distinguish them from benign and malignant neoplasms. A rare exception is contrast enhancement of a hematoma in the setting of active bleeding.

Inflammatory tissue (acute): Inflammatory tissue demonstrates low signal intensity on T1-weighted images and high signal intensity on fat-suppressed T2-weighted images. Early intense enhancement is typical of active inflammation.

Malignant tumor: Malignant tissue typically appears darker on T1-weighted images and brighter on T2-weighted images than the tissue of origin. Exceptions include tumors of the prostate, testes, and seminal vesicles, which appear darker on T2-weighted images than the analogous normal tissue. Malignant tumors may also contain fat, hemorrhage, or cystic elements that alter their signal characteristics. Enhancement of malignant tumors is highly variable.

Mucin: Mucin usually appears relatively dark on T1-weighted images and may appear very bright on T2-weighted images. Therefore, mucin may mimic simple fluid. Mucin within the peritoneal cavity (i.e., pseudomyxoma peritonei) may be distinguished from fluid because bowel loops tend to float in fluid but are displaced by mucin as a result of the mass effect of the latter. Unlike simple fluid, solid tumors containing mucin typically demonstrate enhancement following intravenous gadolinium administration.

Myxoid stroma: Myxoid stroma is rich in mucopolysaccharides and appears very bright on T2-weighted images. Tumors containing myxoid stroma may appear solid on a CT scan and cystic on T2-weighted MR images, providing a clue to their composition. Myxoid tissue is found in a variety of tumors, including some neurogenic tumors and sarcomas.

SUGGESTED READINGS

Nishino M, Hayakawa K, Minami M, et al. Primary retroperitoneal neoplasms: CT and MR imaging findings with anatomic and pathologic diagnostic clues. *Radiographics* 2003;23:45–57.

Siegelman ES, Outwater EK. Tissue characterization in the female pelvis by means of MR imaging. *Radiology* 1999;212:5–218.

Magnetic Resonance Imaging Appearance of 101 Abdominal and Pelvic Abnormalities

GUIDE TO THIS SECTION

This section provides the reader with a quick reference to the typical magnetic resonance imaging (MRI) appearances of some commonly encountered (and a few uncommon) diseases of the abdomen and pelvis. Note that any lesion might have more than one appearance on MRI, and the information contained herein should only be used as a starting point in the development of a differential diagnosis.

The material is organized in the following manner:

T1: *Typical* appearance or signal intensity relative to organ of origin or surrounding structures on a T1-weighted image.

T2: *Typical* appearance or signal intensity relative to organ of origin or surrounding structures on a T2-weighted image.

Enhancement pattern: *Typical* enhancement pattern on dynamic and delayed imaging with intravenous gadolinium (unless otherwise specified).

Characteristic features: Findings that suggest the diagnosis.

Distribution: *Typical* location and multiplicity of abnormalities.

Atypical appearances: Atypical findings that may confuse diagnosis.

Associations: Associated abnormalities or syndromes.

Mimics: Other entities that may have a similar appearance.

Additional comments: Ancillary information.

LIVER, FOCAL ABNORMALITIES

Abscess, Amebic

Description: Abscess caused by the protozoan parasite *Entamoeba histolytica*.

T1: Low signal intensity center.

T2: High signal intensity center. High signal intensity edema may be present around abscess.

Enhancement pattern: Thick enhancing wall.

Characteristic features: Solitary rim-enhancing mass with no central enhancement on delayed contrast-enhanced images in patient with history of fever and diarrhea.

Distribution: Right lobe greater than left. Typically solitary.

Associations: Travel to endemic areas.

Mimics: Pyogenic abscess, necrotic tumor.

Additional comments: May invade and rupture through hemidiaphragm causing empyema (well demonstrated on coronal images).

References: 1, 2

Abscess, Fungal (Fig. 3.4)

Description: Discrete lesions resulting from fungal infection of the liver. Most common offending organism is *Candida albicans*. Other organisms include *Aspergillus* and *Cryptococcus*. Fungal infection of the liver almost always occurs in the setting of a compromised immune system.

T1: Hypointense to mildly hyperintense relative to liver.

T2: High signal intensity.

Enhancement pattern: Usually nonenhancing in immunocompromised patients. Once an immune response can be mounted, lesions may have a more characteristic abscess-like appearance with rim enhancement.

Characteristic features: Lesions often less than 1 cm in diameter and multiple.

Distribution: Multiple. Involves all lobes with some peripheral predilection.

Atypical appearances: In the setting of transfusional hemosiderosis, treated lesions tend to develop a low signal intensity peripheral rim. Healed lesions are low signal intensity on all sequences and do not enhance.

Associations: Involvement of the spleen and kidneys.

Mimics: Multiple pyogenic abscesses, cystic or necrotic metastases, sarcoidosis.

References: 3

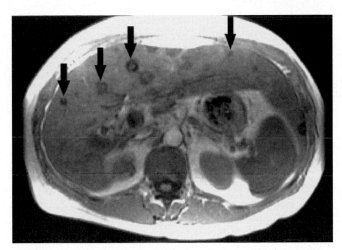

FIG. 3.4. *Candida* abscesses. Axial T1-weighted gradient echo image through liver demonstrates multiple low signal intensity hepatic lesions (*arrows*), some of which have central high signal intensity foci.

Abscess, Pyogenic (Fig. 3.5; see Figs. 3.2, 3.142)

Description: Bacterial infection of the liver characterized by purulent central area surrounded by granulation tissue and inflammation.

T1: Heterogeneous, low signal intensity.

T2: High signal intensity.

Enhancement pattern: Early mural enhancement (typically up to 5 mm) without change in thickness on later images. Perilesional enhancement may be present.

Characteristic features: Septations common. Presence of gas results in areas of signal void, which become more obvious on T2*-weighted images secondary to susceptibility artifact.

Distribution: Solitary or multiple.

Atypical appearances: Infected necrotic tumor may demonstrate thick, irregular wall.

Associations: Ascending cholangitis, diverticulitis, appendicitis, recent biliary procedure, trauma.

Mimics: Necrotic metastases, lymphoma, hydatid disease, necrotic hepatocellular carcinoma (HCC). Necrotic tumors tend to demonstrate thick, irregular walls that enhance in a centripetal manner.

Additional comments: When hepatic abscesses are present, always look for evidence of portal venous gas or thrombus and inflammatory disease elsewhere in the abdomen.

References: 4, 5

Adenoma (Figs. 3.6, 3.7)

Description: Benign epithelial tumor of hepatocellular origin.

T1: Variable signal intensity. Hemorrhage or fat content may cause high signal intensity foci. Areas of fibrosis, necrosis, or calcification may create low signal intensity foci.

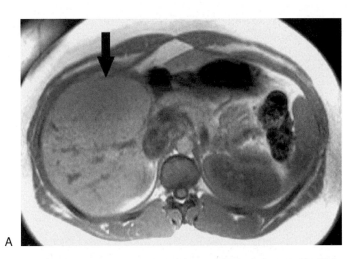

A

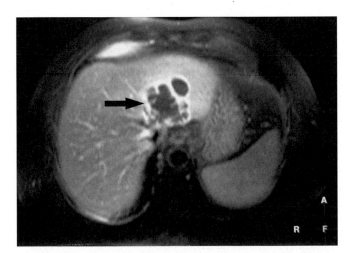

FIG. 3.5. Pyogenic abscess. Fat-suppressed, T1-weighted gradient echo image after intravenous gadolinium administration in same patient as Figure 3.2 shows complex hypointense lesion with rim-enhancement (*arrow*).

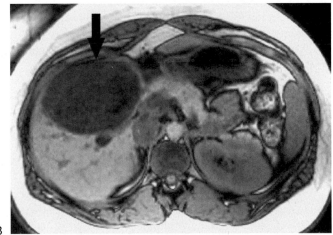

B

FIG. 3.6. Hepatic adenoma. In-phase **(A)** and opposed-phase **(B)** gradient echo images show large mass in right hepatic lobe (*arrow*) that loses signal on opposed-phase image as a result of intracytoplasmic lipid content.

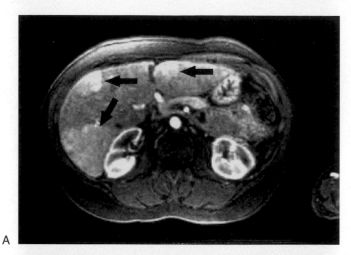

A

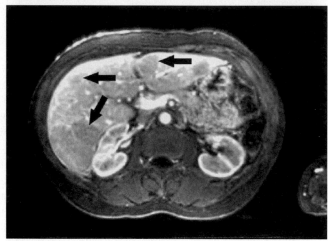

B

FIG. 3.7. Hepatic adenomas. **A:** Arterial phase, fat-suppressed, gradient echo image demonstrates multiple enhancing hepatic lesions (*arrows*). **B:** Portal venous phase image from same dynamic examination shows lesions (*arrows*) are slightly less intense than surrounding liver.

T2: Near isointense to slightly hyperintense relative to liver.

Enhancement pattern: Early enhancement (typically less intense than focal nodular hyperplasia [FNH]).

Characteristic features: Often heterogeneous in appearance due to hemorrhage. May decrease in signal intensity on opposed-phase images as a result of lipid content. Enhances with and retains mangafodipir as a result of functioning hepatocytes.

Distribution: Frequently solitary and variable in location. Multiple (>10) in hepatic adenomatosis.

Atypical appearances: May have low signal intensity pseudocapsule on T1-weighted images. May exhibit central scar.

Associations: Oral contraceptives, anabolic steroids, glycogen storage disease Ia.

Mimics: HCC, atypical FNH, focal fat.

Additional comments: Hepatic adenomas may become complex in appearance as a result of repeated hemorrhage.

Distinction from a well-differentiated HCC may be difficult or impossible. Malignant transformation of hepatic adenoma is rare and is more common in liver adenomatosis.

References: 6, 7

Angiosarcoma

Description: Rare primary malignant mesenchymal tumor of the liver characterized by spindle-shaped cells that form vascular channels.

T1: Low signal intensity with hemorrhagic foci of increased signal intensity.

T2: Heterogeneous, predominantly high signal intensity. Low signal intensity areas may represent fibrous component or hemosiderin. Fluid-fluid levels may be present.

Enhancement pattern: Heterogeneous enhancement early with progressive enhancement on more delayed images.

Characteristic features: Angiosarcoma most commonly appears as multiple nodules or a dominant mass with or without satellite lesions. Tumor is hypervascular but dominant masses enhance heterogeneously with progressive enhancement over time.

Distribution: Frequently, multiple masses are present. Metastases (lung, spleen, bone) are common at presentation.

Associations: Exposure to agents such as thorium dioxide (Thorotrast), arsenic, and vinyl chloride has been associated with angiosarcoma, but cases may occur without known risk factors.

Mimics: Atypical hemangioma, HCC (typically does not demonstrate progressive enhancement or splenic involvement), hypervascular metastases.

References: 8

Bile Duct Hamartoma (Von Meyenburg Complex) (Fig. 3.8; see Fig. 3.143)

Description: Benign malformation of bile duct origin.

T1: Low signal intensity.

T2: Very high signal intensity.

Enhancement pattern: Nonenhancing. May demonstrate a thin rim of apparent contrast enhancement secondary to compressed surrounding parenchyma.

Characteristic features: Multiple, well-defined, cystic-appearing lesions, most measuring less than 1 cm, dispersed throughout the liver.

Distribution: Multiple, diffuse.

Mimics: Caroli's disease, multiple hepatic cysts, cystic metastases.

Additional comments: Commonly confused with simple cysts on imaging.

References: 9

Biliary Cystadenoma and Cystadenocarcinoma (Fig. 3.9)

Description: Rare cystic tumor of biliary origin.

T1: Cysts usually dark but vary in signal characteristics depending on their blood and protein content.

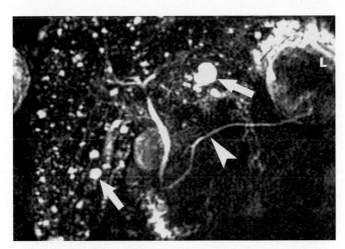

FIG. 3.8. Bile duct hamartomas. Thick-slab magnetic resonance cholangiopancreatography image demonstrates multiple small cystic lesions throughout the liver (*arrows*). *Arrowhead* denotes pancreatic duct.

T2: Cysts typically very bright but may vary in signal intensity.

Enhancement pattern: Cyst walls and septations enhance with intravenous gadolinium chelates. Mural nodules, when present, also enhance.

Characteristic features: Complex multilocular cystic mass with septations and variable mural nodularity. Benign and malignant lesions cannot be reliably distinguished, although mural nodularity favors malignant tumor.

Distribution: No characteristic distribution but more common in right lobe. Typically solitary.

Atypical appearances: Unilocular cystic mass.

Mimics: Complex cystic lesions of the liver such as abscess, echinococcal cysts, necrotic tumors.

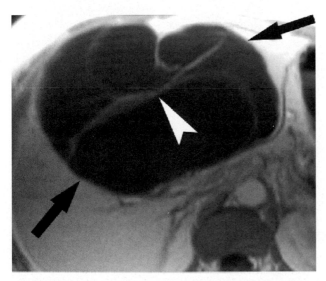

FIG. 3.9. Biliary cystadenoma. T1-weighted image following gadolinium administration demonstrates large cystic mass (*arrows*) in liver with thin septations (*arrowhead*).

Additional comments: Female predominance. Usually age older than 30 years.

References: 10

Cholangiocarcinoma (Figs. 3.10, 3.11; see Fig. 2.37)

Description: The majority of cholangiocarcinomas are sclerosing adenocarcinomas arising from bile duct epithelium. Other histologic types are possible, including anaplastic and squamous. After HCC, second most common primary hepatic malignant tumor.

T1: Hypointense to liver.

T2: Mildly hyperintense to liver.

Enhancement pattern: Delayed enhancement is typical. Early peripheral enhancement may occur. Complete enhancement may take several minutes.

Characteristic features: Delayed enhancement of this tumor distinguishes it from many other focal hepatic masses. Central lesions associated with biliary obstruction, occasionally resulting in parenchymal atrophy of the affected portion of the liver. Tends to extrinsically compress rather than invade portal vessels. Central necrosis, fibrosis, and hyalinization are common in large tumor masses.

Distribution: Peripheral cholangiocarcinomas arise from higher order peripheral ducts and appear as intrahepatic masses. Satellite lesions are common with peripheral cholangiocarcinomas. Tumors arising from the region of the right and left hepatic duct confluence are commonly referred to as hilar (or Klatskin) tumors. Extrahepatic tumors arise from the common hepatic or common bile ducts.

Atypical appearances: Portal vein invasion is uncommon. Calcifications may appear as foci of low signal intensity. A discrete mass may not be visible in some cases despite significant biliary ductal dilatation.

Associations: Primary sclerosing cholangitis, clonorchiasis, recurrent pyogenic cholangitis, choledochal cyst.

Mimics: Metastases (particularly colorectal, sarcomas), atypical HCC, other causes of biliary obstruction.

References: 11, 12

Choledochal Cyst (Figs. 3.12, 3.13; see Figs. 2.33, 3.156)

Description: Congenital cystic dilatation of the bile ducts. An anomalous union of the pancreatic duct and common bile duct more than 1 cm proximal to the ampulla is thought to contribute to choledochal cyst formation by allowing reflux of pancreatic enzymes into the bile duct.

T1: Isointense to bile.

T2: Isointense to bile.

Enhancement pattern: Nonenhancing. Enhancement of thickened wall or soft-tissue nodules should raise concern for development of cholangiocarcinoma.

Characteristic features: Confident diagnosis of choledochal cyst and differentiation from other cystic entities relies on demonstrating direct communication between the

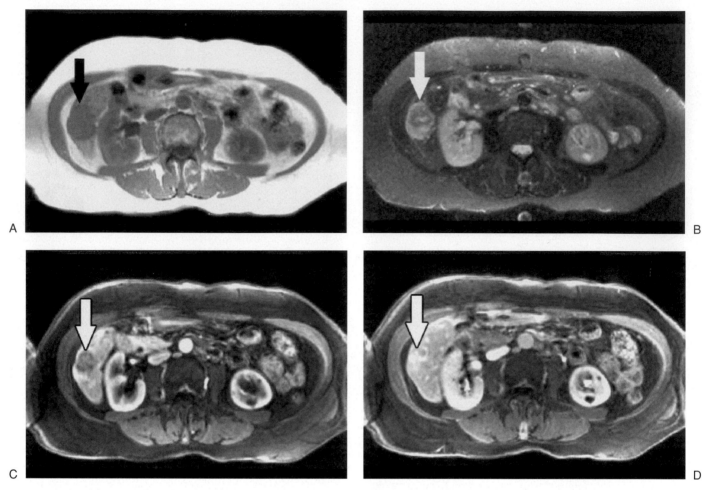

FIG. 3.10. Peripheral cholangiocarcinoma. **A:** T1-weighted gradient echo image shows hypointense mass (*arrow*) in caudal right hepatic lobe. **B:** Mass (*arrow*) is hyperintense on fat-suppressed T2-weighted image. **C:** During arterial phase of dynamic, gadolinium-enhanced sequence, mass (*arrow*) is hypoenhancing relative to liver. **D:** Delayed fat-suppressed T1-weighted gradient echo image obtained after several minutes demonstrates lesion (*arrow*) to be slightly hyperintense to liver.

cyst and the biliary system. A useful diagnostic sign in Caroli disease is the "central dot sign." The central "dot" represents the portal triad vessels surrounded by dilated bile ducts.

Distribution: Type I cysts are most common and consist of dilatation of the common bile duct. Type II cysts are diverticula-like cysts communicating with the common bile duct, often by a stalk. Type III cysts, often referred to as choledochoceles, are characterized by cystic dilatation of the intraduodenal portion of the common bile duct. Type IV cysts are multiple dilatations involving the intrahepatic and extrahepatic ducts (IVA) or extrahepatic ducts (IVB). Type V cysts are usually referred to as Caroli disease and consist of multiple cysts of the intrahepatic bile ducts.

Associations: Cholangiocarcinoma.

Mimics: Other cystic lesions of the liver or periampullary region.

References: 13 to 15

Confluent Hepatic Fibrosis (Fig. 3.14)

Description: Mass-like region of hepatic fibrosis occurring in the setting of cirrhosis.

T1: Hypointense to liver

T2: Hyperintense to liver

Enhancement pattern: Usually progressive enhancement after intravenous gadolinium administration. Arterial phase enhancement may occur.

Characteristic features: Associated with parenchymal atrophy and capsular retraction. Progressive enhancement after contrast administration is typical.

Distribution: Linear or wedge-shaped areas extend from porta hepatis to liver capsule. Commonly involves medial segment of the left lobe and anterior segment of the right lobe.

Associations: Cirrhosis.

Mimics: Cholangiocarcinoma, HCC.

Additional comments: Typical shape, location, and

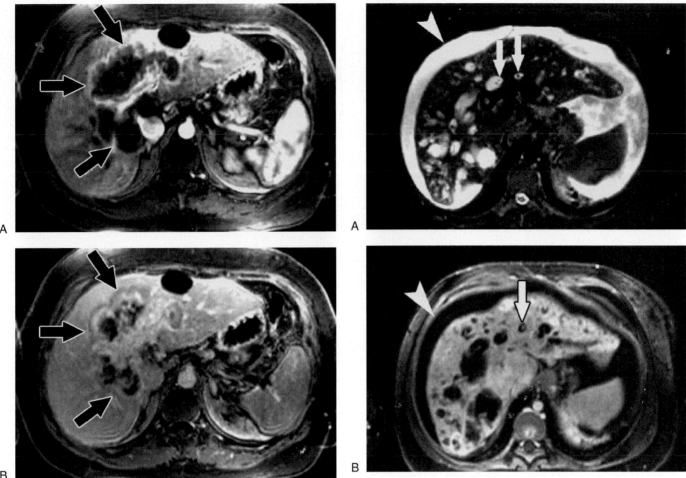

FIG. 3.11. Advanced cholangiocarcinoma. **A:** Early image from fat-suppressed, gadolinium-enhanced dynamic gradient echo sequence shows large hypovascular mass (*arrows*) involving central portion of liver. **B:** Delayed image obtained several minutes later shows progressive enhancement of tumor (*arrows*).

FIG. 3.13. Caroli disease. Fat-suppressed T2-weighted **(A)** and fat-suppressed, gadolinium-enhanced T1-weighted **(B)** images of the liver demonstrate multiple cystic lesions throughout liver, some of which appear tubular with "central dot sign" (*arrows*). Note ascites (*arrowhead*).

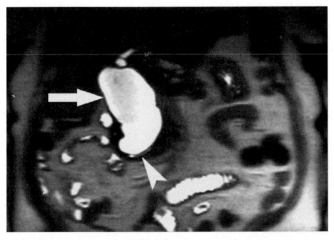

FIG. 3.12. Type I choledochal cyst. Coronal HASTE image demonstrates diffuse dilatation of the common bile duct (*arrow*). *Arrowhead* denotes distal pancreatic duct.

signal intensity or enhancement pattern usually allows a correct diagnosis, but atypical cases may require biopsy or close follow-up to exclude HCC.

References: 16, 17

Cyst, Simple Benign (Fig. 3.15)

Description: Epithelial lined, round or oval shaped, fluid-filled lesion.

T1: Hypointense.

T2: Very hyperintense.

Enhancement pattern: No enhancement.

Characteristic features: Sharply marginated and typically unilocular. Very long T2 relaxation time.

Distribution: Frequently multiple. No particular distribution.

Atypical appearances: Septations may be present. Hemorrhage or proteinaceous material may cause increased signal

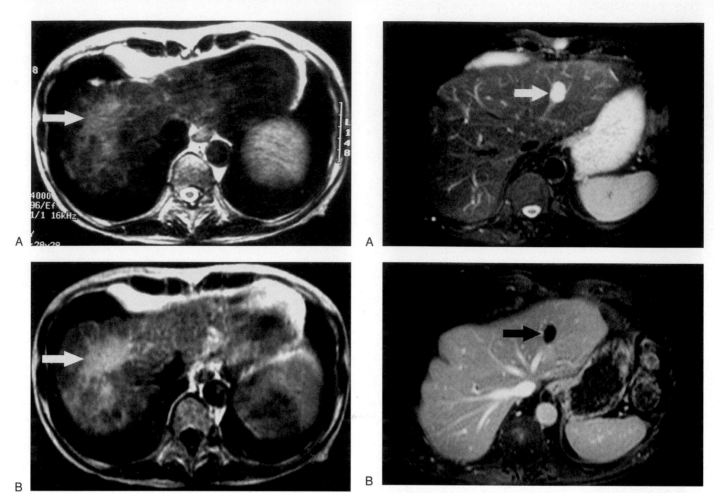

FIG. 3.14. Confluent hepatic fibrosis. **A:** T2-weighted image through liver of cirrhotic patient shows irregular area of high signal intensity (*arrow*) near hepatic dome. **B:** Same area (*arrow*) demonstrates homogeneous enhancement on delayed post-gadolinium T1-weighted image.

FIG. 3.15. Hepatic cyst. **A:** Fat-suppressed T2-weighted image shows cyst (*arrow*) to be of uniform high signal intensity. **B:** Fat-suppressed, gadolinium-enhanced T1-weighted gradient echo image shows no enhancement of cyst (*arrow*).

intensity on T1-weighted images and decreased signal intensity on T2-weighted images.

Associations: Autosomal dominant polycystic kidney disease.

Mimics: Cystic metastases, Caroli disease, bile duct hamartomas, echinococcal disease, abscess.

Dysplastic Nodule (Fig. 3.16)

Description: Dysplastic nodules represent an intermediate step in the continuum from regenerative nodule to HCC in the setting of cirrhosis. They contain abnormal hepatocytes with variable amounts of cytologic atypia but no clear malignancy. Dysplastic nodules are considered premalignant lesions.

T1: Increased signal intensity on T1-weighted images is considered typical. Siderotic dysplastic nodules demonstrate decreased signal intensity.

T2: Hypointense to isointense. On T2*-weighted gradient echo images, iron-containing nodules appear dark. Foci of increased signal intensity should raise concern for HCC.

Enhancement pattern: Variable, but typically enhance less than or equal to liver, because most dysplastic nodules have predominately portal venous blood supply.

Characteristic features: The classically described dysplastic nodule has high signal intensity on T1-weighted and low signal intensity on T2-weighted images without significant arterial phase enhancement.

Distribution: Diffuse and multiple.

Atypical appearances: Some dysplastic nodules may enhance during the arterial phase, making distinction from HCC difficult or impossible.

Associations: Cirrhosis, chronic hepatitis.

Mimics: Well-differentiated HCC, benign regenerative nodules associated with Budd-Chiari syndrome.

Additional comments: Some overlap exists between the imaging appearance of dysplastic nodules and that of well-differentiated HCC. Features that should increase suspicion

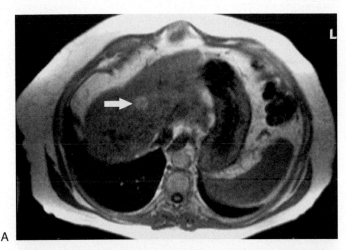

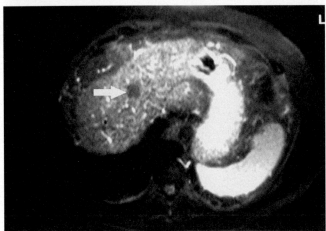

FIG. 3.16. Dysplastic nodule. **A:** T1-weighted gradient echo image of liver in patient with cirrhosis shows high signal intensity hepatic nodule (*arrow*). **B:** Fat-suppressed T2-weighted image shows nodule (*arrow*) to be low in signal intensity. Biopsy revealed atypical cells but no malignancy.

for carcinoma include increased signal intensity on T2-weighted images, arterial phase enhancement, large size, presence of a pseudocapsule, or rapid growth. In addition, a focal region of arterial enhancement or high signal intensity on T2-weighted images in an otherwise typical dysplastic nodule is suspicious for development of a focus of HCC (nodule-within-a-nodule sign). Siderotic regenerative nodules and siderotic dysplastic nodules may be indistinguishable with MRI. High signal intensity nodules are relatively common on T1-weighted images of cirrhotic livers. Not all nodules with increased signal intensity on T1-weighted images are dysplastic.

References: 18, 19

Embryonal Sarcoma (Fig. 3.17)

Description: Uncommon primary hepatic malignant tumor composed of spindle- and stellate-shaped cells in a myxoid background.

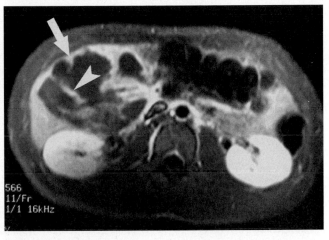

FIG. 3.17. Embryonal sarcoma in teenager. Post-gadolinium, fat-suppressed T1-weighted image shows peripheral enhancement of tumor (*arrow*) with thick internal enhancing tissue septa (*arrowhead*). Lesion was very bright on T2-weighted image (not shown).

T1: Predominantly low signal intensity. Focal areas of high signal intensity represent hemorrhage.

T2: Very high signal intensity approaching that of cerebrospinal fluid.

Enhancement pattern: Enhancement of solid tissue components, mainly involving the tumor periphery and some septum-like areas within the tumor, creating a heterogeneous appearance after gadolinium administration.

Characteristic features: These tumors often appear cyst-like on MR images but appear solid on sonograms. Areas of cystic hemorrhagic degeneration are relatively common (best appreciated on T1-weighted images).

Distribution: Solitary. More commonly described in right hepatic lobe.

Atypical appearances: An intratumoral fluid-debris level may occasionally be seen.

Mimics: Other complex cystic tumors of the liver, including cystic metastases, hepatic abscess, and resolving hematoma.

Additional comments: Occurs mainly in children and young adults.

References: 20

Fatty Infiltration, Focal (Fig. 3.18)

Description: The focal form of hepatic steatosis.

T1: Isointense to slightly hyperintense relative to normal liver.

T2: Isointense to slightly hyperintense on non–fat-saturated images.

Enhancement pattern: Similar to normal liver

Characteristic features: Loss of hepatic signal intensity on opposed-phase gradient echo images. Lacks mass effect on vessels or bile ducts.

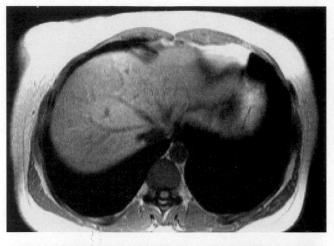
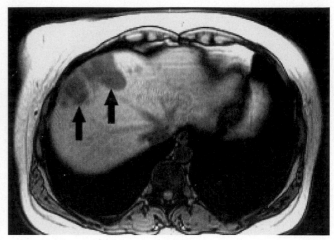
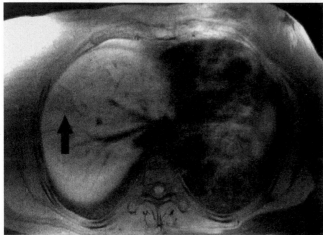

FIG. 3.18. Focal fat. **A:** In-phase T1-weighted gradient echo image shows homogeneous liver. **B:** Opposed-phase gradient echo image shows areas of focal signal loss (*arrows*) consistent with focal steatosis. **C:** T1-weighted gradient echo image with fat saturation in same patient is not nearly as effective at demonstrating areas of steatosis (*arrow*).

Distribution: May be focal, multifocal, or diffuse. Location highly variable, but typical locations include adjacent to falciform ligament, central aspect of medial segment, and adjacent to gallbladder fossa.

Atypical appearances: May appear as multiple discrete nodules

Mimics: Lipid-containing adenoma or HCC.

References: 21

Fibrolamellar Hepatocellular Carcinoma

Description: Desmoplastic malignant tumor of hepatocellular origin. Fibrous septa and central stellate scar are characteristic.

T1: Slightly hypointense, heterogeneous. Low signal intensity central scar.

T2: Variably hyperintense. Low signal intensity central scar.

Enhancement pattern: Enhances early, intensely, and heterogeneously. Central scar poorly enhancing, but may enhance after a delay of several minutes.

Characteristic features: Lobulated mass in noncirrhotic liver of a young adult. Tumor tends to be large at time of diagnosis. A nonenhancing central scar that is hypointense on both T1- and T2-weighted images helps distinguish this entity from FNH. Central scar may be calcified on computed tomography (CT).

Distribution: Typically solitary.

Atypical appearances: May occur in middle-aged and older patients. Central scar may be absent.

Associations: Unlike typical HCC, fibrolamellar HCC is not associated with cirrhosis.

Mimics: FNH.

Additional comments: Alpha-fetoprotein is usually within normal range.

References: 22

Focal Nodular Hyperplasia (Fig. 3.19; see 3.146)

Description: Focal masslike area of hyperplasia composed of hepatocytes, Kupffer cells, and bile ducts. Central scar consists of vascular channels, fibrosis, and bile ducts.

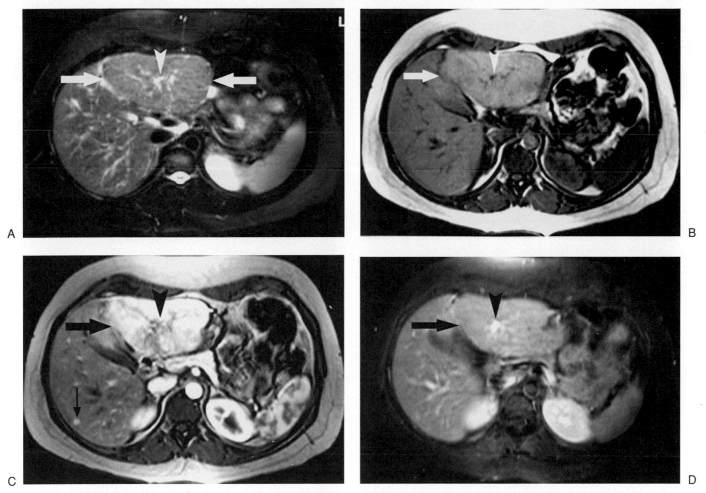

FIG. 3.19. Focal nodular hyperplasia. **A:** Fat-suppressed T2-weighted image through liver shows large mass (*arrows*) in left hepatic lobe that is nearly isointense to liver. High signal intensity central scar is present (*arrowhead*). **B:** Mass (*arrow*) is slightly higher in signal intensity than liver on T1-weighted opposed-phase gradient echo image due to mild hepatic steatosis. Central scar (*arrowhead*) is low signal intensity. **C:** During arterial phase of dynamic gadolinium-enhanced study, mass (*arrow*) is hyper-enhancing, although central scar (*arrowhead*) remains dark. Note incidental second lesion (*thin arrow*). **D:** Delayed gadolinium-enhanced, fat-suppressed T1-weighted image shows the mass (*arrow*) as isointense to liver, although central scar (*arrowhead*) is enhancing.

Once described as rare in the literature, these lesions are commonly discovered on dynamic, contrast-enhanced images.

T1: Nearly isointense to liver with low signal intensity central scar (when present).

T2: Nearly isointense to minimally hyperintense with high signal intensity central scar (when present).

Enhancement pattern: Early intense enhancement. Fades rapidly to become nearly isointense to liver on later images. Delayed enhancement of central scar. Mass enhances with and retains mangafodipir due to presence of functioning hepatocytes. Uptake of ferumoxides is typical due to presence of Kupffer cells. Signal loss of FNH following ferumoxides administration typically exceeds that of other tumors.

Characteristic features: Well marginated lobulated mass, often nearly invisible on precontrast T1- and T2-weighted im-

ages. Typical appearance of stellate central scar very specific for diagnosis. May be associated with abnormal vasculature.

Distribution: Subcapsular location is common. Two or more lesions are present in up to one third of patients with FNH.

Atypical appearances: May be pedunculated. Central scar or early enhancement may be absent. May rarely contain sufficient lipid to lose signal on opposed-phase imaging (see Fig. 3.125). May appear hyperintense on T1-weighted images or moderately bright on T2-weighted images.

Associations: Hepatic hemangioma.

Mimics: Fibrolamellar carcinoma, hepatic adenoma (although FNH shows more exuberant arterial phase enhancement and rarely demonstrates significant intratumoral hemorrhage or steatosis).

Additional comments: No malignant potential. When typical MR findings are present, no further action is indicated.

Ferumoxides may have some utility in confirming diagnosis when typical features are absent.

References: 23, 24

Hemangioma, Hepatic (Fig. 3.20; see Figs. 1.43, 1.44, 3.145)

Description: Common benign vascular tumor. Most hemangiomas are cavernous lesions characterized by large vascular channels. Occasionally, lesions resemble capillary telangiectasias.

T1: Low signal intensity.

T2: Very high signal intensity.

Enhancement pattern: Most typical enhancement pattern is early peripheral nodular enhancement (puddling) with progressive centripetal enhancement of remainder of lesion (type 2 enhancement). Delayed images reveal homogeneous enhancement with retention of contrast (isointense to vessels). Small lesions may demonstrate early intense homogeneous enhancement (type 1 enhancement). Early, transient peritumoral enhancement may also occur (more common with type 1 enhancing lesions).

Characteristic features: Distinct lobular margins, typical centripetal enhancement pattern, and long T2 relaxation time are virtually diagnostic of hemangioma.

Distribution: May occur anywhere in the liver, although most common in right lobe. Frequently multiple.

Atypical appearances: May be pedunculated. May have central scar that fails to enhance with gadolinium (type 3 enhancement). Large lesions (giant hemangioma) may contain fibrous septa or areas of hemorrhage or necrosis. Sclerosing hemangiomas may have only modestly increased signal intensity on T2-weighted images. Arterial-portal shunting may be present on contrast-enhanced images.

Associations: Blue rubber bleb nevus syndrome (see Fig. 3.49), FNH, thrombocytopenia (Kasabach-Merritt syndrome).

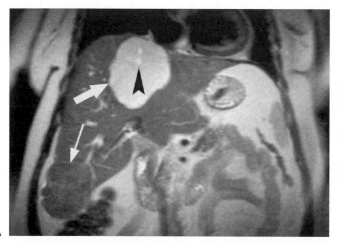

A

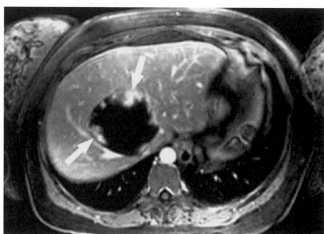

B

C

FIG. 3.20. Hemangioma. **A:** Coronal HASTE image shows large high signal intensity hepatic mass (*arrow*). Note small focus of central higher signal intensity (*arrowhead*). A mass of focal nodular hyperplasia (*thin arrow*) nearly escapes detection on this image. **B:** Portal venous phase image from dynamic fat-suppressed, gadolinium-enhanced sequence shows typical nodular peripheral enhancement (*arrows*). **C:** Note progressive centripetal filling (*arrows*) on delayed contrast-enhanced image.

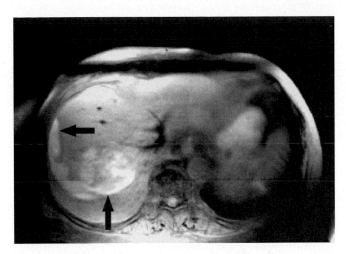

FIG. 3.21. Hepatic hematoma in patient with lymphoma. Fat-suppressed gradient echo T1-weighted image shows high signal intensity mass in right hepatic lobe with hemorrhage extending to liver capsule (*arrows*).

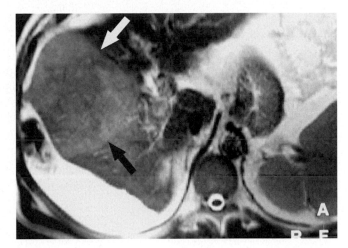

FIG. 3.22. Hepatocellular carcinoma. Axial HASTE image shows high signal intensity mass (*arrows*) in right lobe of cirrhotic liver.

Mimics: Angiosarcoma. Hypervascular or necrotic (postchemotherapy) metastases.

References: 25, 26

Hematoma (Fig. 3.21)

Description: Focal hemorrhage that may occur in intraparenchymal or subcapsular locations.

T1: Mixed signal intensity. Extracellular methemoglobin results in characteristic areas of high signal intensity over the course of several days.

T2: Mixed signal intensity. Soon after hematoma forms, signal intensity is high and subsequently fades and becomes more complex as blood products evolve.

Enhancement pattern: Nonenhancing unless active bleeding is present.

Characteristic features: High signal intensity foci on T1- and T2-weighted images. Size and signal intensity vary over time.

Distribution: Intraparenchymal or subcapsular. May demonstrate fluid-fluid level.

Associations: Trauma, HELLP syndrome (hemolysis, elevated liver enzymes, and low platelet count in women with pregnancy-induced hypertension), hepatic tumors (particularly adenoma).

Mimics: Hemorrhagic cystic tumor. Lesions containing macroscopic fat are rare in the liver but may be distinguished from hemorrhage with use of fat suppression.

Hepatocellular Carcinoma (Figs. 3.22 to 3.25; see Fig. 3.126)

Description: Malignant tumor of hepatocellular origin. Most common primary malignant tumor of the liver.

T1: Variable, but commonly hypointense to isointense to liver. Well-differentiated HCC may be hyperintense to liver.

T2: Variable, but most commonly isointense to hyperintense to liver. Low signal intensity pseudocapsule may be present. Higher signal intensity tumors tend to be less well differentiated.

Enhancement pattern: Early, often intense, heterogeneous enhancement that fades quickly. Small lesions are frequently only visible on arterial phase images of dynamic gadolinium-enhanced study. Pseudocapsule enhancement may be present on delayed images. Well-differentiated tumors may take up and retain mangafodipir or ferumoxides as a result of residual hepatocyte or Kupffer cell function, respectively.

Characteristic features: HCC most frequently occurs in patients with underlying cirrhosis, hemochromatosis, or chronic

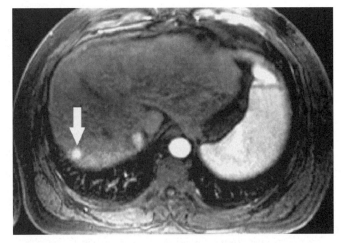

FIG. 3.23. Hepatocellular carcinoma. Axial fat-suppressed, gadolinium-enhanced arterial phase image demonstrates small hypervascular hepatocellular carcinoma (*arrow*). Lesion was inconspicuous on other sequences (not shown).

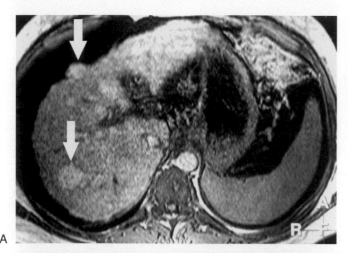

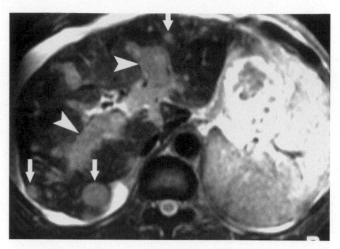

FIG. 3.25. Multifocal hepatocellular carcinoma with portal vein invasion. Fat-suppressed T2-weighted image shows multiple hepatic nodules (*arrows*) and expansion of the portal veins (*arrowheads*) with high signal intensity tumor.

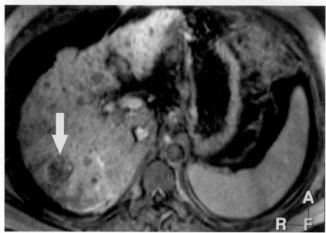

FIG. 3.24. Multifocal hepatocellular carcinoma. **A:** T1-weighted gradient echo image demonstrates multiple high signal intensity hepatic nodules (*arrows*). **B:** Portal venous phase post-gadolinium T1-weighted gradient echo image demonstrates heterogeneous enhancement of largest nodule (*arrow*). Multifocal hepatocellular carcinoma was found at transplantation.

Associations: Cirrhosis, chronic viral hepatitis, hemachromatosis, Wilson disease, alpha$_1$-antitrypsin deficiency, glycogen storage disease.

Mimics: Adenoma, angiosarcoma, arterial-portal shunting, confluent fibrosis, dysplastic nodule, inflammatory pseudotumor.

Additional comments: Leading cause of cancer death in Southeastern Asia and sub-Saharan Africa where chronic hepatitis is endemic. Alpha-fetoprotein levels may be normal in more than one third of patients with HCC.

References: 27 to 29

Lymphoma, Hepatic

Description: Malignant lymphocytic tumor. Lymphoma of the liver most commonly results from secondary infiltration. Primary hepatic lymphoma is rare.

T1: Hypointense to isointense to liver.

T2: Typically isointense to slightly hyperintense to liver, although it can have low signal intensity.

Enhancement pattern: When present, enhancement is typically peripheral.

Characteristic features: A history of lymphoma is helpful, because the diagnosis is difficult based on imaging characteristics alone.

Distribution: Can appear as a focal mass or diffuse infiltrative process. Diffuse disease (hepatomegaly) is more common. Focal disease may be solitary or multiple and is more common with non-Hodgkin lymphoma. Periportal tumor may appear as high signal intensity on fat-suppressed T2-weighted and contrast-enhanced T1-weighted images.

Atypical appearances: Large solitary mass.

Associations: In transplant recipients on immunosuppressive therapy, posttransplant lymphoproliferative disorder affecting the liver may develop.

viral hepatitis. Portal or hepatic vein invasion presents as tumor thrombus with similar enhancement characteristics to primary tumor. Nodule-within-a-nodule appearance may be seen on T1-weighted images when low signal intensity HCC develops in a high signal intensity dysplastic nodule. Nodule-within-a-nodule appearance can also occur when a high signal intensity focus of HCC develops in a low signal intensity dysplastic nodule on T2-weighted images or a focus of enhancement is seen in a cirrhotic nodule after gadolinium administration.

Distribution: Anywhere in the liver. May be solitary (approximately half of cases), multiple, or diffuse. Satellite lesions are common. Most common sites of extrahepatic metastases are lymph nodes, lungs, and bone.

Atypical appearances: May contain fat or invade bile ducts. Well-differentiated tumors may appear relatively hypovascular.

Mimics: Hepatic metastases.

Additional comments: Most cases of hepatic lymphoma are of the secondary, infiltrative variety. Therefore, detection may be difficult with MRI. Primary lymphoma of the liver is extremely rare.

References: 30

Metastasis, Hepatic (Figs. 3.26 to 3.28; see Figs. 3.144, 3.158)

Description: Malignant tumor within the liver of extrahepatic origin. Metastases are more common than primary hepatic malignant tumors. A great variety of primary malignant tumors can metastasize to the liver. However, the most common sites of origin are the gastrointestinal tract, breast, and lung.

T1: Hypointense to isointense. Uncommonly, metastases can be hyperintense relative to liver as a result of hemorrhage, melanin, or protein content.

T2: Isointense to hyperintense. Cystic (typical of ovarian cancer), mucinous, hypervascular, or necrotic metastases may be very hyperintense.

Enhancement pattern: Variable. A pattern of early ring enhancement with progressive central filling is relatively common. Delayed images may reveal peripheral washout of contrast. Perilesional enhancement may occur. Small hypervascular metastases may enhance early, intensely, and homogeneously, fading relative to hepatic parenchyma on more delayed images. Hypervascular metastases classically occur with renal cell carcinoma, melanoma, and endocrine or neuroendocrine tumors such as islet cell tumor and carcinoid. Hypervascular metastases occur less commonly with carcinoma of the breast, pancreas, colon, and lung. Most adenocarcinoma metastases are hypovascular relative to liver. With rare exceptions, metastases do not accumulate mangafodipir or ferumoxides.

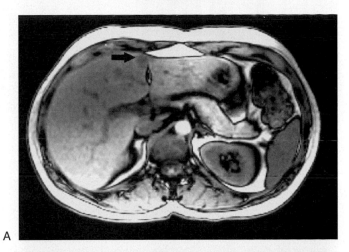

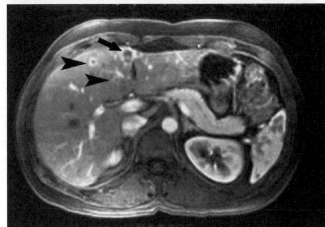

FIG. 3.27. Liver metastases, breast carcinoma. **A:** Opposed-phase T1-weighted gradient echo image of liver shows low signal intensity focus (*arrow*) adjacent to falciform ligament. On this image alone, this could be confused with focal fat. **B:** Following administration of intravenous gadolinium, ring enhancement is demonstrated (*arrow*). Two additional lesions also demonstrating ring enhancement (*arrowheads*) are better appreciated on enhanced study.

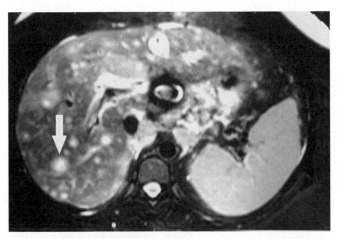

FIG. 3.26. Liver metastases, adenocarcinoma of unknown primary. Fat-suppressed T2-weighted image through liver shows multiple high signal intensity masses (*arrow*).

Characteristic features: Metastases have a wide range of appearances. The presence of multiple hepatic lesions with irregular or ill-defined borders demonstrating uninterrupted ring enhancement with progressive central filling and delayed peripheral washout is virtually pathognomonic for metastases.

Distribution: Anywhere. Most often multiple. Solitary metastases most common with colorectal carcinoma.

Atypical appearances: The range of appearances for liver metastases is so varied that it is difficult to define an atypical case. Treated diffuse breast cancer metastases may simulate the appearance of macronodular cirrhosis.

Associations: Primary malignant tumor.

Mimics: Atypical hemangioma, adenoma, FNH (particularly when multiple), multifocal HCC, multiple hepatic abscesses.

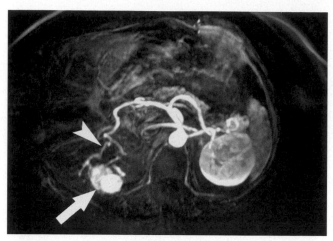

FIG. 3.28. Liver metastasis, renal cell carcinoma. Maximum intensity projection of arterial phase image from digital subtraction three-dimensional gadolinium-enhanced dynamic examination of the liver. Note briskly enhancing lesion (*arrow*) in right hepatic lobe supplied by large branches of the hepatic artery (*arrowhead*).

Additional comments: Mangafodipir or ferumoxides-enhanced imaging has been advocated to improve detection of hepatic metastases. However, the majority of liver MRI examinations for evaluation of known or suspected metastatic disease are performed with gadolinium chelates.

References: 31

Regenerative Nodule

Description: Regenerative nodules are benign nodular collections of histologically normal hepatocytes between areas of fibrosis within a cirrhotic liver. Regenerative nodules should be distinguished from dysplastic nodules, which are considered premalignant.

T1: Variable but most often hypointense to isointense. Regenerative nodules often have high iron content, resulting in very low signal intensity on gradient echo images.

T2: Hypointense to isointense. On T2*-weighted gradient echo images, iron-containing nodules appear very dark.

Enhancement pattern: A cirrhotic liver is essentially composed of regenerative nodules separated by bands of fibrosis. Therefore, most regenerative nodules enhance similarly. Focal lesions that enhance significantly more than other surrounding nodules should be viewed with suspicion.

Characteristic features: Multiple small nodules of low signal intensity on both T1- and T2-weighted images are typical of regenerative nodules. Siderotic nodules are more pronounced on T2*-weighted (long echo time [TE] gradient echo) images because of the magnetic susceptibility effects of iron.

Distribution: Diffuse and multiple.

Atypical appearances: Regenerative nodules may contain lipid (Fig. 3.29). In the setting of Budd-Chiari syndrome, re-

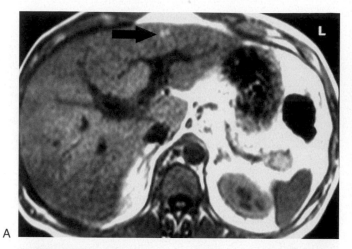

A

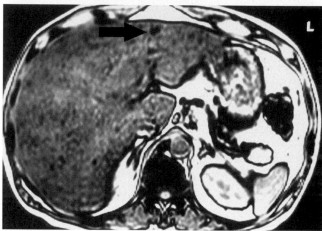

B

FIG. 3.29. Regenerative nodules. **A:** In-phase T1-weighted gradient echo image demonstrates multiple tiny nodules throughout the liver in patient with cirrhosis. Many nodules are increased in signal intensity (*arrow*). **B:** Opposed-phase image shows many of the nodules lose signal intensity (*arrow*), consistent with lipid content. Siderotic nodules would have demonstrated loss of signal intensity on in-phase image due to susceptibility effects.

generative nodules may have increased signal intensity on T1 or T2-weighted images and enhance considerably with contrast. Infarcted regenerative nodules may demonstrate increased signal intensity on T2-weighted images.

Associations: Cirrhosis, Budd-Chiari syndrome.

Additional comments: Available data do not strongly support a direct causative relationship between siderotic nodules and dysplasia or HCC.

References: 32 to 35

LIVER, DIFFUSE ABNORMALITIES

Cirrhosis (Figs. 3.30 to 3.32)

Description: Hepatic parenchymal cell injury associated with nodular regeneration, fibrosis, and architectural distortion.

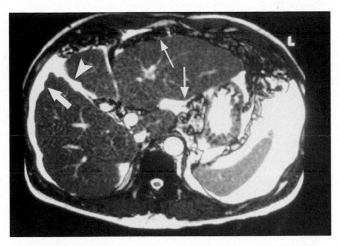

FIG. 3.30. Morphologic changes of cirrhosis. Axial steady-state gradient echo image (balanced-FFE) demonstrates nodular liver contour (*arrow*), widening of the interlobar fissure (*arrowhead*), and hypertrophy of the lateral segment (*thin arrows*).

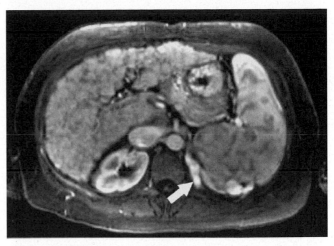

FIG. 3.32. Cirrhosis with regenerative nodules. Axial fat-suppressed, gadolinium-enhanced gradient echo image shows multiple small regenerative nodules throughout the liver associated with splenomegaly and varices (*arrow*).

T1: Regenerative nodules of variable signal intensity. Low signal intensity intervening fibrosis.

T2: Regenerative nodules are usually hypointense relative to surrounding fibrosis.

Enhancement pattern: Frequently heterogeneous during the arterial phase of enhancement with increasing homogeneity on subsequent postcontrast images. Confluent hepatic fibrosis often shows progressive or delayed enhancement.

Characteristic features: Nodular liver contour that may vary from micronodular to macronodular depending on the size of the regenerative nodules. Varying degrees and locations of parenchymal atrophy and hypertrophy may result in a lobulated contour that is relatively common with pri-

mary sclerosing cholangitis but uncommon with primary biliary cirrhosis. Fibrosis forms a reticular pattern of decreased (T1-weighted images) or increased (T2-weighted images) signal intensity between regenerative nodules. Siderotic regenerative nodules become more apparent on T2*-weighted images.

Distribution: A pattern of right lobe and medial segment atrophy with caudate and lateral segment preservation or hypertrophy is relatively common with cirrhosis. Expansion of the hilar periportal space and interlobar fissure is also common. Approximately one third of end-stage cirrhotic livers demonstrate diffuse atrophy. Diffuse hypertrophy of the liver and hypertrophy of the right posterior segment are rare.

Atypical appearances: Diffuse hepatic steatosis results in parenchymal signal loss on opposed-phase gradient echo images relative to in-phase images. This is in contrast to hepatic siderosis, which causes relative signal loss on the in-phase images (due to the longer TE). Small peribiliary cysts exhibiting decreased signal intensity on T1-weighted images and increased signal intensity on T2-weighted images may be present in some cases.

Associations: Ethanol abuse, viral hepatitis, primary biliary cirrhosis, primary sclerosing cholangitis, hepatic vein occlusion, Wilson disease, hemochromatosis, autoimmune disease.

Mimics: Treated breast carcinoma.

Additional comments: The process of fibrosis alters the imaging appearance of hemangiomas, preventing definitive diagnosis in some cases. Small arterially enhancing nodules are common in the cirrhotic liver with high-resolution, dynamic, gadolinium-enhanced MRI (Fig. 3.33). Most lesions less than 1 cm in diameter are benign but often cannot be reliably distinguished from HCC. Therefore, close imaging follow-up of small, arterially enhancing lesions is

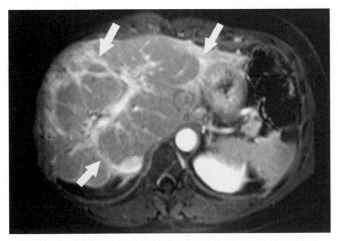

FIG. 3.31. Cirrhosis secondary to sclerosing cholangitis. Axial fat-suppressed, gadolinium-enhanced gradient echo image demonstrates findings typical of sclerosing cholangitis with large regenerative nodules surrounded by bands of fibrosis (*arrows*) resulting in a lobulated appearance of the liver.

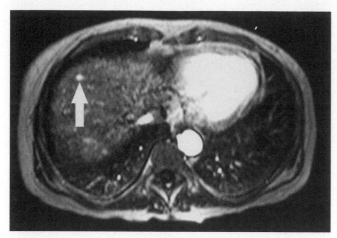

FIG. 3.33. Small hypervascular lesion in cirrhotic liver. Arterial phase image from dynamic three-dimensional gadolinium-enhanced study of patient with cirrhosis shows small enhancing lesion in dome of liver. Lesions such as this are common in cirrhosis and should be followed closely.

appropriate, and any evidence of growth should be considered a sign of malignancy.

References: 36 to 38

Fatty Infiltration, Diffuse (Steatosis) (Fig. 3.34)

Description: Hepatocellular lipid accumulation

T1: Diffuse increased signal intensity (altered signal intensity may be subtle or absent with mild degrees of steatosis).

T2: Slightly hyperintense on non–fat-saturated fast spin echo images (altered signal intensity may be subtle or absent with mild degrees of steatosis).

Enhancement pattern: normal.

Characteristic features: Diffuse loss of signal intensity on opposed-phase (relative to in-phase) gradient echo images. Lacks mass effect on vessels or bile ducts, which can be seen coursing normally through the fatty liver.

Distribution: Diffuse with areas of focal sparing. Sparing is common around the gallbladder fossa or adjacent to the left portal vein in the medial segment.

Associations: Pregnancy, diabetes, alcohol abuse, obesity, hyperlipidemia, glycogen storage disease, steroids, chemotherapy.

Mimics: A focal hepatic mass may mimic an area of focal fatty sparing.

Additional comments: Because lipid is delivered to the liver via the portal vein, portions of the liver with diminished portal blood flow may demonstrate sparing in the setting of hepatic steatosis. Therefore, a pattern of segmental fatty sparing should prompt a search for abnormality of the feeding portal branch. MR spectroscopy may have utility in quantifying intracellular lipid in hepatic steatosis. Although fatty infiltration is often thought of as a benign condition, steatohepatitis can progress to cirrhosis in some patients. Obese,

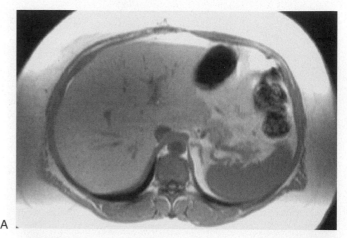

A

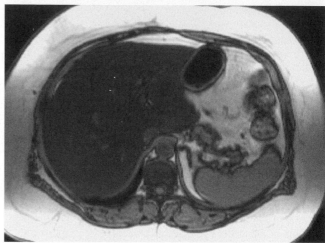

B

FIG. 3.34. Diffuse hepatic steatosis. **A:** In-phase T1-weighted gradient echo image demonstrates homogeneous, slightly increased signal intensity of liver. Note liver is hyperintense relative to spleen. **B:** Opposed-phase image obtained during same sequence shows diffuse loss of hepatic signal intensity. Liver is hypointense relative to spleen.

type II diabetics appear to be at particular risk for this complication.

References: 39

Hepatic Vein Thrombosis or Occlusion (Budd-Chiari Syndrome) (Figs. 3.35, 3.36)

Description: Thrombosis of one or more of the hepatic veins.

T1: Peripheral hepatic edema may manifest as decreased signal intensity in the acute phase.

T2: Peripheral hepatic edema manifests as increased signal intensity in the acute phase.

Enhancement pattern: Heterogeneous, with diminished enhancement of the liver periphery and preferential enhancement of caudate lobe in acute hepatic vein occlusion. As intrahepatic venous collaterals develop over time, heterogeneous peripheral enhancement occurs.

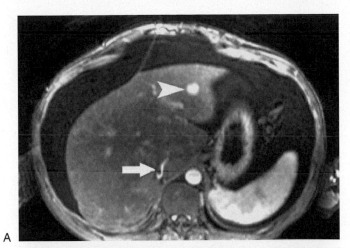

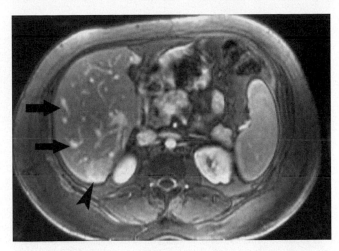

FIG. **3.36.** Hepatic vein obstruction. Fat-suppressed, gadolinium-enhanced T1-weighted image in patient with large focal nodular hyperplasia (FNH) (not shown) obstructing hepatic veins near confluence. Note abnormal comma-shaped veins (*arrows*) at liver periphery. Incidental note is made of presumed second FNH (*arrowhead*).

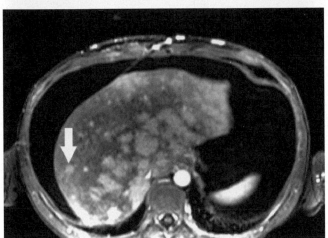

FIG. **3.35.** Hepatic vein thrombosis. **A:** Fat-suppressed, gadolinium-enhanced T1-weighted image shows filling defect in inferior vena cava (*arrow*) and enhancing nodule in left lateral segment (*arrowhead*). Normal hepatic veins could not be detected on any image. **B:** More delayed image cephalad to **(A)** shows heterogeneous enhancement with diminished enhancement of liver periphery. Persistent enhancing nodule is also present (*arrow*). Nodules such as these are typical for regenerative nodules of Budd-Chiari syndrome.

Characteristic features: Nonvisualization of the hepatic veins. Disorganized hepatic venous collaterals sometimes resembling "comma" shapes may become visible over time (see Fig. 3.36). Hypertrophy of the caudate lobe and central liver, ascites, and portal hypertension occur with longstanding hepatic vein occlusion. Regenerative nodules in chronic Budd-Chiari syndrome typically are isointense or hyperintense on T1-weighted images and have variable signal intensity on T2-weighted images. These nodules tend to enhance considerably on early gadolinium-enhanced images, and enhancement may persist into the portal venous phase (see Fig. 3.35).

Distribution: Hepatic vein occlusion may involve one or more hepatic veins or the suprahepatic inferior vena cava (IVC).

Associations: Oral contraceptive use, myeloproliferative disorders, antiphospholipid syndrome, antithrombin III deficiency, factor V Leiden, paroxysmal nocturnal hemoglobinuria, protein C deficiency, protein S deficiency, other hypercoagulable states.

Mimics: Elevated right heart pressure may result in delayed enhancement of enlarged hepatic veins and mosaic enhancement of the hepatic parenchyma. Hepatic veins and IVC may be attenuated and poorly visualized in cirrhosis.

Additional comments: Regenerative nodules associated with Budd-Chiari syndrome may be indistinguishable from HCC by imaging alone. Most hepatic nodules associated with Budd-Chiari syndrome are benign, although HCC may occur, particularly if risk factors for HCC exist (e.g., viral hepatitis).

References: 40 to 42

Iron Deposition (Fig. 3.37)

Description: Occurs with primary hemochromatosis and transfusional hemosiderosis.

T1: Signal intensity of liver decreased or normal.

T2: Signal intensity of liver decreased. Mild iron deposition may be evident on T2 or T2*-weighted images when signal intensity on T1-weighted images is normal.

Enhancement pattern: Normal.

Characteristic features: As a rule of thumb, abnormal iron deposition is characterized by liver parenchyma that appears darker than skeletal muscle on all pulse sequences. Hepatic signal loss is exacerbated on T2*-weighted (long TE) gradient echo sequences. Primary hemochromatosis eventually leads to cirrhosis (rare with transfusional iron overload).

Distribution: Entire liver.

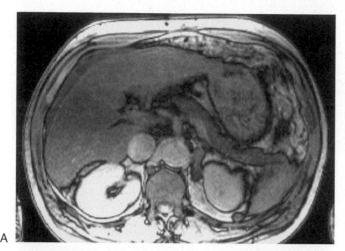

A

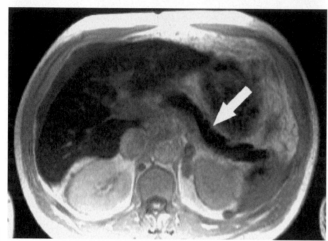

B

FIG. 3.37. Hepatic iron deposition. Opposed-phase (A) and in-phase (B) gradient echo images of patient with primary hemochromatosis demonstrate signal loss in liver and pancreas (*arrow*) on in-phase image (B).

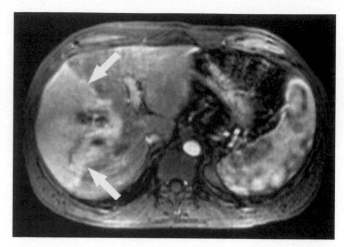

FIG. 3.38. Acute thrombosis of the anterior segment branch of right portal vein. Note wedge-shaped enhancement (*arrows*) of territory supplied by thrombosed portal branch.

Associations: Primary (genetic) hemochromatosis, cirrhosis, multiple blood transfusions, paroxysmal nocturnal hemoglobinuria, thalassemia, Bantu siderosis.

Additional comments: Primary hemochromatosis is a genetic abnormality resulting in excessive gastrointestinal absorption of iron and iron deposition in various organs including liver, pancreas, skin, heart, and pituitary. In hemochromatosis, hepatic iron deposition is primarily within hepatocytes. Transfusional iron overload results in iron deposition in the reticuloendothelial system (Kupffer cells) as a result of multiple blood transfusions. Splenic accumulation of iron is typical of transfusional iron overload, but not primary hemochromatosis.

References: 43

Portal Vein Thrombosis (Fig. 3.38)

Description: Occlusion of the main portal vein or a portal vein branch by clot or tumor.

T1: Most commonly intermediate signal intensity with loss of flow void or flow related enhancement (gradient echo sequences). Subacute thrombus may appear as high signal intensity (see Fig. 2.21A).

T2: Intermediate to high signal intensity of thrombus with loss of flow void in affected vein. Liver parenchyma supplied by thrombosed vessel may show increased signal intensity on T2-weighted images.

Enhancement pattern: May be associated with increased enhancement of the involved segments during the arterial phase, particularly in the periphery, related to a compensatory increase in arterial flow. Pattern may appear as the opposite of hepatic vein thrombosis, in which enhancement tends to be central. Abnormal venous mural enhancement may be present with septic thrombophlebitis.

Characteristic features: Bland thrombus typically does not enhance after contrast injection. Tumor thrombus often enhances in a similar manner to the primary tumor. HCC has a predilection for invading the portal venous system and, less commonly, the hepatic venous system. Tumor thrombus tends to expand the vessel lumen, whereas bland thrombus typically does not. The chronic form of portal vein thrombosis manifests as multiple collateral veins in the porta hepatis and periportal regions (referred to as cavernous transformation) (see Fig. 2.22). Stigmata of portal hypertension (e.g., varices, splenomegaly) may be present with the chronic form.

Distribution: May involve main, right, left, or segmental veins. Involvement by tumor is typically contiguous with the primary lesion with retrograde growth into the more central portal veins.

Associations: Hypercoagulable states, malignant tumors (most commonly HCC), cirrhosis.

Mimics: Flow artifact.

References: 44

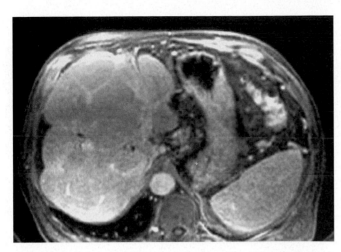

FIG. 3.39. Primary sclerosing cholangitis. Fat-suppressed, gadolinium-enhanced T1-weighted image of the liver in patient with sclerosing cholangitis demonstrates typical lobular pattern of fibrosis and liver regeneration. This is same patient as in Figure 2.36.

Primary Sclerosing Cholangitis (Fig. 3.39; see Fig. 2.36)

Description: Chronic, progressive inflammatory and fibrotic disease of the intrahepatic and extrahepatic bile ducts.

T1: Fibrosis may appear as low signal intensity bands.

T2: Peripheral wedge-shaped or reticular areas of increased signal intensity are relatively common, presumably the result of fibrosis. Periportal inflammation and edema may result in periportal increased signal intensity on T2-weighted images.

Enhancement pattern: Increased arterial phase enhancement may be present in the periphery of the liver. Bile duct wall enhancement is typical. A modest degree (3 to 4 mm) of bile duct wall thickening may be present, particularly on gadolinium-enhanced T1-weighted images. However, bile duct wall thickening greater than 5 mm suggests the presence of cholangiocarcinoma.

Characteristic features: Primary sclerosing cholangitis is characterized on magnetic resonance cholangiopancreatography (MRCP) by multiple strictures of the intrahepatic and extrahepatic bile ducts due to progressive periductal fibrosis. Biliary dilatation may be present between strictures, creating a characteristic beaded appearance of the ducts. However, because of the periductal inflammation and fibrosis present with this disease, the intrahepatic bile ducts may not dilate to the extent typical of more focal causes of biliary obstruction. Eventually, the fibrotic process obliterates the peripheral duct lumens, resulting in the appearance of pruning. Cirrhosis develops as a late sequela of sclerosing cholangitis, resulting in a lobulated liver contour with caudate lobe hypertrophy. Lateral and posterior segment atrophy may also be present more commonly than in other forms of cirrhosis. Associated periportal lymphadenopathy is common.

Distribution: Involves intrahepatic ducts, extrahepatic ducts, or both.

Atypical appearances: Intraductal stones are uncommon.

Associations: Most cases of primary sclerosing cholangitis occur in patients with inflammatory bowel disease (up to three fourths of patients, most commonly with ulcerative colitis). However, primary sclerosing cholangitis never develops in the great majority of patients with inflammatory bowel disease. Between 5% and 15% of patients with primary sclerosing cholangitis develop cholangiocarcinoma.

Mimics: Infectious cholangitis (including human immunodeficiency virus-associated cholangiopathy), biliary ischemia.

References: 45 to 47

Sarcoidosis (Fig. 3.40)

Description: Systemic disease of unknown etiology characterized by noncaseating granulomas. Liver involvement is common histologically.

T1: Typically low signal intensity.

T2: Typically low signal intensity.

Enhancement pattern: Diminished enhancement relative to normal liver parenchyma.

Characteristic features: Multiple, subcentimeter low signal intensity nodules throughout the liver. Abdominal lymphadenopathy and splenomegaly may be present.

Distribution: Diffuse.

Mimics: Other granulomatous processes, regenerative nodules.

Additional comments: Focal splenic lesions of sarcoidosis resemble hepatic sarcoid lesions.

References: 48

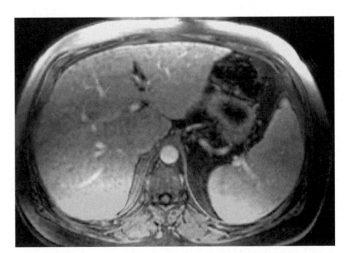

FIG. 3.40. Hepatic sarcoidosis. T1-weighted gradient echo image demonstrates multiple low signal intensity nodules throughout the liver. Biopsy revealed typical noncaseating granulomas.

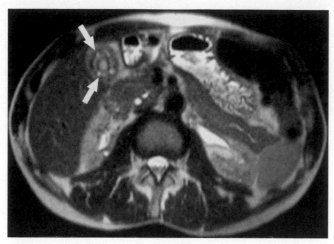

FIG. 3.41. Adenomyomatosis of gallbladder. Axial HASTE image demonstrates thickening of the gallbladder wall with multiple high signal intensity cystic spaces (*arrows*).

GALLBLADDER

Adenomyomatosis (Fig. 3.41)

Description: A hyperplastic cholecystosis characterized by intramural diverticula (Rokitansky-Aschoff sinuses) extending into the thickened muscular layer.

T1: Diverticula may be of variable signal intensity depending on cholesterol content.

T2: Diverticula may be visible as high signal intensity foci within the gallbladder wall.

Enhancement pattern: Diverticula do not enhance with intravenous gadolinium but may fill with hepatobiliary agents.

Characteristic features: Thickened gallbladder wall with intramural diverticula.

Distribution: May be focal, diffuse, or annular.

Atypical appearances: Annular form may obstruct a portion of the gallbladder, resulting in cholecystitis (Fig. 3.42).

Associations: Cholesterolosis, cholelithiasis.

Mimics: Other causes of gallbladder wall thickening, including cholecystitis and carcinoma.

Additional comments: MRI has been shown to be more accurate than CT or ultrasound for the diagnosis of adenomyomatosis of the gallbladder. HASTE sequences are particularly useful in this regard.

References: 49, 50

Cholecystitis (Acute) (Fig. 3.43)

Description: Inflammation of the gallbladder, usually caused by obstruction of the cystic duct.

T1: Signal intensity on non–contrast-enhanced images usually unremarkable.

T2: Pericholecystic fluid and edema manifest as increased signal intensity adjacent to the gallbladder. Edema may extend to the periportal regions. High signal intensity within

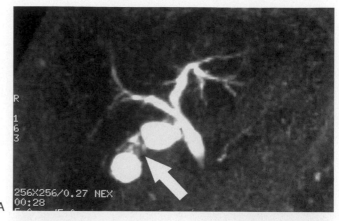

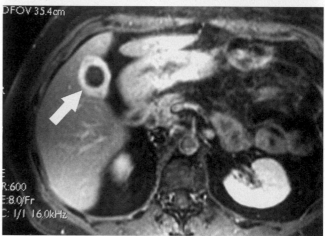

FIG. 3.42. Adenomyomatosis of gallbladder with acute cholecystitis. **A:** Coronal magnetic resonance cholangiopancreatography image demonstrates stenosing adenomyomatosis of the gallbladder (*arrow*) obstructing gallbladder fundus. **B:** Fat-suppressed, gadolinium-enhanced T1-weighted image of same patient as in **(A)** shows thickened, enhancing gallbladder fundus (*arrow*). Cholecystitis of gallbladder fundus was found at surgery.

the gallbladder wall may be seen as a result of intramural edema. Very bright intramural fluid collections may signify gallbladder wall necrosis.

Enhancement pattern: Markedly enhancing, thickened gallbladder wall. Mucosa typically enhances first. Early, transiently increased enhancement of adjacent liver may occur as a result of hyperemia.

Characteristic features: Uniformly thickened and enhancing gallbladder wall with surrounding edema or fluid. Gallstones usually present. With emphysematous cholecystitis, gas within the gallbladder wall or lumen is most conspicuous on T2*-weighted images.

Distribution: Diffuse mural involvement.

Atypical appearances: Stones absent in acalculous cholecystitis (severely ill patients). Hemorrhagic cholecystitis may demonstrate a complex thickened wall of variable signal intensity on T1- and T2-weighted images.

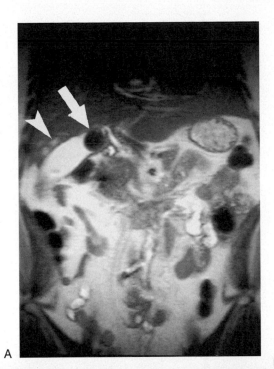

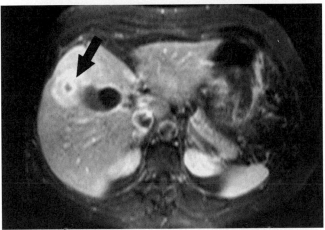

FIG. 3.43. Acute cholecystitis. **A:** Coronal HASTE image of patient with fever and right upper quadrant pain shows large stone (*arrow*) impacted in gallbladder neck. Note abnormal high signal foci in adjacent liver (*arrowhead*). **B:** Fat-suppressed T1-weighted image of liver demonstrates gallbladder wall enhancement and adjacent abnormal enhancement of liver (*arrow*). Pericholecystic abscess was found at surgery.

Associations: Cholelithiasis, cystic duct obstruction of any cause, interruption of blood supply via cystic artery (e.g., embolization). Most common in obese middle-aged women.

Mimics: Diffuse carcinoma and diffuse adenomyomatosis of the gallbladder can usually be distinguished from cholecystitis clinically, although these entities may coexist with cholecystitis (see Fig. 3.42). Gallbladder enhancement is usually less marked in other entities that cause gallbladder

wall thickening. Chronic cholecystitis results in fibrosis and relatively less mural enhancement. Xanthogranulomatous cholecystitis, hepatitis, cirrhosis, hypoalbuminemia, portal hypertension, acquired immunodeficiency syndrome cholangiopathy, and graft-versus-host disease are additional causes of gallbladder wall thickening. However, wall enhancement and transient hepatic enhancement in these entities are absent or decreased relative to acute cholecystitis.

References: 51, 52

Cholelithiasis (Fig. 3.44)

Description: Stones within the gallbladder consisting of variable amounts of cholesterol, calcium carbonate, and pigment (bilirubin).

T1: Stones have variable signal intensity from dark to bright.

T2: Variable, but most commonly dark relative to bile. May have central area of increased signal intensity.

Enhancement pattern: None.

Characteristic features: Stones may be round, faceted, or laminated and show no enhancement after intravenous contrast injection.

Distribution: Single or multiple. Usually layer dependently but may float when specific gravity of stone is lower than bile.

Atypical appearances: May contain gas.

Associations: Cholestasis, inflammatory bowel disease, hemolytic diseases (pigment stones), metabolic disorders, familial predisposition.

Mimics: Gallbladder polyp (contrast enhancement excludes a stone). Gallbladder air.

Additional comments: Normal bile within the gallbladder has variable signal intensity on MR images. MR appearance of gallstones may provide a clue to their composition.

References: 53

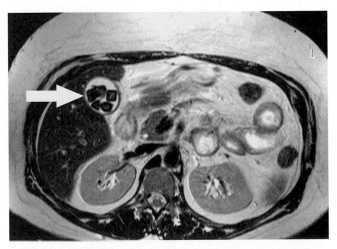

FIG. 3.44. Cholelithiasis. Multiple faceted stones are present within gallbladder (*arrow*) on respiratory-triggered T2-weighted image.

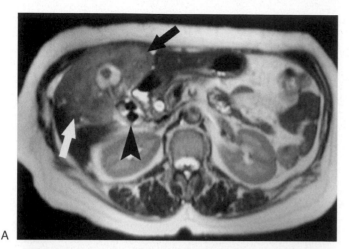

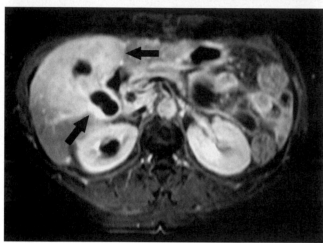

FIG. 3.45. Gallbladder carcinoma. **A:** Axial T2-weighted image shows large mass (*arrows*) originating from stone-filled gallbladder (*arrowhead*) and invading adjacent liver. **B:** Fat-suppressed, gadolinium-enhanced T1-weighted image shows enhancement of gallbladder and mass (*arrows*).

Gallbladder Carcinoma (Fig. 3.45)

Description: Malignant tumor of gallbladder origin, most commonly scirrhous adenocarcinoma.

T1: Intermediate signal intensity. Invasive tumor appears hypointense to liver.

T2: Hypointense to bile, hyperintense to liver.

Enhancement pattern: Heterogeneous early enhancement that persists on later images.

Characteristic features: Gallbladder wall thickening greater than 1 cm, a polyp greater than 2 cm, or a gallbladder mass that invades nearby structures suggest carcinoma. Direct extension into the adjacent liver is common.

Distribution: Most common in body and fundus of gallbladder. May appear as focal or diffuse thickening of the gallbladder or as a polypoid mass. Most common patterns of regional spread are direct liver invasion, lymph node metastases, and bile duct invasion. Omental or peritoneal metastases occur but may be difficult to detect.

Atypical appearances: Complete replacement of gallbladder by carcinoma.

Associations: Gallstones, chronic cholecystitis, ulcerative colitis, porcelain gallbladder.

Mimics: Acute or chronic cholecystitis (may coexist with carcinoma), xanthogranulomatous cholecystitis, gallbladder involvement by tumors not of biliary origin, adenomyomatosis.

References: 54, 55

SPLEEN

Cyst (Fig. 3.46)

Description: Splenic cysts include true (developmental) cysts, pseudocysts, and hydatid cysts. True cysts are epithelial lined. Pseudocysts are posttraumatic or postinflammatory in nature and are far more common.

T1: Low signal intensity unless associated with hemorrhage.

T2: Very high signal intensity.

Enhancement pattern: Nonenhancing.

Characteristic features: Similar to cysts occurring in the liver. Most often unilocular.

Distribution: Usually solitary, but multiple cysts may occur.

Atypical appearances: May appear multilocular or septated.

Associations: History of trauma or inflammation.

References: 56

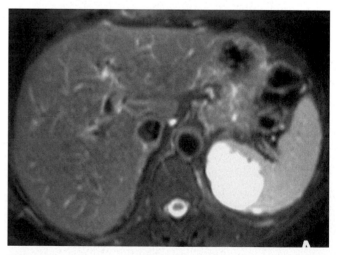

FIG. 3.46. Splenic cyst. Very high signal intensity lesion in medial spleen that showed no enhancement with contrast (not shown). This likely represents a pseudocyst rather than a true cyst.

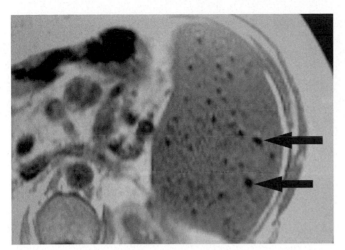

FIG. 3.47. Gamna-Gandy bodies. T1-weighted in-phase gradient echo image of the spleen in patient with cirrhosis and portal hypertension shows multiple dark (siderotic) nodules (*arrows*) within the spleen.

Gamna-Gandy Bodies (Fig. 3.47)

Description: Siderotic foci within the spleen.

T1: Very low signal intensity. Lesions become more conspicuous on gradient echo images with increasing echo time (blooming effect).

T2: Very low signal intensity.

Enhancement pattern: Nonenhancing.

Characteristic features: Multiple subcentimeter foci of very low signal intensity commonly seen in the setting of cirrhosis and chronic portal hypertension.

Distribution: Multiple, diffuse.

Associations: Cirrhosis and chronic portal hypertension.

Mimics: Calcified granulomas.

References: 57, 58

Hamartoma, Splenic (Fig. 3.48)

Description: Benign splenic mass consisting of disorganized splenic tissue.

T1: Mildly hypointense to isointense compared with spleen.

T2: Isointense to mildly hyperintense compared with spleen.

Enhancement pattern: Enhances early, diffusely, and somewhat heterogeneously and becomes more homogeneous with time. Enhancement may persist. May exhibit central area of nonenhancement.

Characteristic features: An incidentally found, solitary, well-circumscribed and spherical lesion that is only mildly or moderately different in signal intensity from spleen on all pulse sequences suggests the diagnosis.

Distribution: Usually solitary. Occurs anywhere in the spleen.

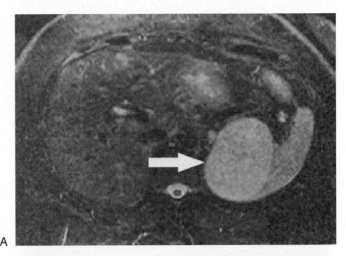

A

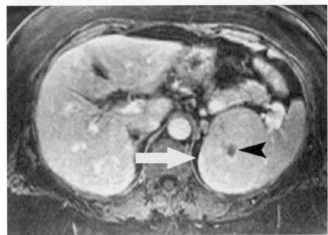

B

FIG. 3.48. Splenic hamartoma. **A:** Fat-suppressed T2-weighted image demonstrates mass (*arrow*) arising from and slightly hyperintense to spleen. **B:** Fat-suppressed, gadolinium-enhanced T1-weighted gradient echo image shows mass (*arrow*) to enhance similarly to spleen. Note central scar (*arrowhead*).

Atypical appearances: May appear as a low signal intensity mass on T2-weighted images.

Mimics: Solitary mass of lymphoma, sarcoma.

References: 59

Hemangioma, Splenic (Fig. 3.49)

Description: Benign vascular neoplasm similar to hemangioma of the liver. Most common benign splenic tumor.

T1: Hypointense to isointense relative to spleen.

T2: Hyperintense relative to spleen. Contrast between hemangioma and normal spleen not as striking as with liver hemangiomas due to relatively high signal intensity of normal splenic tissue.

Enhancement pattern: Spectrum of enhancement similar to hepatic hemangiomas, but peripheral nodularity may not be as well-defined.

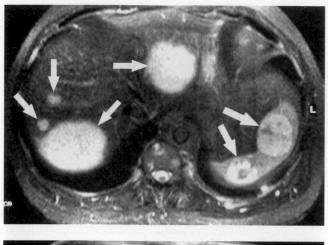

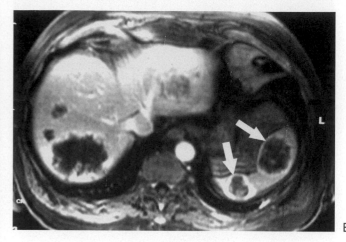

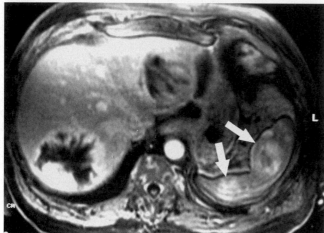

FIG. 3.49. Splenic hemangiomas in patient with blue rubber bleb nevus syndrome. **A:** Fat-suppressed T2-weighted image shows multiple high signal intensity masses (*arrows*) in liver and spleen. Early **(B)** and delayed **(C)** images from fat-suppressed, dynamic gadolinium-enhanced sequence show progressive enhancement of liver and splenic (*arrows*) lesions.

Characteristic features: Similar to hepatic hemangiomas.

Distribution: Solitary or multiple. Anywhere in the spleen.

Atypical appearances: May have central scar of lower signal intensity on T2-weighted images that enhances weakly after gadolinium administration. Sclerosing hemangioma may have relatively low signal intensity on T2-weighted images.

Mimics: Angiosarcoma.

References: 59

Infarct, Splenic (Fig. 3.50)

Description: Devitalized splenic tissue, most commonly the result of interruption of the blood supply related to trauma, thrombosis, or embolization of the splenic artery or one of its branches.

T1: Variable depending on the presence or absence of associated hemorrhage.

T2: Often increased in signal intensity.

Enhancement pattern: Areas of infarction do not enhance. Often, splenic capsular enhancement is present at the periphery of the infarct.

Characteristic features: Wedge-shaped, subcapsular, nonenhancing lesions with enhancement of the adjacent splenic capsule.

Distribution: Subcapsular. Frequently multiple but may be solitary.

Associations: Embolic disease, vasculitis, recent surgery or intervention.

Mimics: Septic emboli.

Lymphoma, Splenic

Description: Malignant tumor of lymphocytes (Hodgkin or non-Hodgkin). Most common malignant lesion of the spleen.

T1: Frequently isointense.

T2: Frequently isointense. Focal or multifocal disease may appear as low signal intensity nodules.

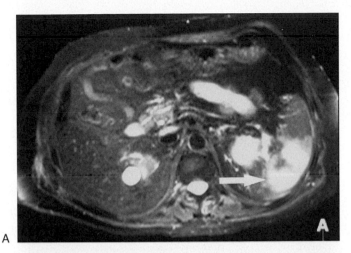

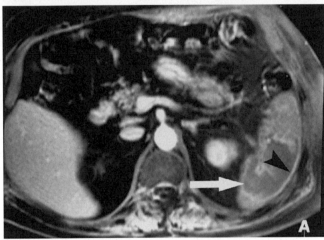

FIG. 3.50. Splenic infarct. **A:** Fat-suppressed T2-weighted image shows large high signal intensity region (*arrow*) in spleen. **B:** Fat-suppressed T1-weighted image following administration of intravenous gadolinium shows diminished enhancement of infarcted tissue (*arrow*). Note capsular enhancement is present (*arrowhead*).

Enhancement pattern: Focal lesions may appear hypointense on early contrast-enhanced images. Lesions tend to match surrounding splenic parenchyma on later images.

Characteristic features: Splenomegaly and lymphadenopathy are common but may be absent in some cases. Lymphoma tends to be inconspicuous on unenhanced images.

Distribution: Diffuse involvement is common and may be difficult to detect. Multifocal disease may be easier to detect but is relatively uncommon.

Atypical appearances: Solitary mass.

Mimics: Metastases may simulate lymphoma, although lymphoma tends to be lower in signal intensity on T2-weighted images. Other causes of splenomegaly and lymphadenopathy (e.g., sarcoidosis, human immunodeficiency virus) may mimic lymphoma.

Additional comments: Superparamagnetic iron oxide particles are not taken up by lymphoma, causing focal lesions

to appear brighter than the normal spleen on ferumoxides-enhanced images. After treatment, lesions may become hypointense on T1- and T2-weighted images and may enhance weakly.

References: 60

Lymphangioma, Splenic

Description: A focal collection of dilated lymphatic channels.

T1: Low signal intensity.

T2: Very high signal intensity.

Enhancement pattern: Bulk of lesion is nonenhancing. Septations may enhance.

Characteristic features: Multilocular lesions with signal characteristics closely resembling those of a cyst.

Distribution: No specific distribution. Often multiple.

Atypical appearances: Some areas of high signal intensity may be present on T1-weighted images, representing proteinaceous fluid or blood products.

Mimics: Cyst.

References: 56, 61

Metastasis, Splenic

Description: Hematogenous spread of extrasplenic malignant tumor to the spleen. Most splenic metastases originate from breast cancer, lung cancer, or melanoma. In general, splenic metastases are rare, and the primary tumor is usually widely disseminated by the time splenic involvement is detected.

T1: Metastases tend to have similar signal intensity to spleen on T1-weighted images. Melanin-containing melanoma metastases may be relatively hyperintense to spleen as a result of the paramagnetic qualities of melanin.

T2: Metastases are often similar to spleen in signal intensity.

Enhancement pattern: Dynamic, contrast-enhanced imaging improves conspicuity of splenic metastases over noncontrast images. Lesions may enhance more or less than the surrounding splenic parenchyma at various time points after injection.

Characteristic features: Metastases to the spleen usually occur in the setting of a widely disseminated primary tumor.

Distribution: Occur throughout the spleen. Frequently multiple.

Mimics: Lymphomatous involvement of the spleen.

Additional comments: Metastases may be more conspicuous after superparamagnetic iron oxide administration. Because splenic metastases often occur in the setting of widespread metastatic disease elsewhere, the detection of splenic metastases is rarely critical.

References: 62, 63

Sarcoma, Splenic (Fig. 3.51)

Description: Aggressive primary splenic malignant tumor. Although rare compared with other splenic lesions,

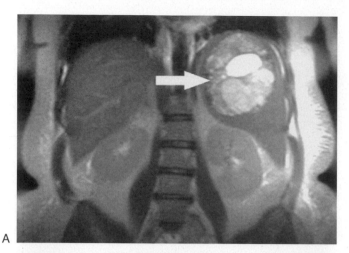

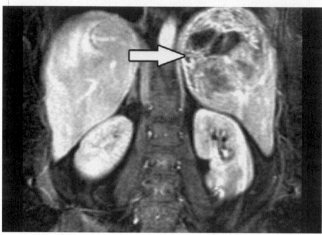

FIG. 3.51. Splenic sarcoma. **A:** Coronal HASTE image of spleen shows large heterogeneous high signal intensity mass (*arrow*). **B:** Coronal fat-suppressed, gadolinium-enhanced T1-weighted image shows heterogeneous enhancement of mass (*arrow*)

Associations: Thorotrast exposure.

Mimics: Splenic metastases, lymphoma.

Additional comments: Spontaneous rupture may occur.

References: 64 to 67

PANCREAS

Acute Pancreatitis (Figs. 3.52, 3.53; see Fig. 3.160)

Description: Acute inflammation of the pancreas due to a variety of causes.

T1: Normal signal intensity in uncomplicated acute pancreatitis. May become heterogeneous and lower in signal intensity as inflammation becomes more severe. Areas of pancreatic necrosis and uncomplicated peripancreatic fluid collections appear dark. Hemorrhagic fluid collections have increased signal intensity.

T2: Early inflammatory changes are best demonstrated on fat-suppressed images. Peripancreatic inflammation and fluid are of very high signal intensity. The pancreatic duct may be narrowed due to surrounding inflammation.

Enhancement pattern: The pancreas enhances normally in mild cases, although early enhancement may be diminished as inflammation becomes more severe. Heterogeneous enhancement with areas of nonenhancing necrosis occurs in more severe cases.

Characteristic features: Enlargement of the pancreas with peripancreatic edema or fluid. Gallstones or pancreatic duct anomalies may be noted.

Distribution: Most commonly involves entire organ, although focal pancreatitis can occur.

Associations: Ethanol abuse, gallstones, pancreatic duct anomalies, hereditary pancreatitis, metabolic disorders, viral agents, trauma, medications. Pancreatic inflammation may occur as a result of adenocarcinoma.

angiosarcoma is the most common primary splenic malignant tumor.

T1: Often low signal intensity relative to spleen due to iron accumulation. Hemorrhagic areas may demonstrate increased signal intensity.

T2: Often low signal intensity relative to spleen due to iron accumulation. Necrotic areas may show increased signal intensity.

Enhancement pattern: Typically hypervascular with heterogeneous enhancement due to presence of necrosis and hemorrhage.

Characteristic features: Hemorrhage, necrosis, and hemosiderin deposits often present.

Distribution: May appear as solitary splenic mass, multiple masses, or diffuse enlargement or replacement of spleen. Metastases are common. Liver represents most common site of metastatic disease.

Atypical appearances: May calcify.

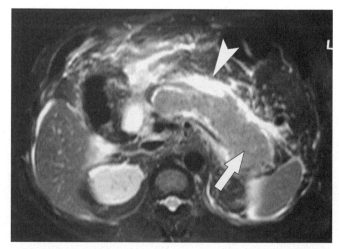

FIG. 3.52. Acute pancreatitis. Fat-suppressed T2-weighted image demonstrates enlargement and edema of pancreatic body and tail (*arrow*) with peripancreatic fluid (*arrowhead*).

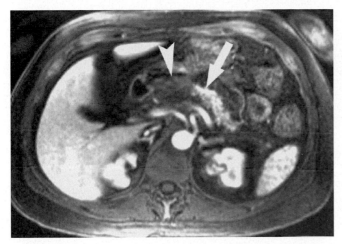

FIG. 3.53. Pancreatic necrosis secondary to acute pancreatitis. Fat-suppressed, gadolinium-enhanced gradient echo image of patient with acute pancreatitis shows abrupt transition between enhancing viable pancreatic parenchyma (*arrow*) and necrotic pancreatic tissue (*arrowhead*).

Mimics: Autoimmune pancreatitis (Fig. 3.54). Pancreatic adenocarcinoma may mimic pancreatitis, although acute pancreatitis does not typically encase vessels or cause dilatation of the pancreatic duct. Pancreatitis may coexist with adenocarcinoma.

Additional comments: The diagnosis of acute pancreatitis is often known or suspected before imaging due to typical presentation of severe midepigastric pain and elevated pancreatic amylase and lipase. Imaging is most useful for determining underlying causes, assessing severity, and detecting complications. In contrast to chronic pancreatitis and pancreatic cancer, the pancreatic duct is typically smooth and of normal caliber in the setting of acute pancreatitis. However, compression of the duct by adjacent inflammation and edema may occur. MRCP may demonstrate widening of the duodenal c-loop and duodenal fold thickening. High signal intensity peripancreatic fluid collections are clearly depicted on heavily T2-weighted images and, when extensive, may interfere with visualization of ductal structures.

References: 68, 69

Adenocarcinoma of the Pancreas (Fig. 3.55; see Figs. 2.43, 4.17)

Description: Malignant tumor of pancreatic ductal origin. Tends to be scirrhous and infiltrative. Most patients have advanced local disease at the time of diagnosis.

T1: Low signal intensity relative to pancreas. Fat-suppressed T1-weighted images often demonstrate the lesion well.

T2: Isointense to slightly hyperintense relative to normal pancreas.

Enhancement pattern: Enhances less than pancreatic parenchyma on early post-gadolinium images. Typically en-

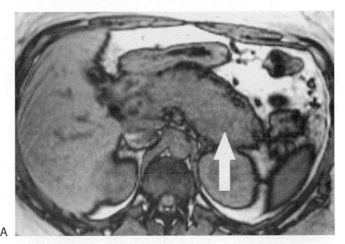

A

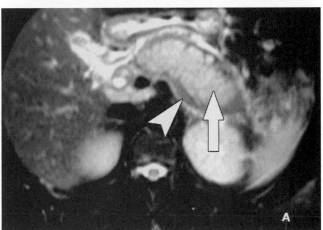

B

FIG. 3.54. Autoimmune pancreatitis. T1-weighted gradient echo (**A**) and fat-suppressed T2-weighted (**B**) images of the abdomen show diffuse enlargement of the pancreas (*arrows*) with low-signal intensity rim (*arrowhead*) on T2-weighted image. Appearance of pancreas returned to normal following steroid therapy (not shown).

hances gradually to become isointense or even hyperintense to normal pancreas on delayed postcontrast images. Large lesions may have central necrosis with little or no enhancement. Enhancement characteristics may overlap with those of chronic pancreatitis.

Characteristic features: Pancreatic adenocarcinoma is typically low signal intensity relative to normal pancreas on T1-weighted images and demonstrates delayed enhancement following gadolinium administration. Obstruction of the common bile duct and pancreatic duct produces the classic double duct sign, although isolated dilatation of the pancreatic duct occurs with tumor of the pancreatic body or tail. Tumor often encases, invades, and obstructs vessels.

Distribution: Most common in the pancreatic head (roughly two thirds) and least common in the pancreatic tail.

Atypical appearances: May present as an infiltrating perivascular abnormality or as obstruction of the pancreatic duct without a detectable mass within the pancreas. Dilatation

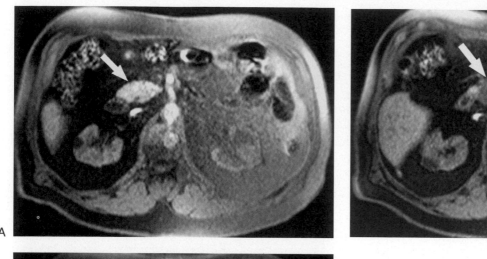

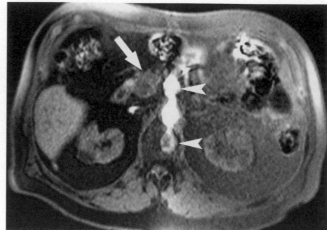

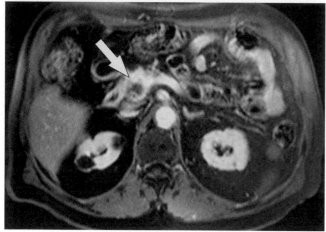

FIG. 3.55. Adenocarcinoma of pancreas. **A:** Fat-suppressed T1-weighted gradient echo image shows normal signal intensity of pancreatic head (*arrow*). **B:** Image from same sequence a few slices cephalad to **(A)** shows mass (*arrow*) in region of pancreatic neck with lower signal intensity than normal pancreas. Note phase ghosts from aorta (*arrowheads*). **C:** Fat-suppressed, gadolinium-enhanced gradient echo image shows heterogeneous enhancement of mass (*arrow*).

of the common bile duct can occur in the absence of pancreatic duct dilatation.

Mimics: Focal pancreatitis, metastasis, periampullary or ampullary carcinoma.

Additional comments: Tends to be infiltrating and locally invasive. Most common sites of spread include direct extension into peripancreatic tissues and metastases to the regional lymph nodes, liver, peritoneal surfaces, and lungs. MRI is usually performed to detect a pancreatic mass in a patient with suspicious signs or symptoms (e.g., painless jaundice) or to assess resectability in a patient with a known pancreatic tumor. MRI has been reported to have positive and negative predictive values for nonresectability of 90% and 83%, respectively. Acute or chronic pancreatitis often coexists with pancreatic cancer, making it difficult to accurately determine extent of disease. Preoperative assessment of pancreatic adenocarcinoma is discussed in more detail in Section 3.4.

References: 70

Chronic Pancreatitis (Fig. 3.56; see Fig. 3.167)

Description: Recurring or persistent inflammation of the pancreas resulting in irreversible parenchymal damage.

T1: Pancreatic parenchymal signal intensity is typically decreased due to fibrosis.

T2: Fluid-containing structures, such as pancreatic pseudocysts and dilated main and branch ducts, are well demonstrated as very high signal intensity structures. Pseudocysts containing proteinaceous or hemorrhagic debris may appear heterogeneous and less bright than simple cysts.

Enhancement pattern: Pancreatic parenchymal enhancement is typically diminished and tends to occur more gradually than normal. There is overlap between enhancement of inflammatory masses of chronic pancreatitis and adenocarcinoma.

Characteristic features: Pancreatic parenchymal atrophy, dilatation and strictures of the main pancreatic duct

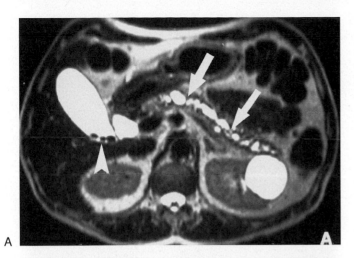

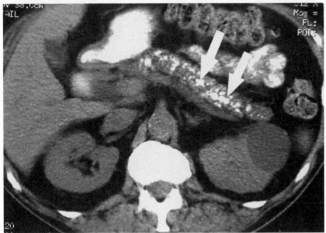

FIG. 3.56. Chronic pancreatitis. **A:** Heavily T2-weighted axial HASTE image through pancreatic body and tail clearly demonstrates parenchymal atrophy and dilated pancreatic duct (*arrows*) with multiple strictures. Note gallstones (*arrowhead*). **B:** Noncontrast computed tomography scan in same patient as **(A)** more clearly demonstrates pancreatic calcifications (*arrows*), but pancreatic duct is poorly seen.

with branch duct ectasia, and pancreatic duct stones are all characteristic. Pseudocysts or splenic vein thrombosis may be present. Pancreatic calcification, readily detected with CT, may be missed or underestimated with MRI.

Distribution: Usually diffuse, although focal pancreatic changes may occur and simulate pancreatic adenocarcinoma.

Atypical appearances: Obstruction of the common bile duct. Focal involvement simulating a pancreatic tumor. The presence of a capsule-like rim that is low signal intensity on T1- and T2-weighted images in the setting of a diffusely enlarged pancreas suggests autoimmune pancreatitis (see Fig. 3.54).

Associations: See acute pancreatitis. Autoimmune pancreatitis may be associated with autoimmune disorders such as Sjögren syndrome and a sclerosing cholangitis-like abnormality of the bile ducts.

Mimics: Intraductal papillary mucinous tumor (strictures of the pancreatic duct are not typical of intraductal papillary mucinous tumor [IPMT] and enhancing soft tissue nodules may be present), pancreatic adenocarcinoma with pancreatic duct obstruction (ductal adenocarcinoma typically causes abrupt cutoff of the pancreatic duct, whereas the pancreatic duct may be seen to penetrate an inflammatory mass).

References: 71 to 73

Intraductal Papillary Mucinous Tumor (Fig. 3.57; see Figs. 2.44, 2.45, 3.168)

Description: Papillomatous, mucin-producing tumor of the pancreas originating from duct epithelium. Generally low, but not insignificant, malignant potential.

T1: Most often, the solid components of the tumor are not well visualized. Occasionally, intermediate signal intensity tumor nodules are present.

T2: Mucin has a T2 value similar to simple fluid. Therefore, these lesions most commonly appear as very high signal intensity cystic masses or dilatations of the pancreatic duct.

Enhancement pattern: Intraductal mucin does not enhance, but the papillary nodules do demonstrate enhancement when present.

Characteristic features: Classic appearance of main duct type includes diffuse dilatation of the pancreatic duct with ectatic branch ducts and bulging ampulla. Also commonly appears as a unilocular or multilocular cystic-appearing lesion of the pancreas that communicates with a normal or dilated main pancreatic duct. May resemble a cluster of grapes.

Distribution: A simple classification system for IPMT divides this entity into a main duct type and a branch duct type, although features of both types may coexist in a single patient. The main duct type manifests as diffuse, or uncommonly focal, dilatation of the main pancreatic duct. The branch duct

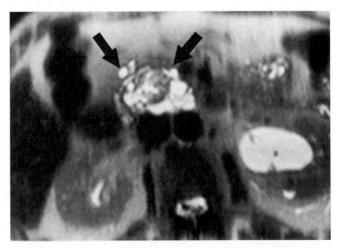

FIG. 3.57. Intraductal papillary mucinous tumor (IPMT). Axial HASTE image shows a large complex cystic mass (*arrows*) in region of pancreatic head.

type occurs most often in the uncinate process, although additional cystic dilatations of the branch ducts are commonly present elsewhere in the pancreas.

Atypical appearances: Rarely, malignant IPMT may obstruct the common bile duct, resulting in a double duct sign.

Associations: Association with familial adenomatous polyposis has been reported.

Mimics: IPMT may be difficult to distinguish from chronic pancreatitis, although the latter entity is typically associated with duct strictures and calcifications (calcifications may be difficult to appreciate with MRI). Chronic pancreatitis and IPMT may coexist in the same patient. Pancreatic adenocarcinoma typically demonstrates a pancreatic duct cutoff sign (as opposed to a bulging ampulla) and more commonly results in common bile duct obstruction. Unlike adenocarcinoma, parenchymal or extrapancreatic extension of an IPMT is rare. Branch duct IPMT may be difficult to distinguish from mucinous cystadenoma or cystadenocarcinoma, although the latter entities infrequently communicate with the pancreatic duct.

Additional comments: It is important to accurately distinguish these tumors from chronic pancreatitis and adenocarcinoma, because management of these entities differs significantly. Definitive diagnosis usually requires endoscopic retrograde cholangiopancreatography or surgery.

References: 74 to 76

Islet Cell Tumor (Fig. 3.58; see Fig. 3.164)

Description: Neuroendocrine tumor of the pancreas of islet cell origin. Tumors may be hormonally active or nonfunctioning. Nonfunctioning tumors tend to be larger at presentation, because symptoms are more likely to be the result of mass effect. The most common islet cell tumors in order of decreasing incidence are insulinomas, gastrinomas and nonfunctioning tumors. Most insulinomas are benign; slightly more than half of gastrinomas are malignant at presentation, and the vast majority of other islet cell tumors are malignant, often with metastases, at the time of diagnosis.

T1: Low signal intensity relative to pancreas.

T2: High signal intensity relative to pancreas.

Enhancement pattern: Early homogeneous or heterogeneous enhancement typical. Enhancement may be ringlike.

Characteristic features: Typically appears as a well-defined hypervascular mass of increased signal intensity on T2-weighted images. Pancreatic duct obstruction and vascular encasement are unusual.

Distribution: Most islet cell tumors occur as solitary pancreatic masses, but they may be multiple or occur in ectopic locations. Gastrinomas tend to occur between the porta hepatis and the second and third portions of the duodenum (gastrinoma triangle).

Atypical appearances: Tumors may be low signal intensity on T2-weighted images or high signal intensity on T1-weighted images. Pancreatic duct obstruction may occur. Tumors may be cystic or exhibit calcifications, features more

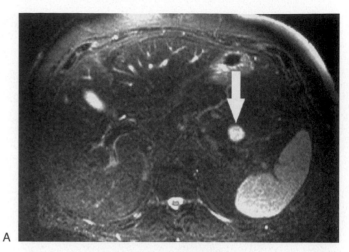

A

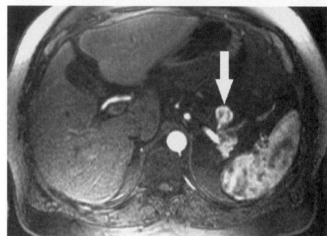

B

FIG. 3.58. Islet cell tumor. **A:** Fat-suppressed T2-weighted image shows small high signal intensity mass (*arrow*) involving tail of pancreas. **B:** Arterial phase fat-suppressed gradient echo image from dynamic examination reveals mass (*arrow*) to be hypervascular.

common with large nonfunctioning tumors. Large islet cell tumors may exhibit necrosis.

Associations: Multiple endocrine neoplasia syndrome (MEN I), von Hipple-Lindau disease.

Mimics: Renal cell carcinoma metastasis to pancreas.

Additional comments: Gastrinomas may present as Zollinger-Ellison syndrome with hypertrophic gastropathy and postbulbar duodenal ulcers (Fig. 3.127). Thickening of the gastric rugae and duodenum may be evident on MR images.

References: 77 to 79

Mucinous Cystadenoma and Cystadenocarcinoma (Macrocystic Adenoma, Mucinous Cystic Neoplasm) (Fig. 3.59)

Description: Mucinous cystic neoplasm of the pancreas that ranges from benign to malignant. Benign cystadenomas are considered premalignant.

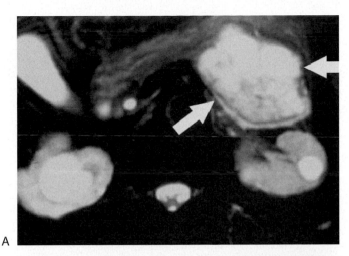

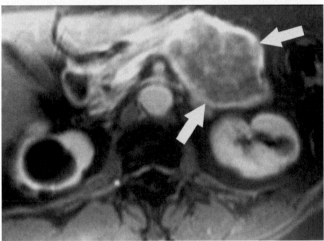

FIG. 3.59. Mucinous cystadenoma. **A:** Axial, heavily T2-weighted, fat-suppressed image demonstrates a complex cystic mass (*arrows*) in tail of pancreas. **B:** Fat-suppressed, gadolinium-enhanced gradient echo image shows faint enhancement of internal architecture of mass (*arrows*).

T1: Low to high signal intensity, depending on fluid content.

T2: Very high signal intensity.

Enhancement pattern: Enhancing septations.

Characteristic features: A unilocular or multilocular macrocystic (cysts > 2 cm) pancreatic lesion in the tail of the pancreas in a middle-aged woman is classic but not specific. There is typically no communication with the pancreatic duct. Mural soft tissue nodules or papillary excrescences and invasion of adjacent structures suggest malignancy.

Distribution: Usually arise from the pancreatic body and tail. Typically solitary.

Atypical appearances: Rarely may communicate with pancreatic duct, likely a result of fistula formation.

Mimics: Pancreatic pseudocyst, atypical serous cystadenoma, IPMT (communicates with pancreatic duct), ductal adenocarcinoma with markedly dilated pancreatic duct, solid and papillary epithelial neoplasm, other cystic lesions of the pancreas.

Additional comments: Females much more commonly affected. Most occur in patients 40 to 60 years old. Mucinous cystadenomas contain ovarian-type stroma. Elevated serum CA 19-9 is concerning for malignancy. Tumors are rarely hormonally active.

References: 80, 81

Pseudocyst (Fig. 3.60)

Description: A cystic-appearing collection of pancreatic secretions with a fibrous wall, usually resulting from pancreatitis or trauma.

T1: Low signal intensity unless complicated by hemorrhage or infection.

T2: Typically high signal intensity. Debris may be evident as low signal intensity filling defects.

Enhancement pattern: Nonenhancing internal components. Variable rim enhancement.

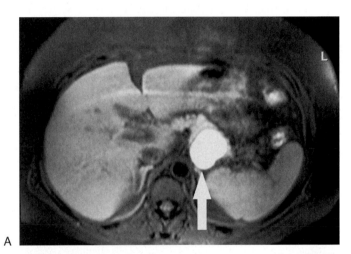

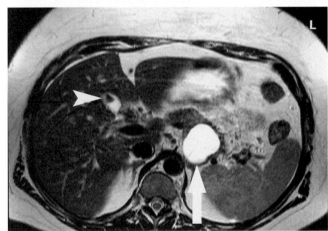

FIG. 3.60. Pancreatic pseudocyst. **A:** Fat-suppressed, non–contrast-enhanced T1-weighted image shows high signal intensity collection (*arrow*) near tail of pancreas consistent with fluid containing blood products. **B:** Respiratory triggered T2-weighted image shows collection (*arrow*) to be very high signal intensity. Note gallstone (*arrowhead*). Hemorrhagic pseudocyst found at surgery.

Characteristic features: Well-defined cystic pancreatic or peripancreatic collection without enhancing soft tissue elements. A history of pancreatitis is usually, but not always, elicited. Communication with the pancreatic duct may be evident.

Distribution: May occur anywhere in the pancreas or peripancreatic tissues. Pseudocysts may occur remote from the pancreas, in sites such as the pelvis or mediastinum, as a result of pancreatic secretions dissecting along tissue planes. Pseudocysts may also involve solid organs such as the liver and spleen.

Atypical appearances: Septations are unusual but may occur.

Associations: Pancreatitis, pancreatic trauma.

Mimics: Cystic lesions of the pancreas, including branch duct IPMT, mucinous cystic tumor, epithelial cyst, and duodenal diverticulum.

Serous Cystadenoma (Microcystic Adenoma) (Fig. 3.61; see Fig. 3.163)

Description: Benign microcystic pancreatic tumor with glycogen-rich cyst fluid and no malignant potential.

T1: Low signal intensity.

T2: Very high signal intensity.

Enhancement pattern: Septations and central scar may enhance.

Characteristic features: Lobulated mass consisting of multiple small cysts. Cysts range from microscopic (too small to be resolved on imaging studies) to 2 cm in diameter. Stellate central scar may be present and may contain calcifications (better appreciated with CT).

Distribution: Occur throughout the pancreas but are more common in the pancreatic head and body. Solitary.

Atypical appearances: Cysts larger than 1 cm (macrocystic variant), unilocular appearance. Pancreatic duct may rarely be obstructed.

Associations: Von Hippel-Lindau disease.

Mimics: Mucinous cystic tumors may overlap in appearance with macrocystic serous cystadenomas. Other cystic lesions of the pancreas should be included in the differential diagnosis when characteristic features of serous cystadenoma are lacking.

Additional comments: Tend to occur in older women (age older than 60 years).

References: 82

Solid and Papillary Epithelial Neoplasm (Cystic and Papillary Epithelial Neoplasm) (Fig. 3.62)

Description: Pancreatic mass of low-grade malignant potential.

T1: Variable signal intensity. High signal intensity areas may be present due to hemorrhage.

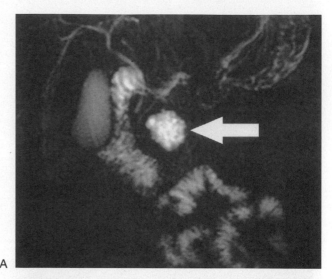

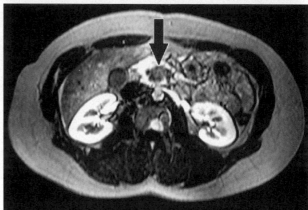

FIG. 3.61. Serous cystadenoma of pancreas. A: Thick slab magnetic resonance cholangiopancreatography image demonstrates high signal intensity lesion (*arrow*) in region of pancreatic head and uncinate process consisting of multiple tiny cysts. B: Arterial phase image from dynamic gadolinium-enhanced gradient echo sequence shows low signal intensity mass in head and uncinate process of pancreas with faint enhancement of internal septations.

T2: Heterogeneous with high signal intensity cystic areas.

Enhancement pattern: Solid components enhance, predominantly peripherally.

Characteristic features: Well-encapsulated solid and cystic mass. Cystic areas may contain blood products and fluid-debris levels.

Distribution: Solitary with some preference for pancreatic tail.

Mimics: Microcystic adenoma, mucinous cystic neoplasm, IPMT, nonfunctioning islet cell tumor, complex pancreatic pseudocyst, other unusual pancreatic masses.

Additional comments: Most common in young women. These tumors rarely metastasize and are typically cured by surgical excision.

References: 83

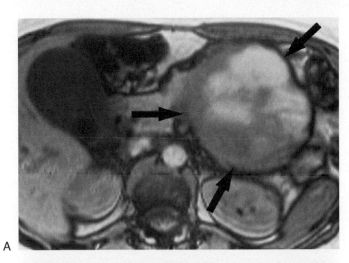

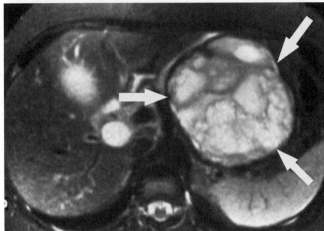

FIG. 3.62. Solid and papillary epithelial neoplasm. **A:** T1-weighted gradient echo image shows large mass in tail of pancreas (*arrows*) with areas of high signal intensity corresponding to hemorrhage. **B:** Fat-suppressed T2-weighted image shows heterogeneous mass (*arrows*) with multiple cystic areas.

ADRENALS

Adrenal Adenoma (Fig. 3.63)

Description: Benign tumor of the adrenal cortex. Most common adrenal mass. May be non-hyperfunctioning or hyperfunctioning.

T1: Variable signal intensity but usually of homogeneous intermediate signal intensity on in-phase gradient echo images.

T2: Variable signal intensity but usually of intermediate to moderately high signal intensity on fat-suppressed images.

Enhancement pattern: Homogeneous rapid enhancement with rapid washout.

Characteristic features: Signal loss on opposed-phase T1-weighted gradient echo images. A signal intensity loss of at least 20% relative to the signal on in-phase images should be present to diagnose adenoma.

Distribution: Usually solitary but may be multiple and bilateral.

Atypical appearances: Heterogeneous signal intensity, representing cystic change or hemorrhage, may be present on precontrast images (see Fig. 4.15). May demonstrate heterogeneous enhancement. Lipid-poor adenomas may demonstrate little or no signal loss on opposed-phase images. Rarely, a metastatic lesion may coexist with an adrenal adenoma (collision tumor) and manifest as a focal area that does not change in signal intensity with in-phase and opposed-phase imaging (see Fig 4.16).

Associations: Conn's syndrome (aldosteronoma), Cushing's syndrome, virilism.

Mimics: Metastases may mimic lipid-poor adenoma. Very rarcly, a lipid-rich metastasis, such as from renal cell (clear cell) carcinoma, may demonstrate signal loss on opposed-phase images.

Additional comments: When trying to determine whether an adrenal mass loses signal between in-phase and opposed-phase images, it is best to compare the adrenal mass with an internal standard of reference. The liver is a poor choice, because it is susceptible to fatty infiltration. It may be helpful to determine whether the mass parallels the signal intensity of bone marrow, which also contains fat and water, or loses signal relative to the spleen or renal cortex, which should not contain intracytoplasmic lipid. If using the spleen or renal cortex as a reference, be certain they do not contain excess iron.

References: 84 to 87

Adrenal Cortical Carcinoma

Description: Rare malignant neoplasm of the adrenal cortex.

T1: Heterogeneous with hyperintense areas (hemorrhage).

T2: Heterogeneous with hyperintense areas (necrosis).

Enhancement pattern: Nonnecrotic portions of the tumor enhance with gadolinium. Peripheral enhancing nodules have been described.

Characteristic features: Tumors tend to be large at diagnosis, with areas of necrosis and hemorrhage. IVC invasion may be present. Intracytoplasmic lipid may be present, resulting in signal loss on opposed-phase gradient echo images.

Distribution: Unilateral, solitary.

Atypical appearances: Rarely, well-differentiated tumor may have benign imaging characteristics similar to adrenal adenoma.

Mimics: Adrenal hemangioma, neuroblastoma, metastasis, degenerated adrenal adenoma.

Additional comments: May be hyperfunctioning in up to 50% of cases.

References: 88

Cyst or Pseudocyst (Fig. 3.64)

Description: Cystic lesion of the adrenal gland that may be endothelial, parasitic, epithelial, or a pseudocyst resulting from hemorrhage.

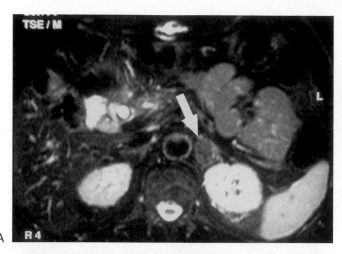
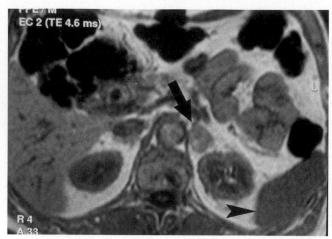
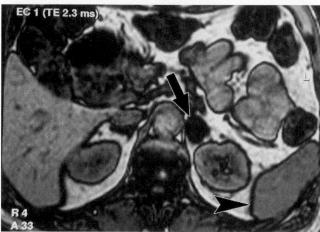

FIG. 3.63. Adrenal adenoma. **A:** Fat-suppressed T2-weighted image shows intermediate signal intensity left adrenal mass (*arrow*). **B:** In-phase T1-weighted gradient echo image shows mass (*arrow*) to be slightly higher in signal intensity than spleen (*arrowhead*). **C:** Opposed-phase gradient echo image shows adrenal mass (*arrow*) to now be significantly lower in signal intensity than spleen (*arrowhead*).

T1: Low signal intensity (unless complicated by hemorrhage or infection).

T2: Very high signal intensity.

Enhancement pattern: Nonenhancing.

Characteristic features: Well demarcated, nonenhancing lesion that follows signal intensity of water on all sequences. Hydatid cyst may show septations or separated membrane (water lily sign). Septations may also be present in lymphangiomatous cysts and pseudocysts.

Distribution: Usually solitary.

Atypical appearances: The presence of blood products may result in increased signal intensity on T1-weighted and decreased signal intensity on T2-weighted images. Thin septations may be present. Punctate or rim calcification may be present but difficult to appreciate on MRI.

Associations: History of adrenal hemorrhage or trauma.

Mimics: Cystic pheochromocytoma, necrotic tumor.

References: 89

Hemangioma

Description: These benign vascular tumors, although common in the liver and spleen, very rarely affect the adrenal glands.

T1: Low signal intensity.

T2: High signal intensity.

Enhancement pattern: Peripheral enhancement. Center may not enhance because of necrosis or fibrosis.

Characteristic features: Peripheral nodular enhancement with incomplete centripetal filling is helpful when present. Phleboliths may be seen with CT.

Distribution: Unilateral, solitary.

Atypical appearances: centripetal enhancement may be absent.

Mimics: Pheochromocytoma also may demonstrate very high signal intensity on T2-weighted images and is much more common. Other necrotic tumors, both benign and malignant, may have a similar appearance.

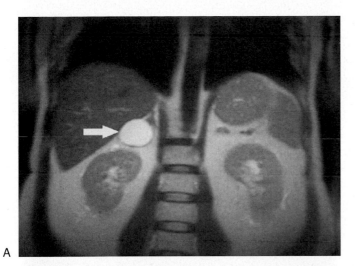

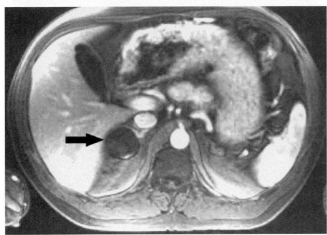

FIG. 3.64. Adrenal cyst. **A:** Coronal HASTE image shows round high signal intensity adrenal cyst (*arrow*). **B:** Fat-suppressed, gadolinium-enhanced, three-dimensional gradient echo image demonstrates no enhancement of cyst (*arrow*).

Additional comments: Surgical removal is typically recommended because of difficulty in distinguishing hemangiomas from malignant adrenal lesions.

References: 89, 90

Metastasis (Fig. 3.65)

Description: Malignant tumor of extraadrenal origin. Most common primary sites include lung, breast, kidney, skin (melanoma), and gastrointestinal tract. Although few incidentally discovered adrenal masses are metastases, adrenal metastases are relatively common in the setting of a known malignant tumor elsewhere.

T1: Variable, but often intermediate, signal intensity (if not cystic or hemorrhagic).

T2: Metastases tend to be moderately high in signal intensity, but considerable overlap exists with other entities, both malignant and benign. Therefore, signal intensity on T2-weighted images should not be relied upon to diagnose adrenal metastases.

Enhancement pattern: Often heterogeneous with progressive filling from the periphery. As opposed to adenomas, metastases tend to retain contrast or washout only mildly on delayed images.

Characteristic features: With very rare exceptions, metastases do not lose signal on opposed-phase gradient echo images.

Distribution: Frequently bilateral but may be unilateral.

Atypical appearances: May occur in an adrenal gland already occupied by an adenoma (collision tumor). Very rarely, metastasis from a lipid-containing tumor (e.g., clear cell carcinoma) may lose signal on an opposed-phase image.

Associations: Primary malignant tumor elsewhere.

Mimics: Adrenal cortical carcinoma, pheochromocytoma, atypical adrenal adenoma, adrenal hemangioma.

References: 86, 91

Myelolipoma (Fig. 3.66)

Description: Benign tumor containing both adipose tissue and hematopoietic elements.

T1: Fat-containing elements are bright on non–fat-suppressed images and suppress with application of fat suppression. Focal areas of hematopoietic tissue remain intermediate in signal intensity before and after application of fat suppression.

T2: Fatty elements parallel the signal intensity of retroperitoneal fat. The presence of hematopoietic tissue may complicate the appearance.

Enhancement pattern: Fatty elements fail to show significant enhancement. Rim of enhancing normal adrenal tissue may be present. Myeloid elements may be evident as foci of enhancement.

Characteristic features: Round, well-marginated, predominantly nonenhancing mass with elements that parallel retroperitoneal fat on all sequences. Most often does not lose signal on opposed-phase images due to insufficient water content. Nonfatty foci of myeloid tissue may be present.

Distribution: Most often unilateral and solitary but may rarely be bilateral. Extraadrenal myelolipoma may occur.

Atypical appearances: May spontaneously hemorrhage, resulting in presence of blood products. Some lesions may contain very little fat. May lose signal on opposed-phase images, simulating the appearance of an adenoma. Myelolipoma may rarely coexist with other adrenal lesions.

Mimics: Liposarcoma.

Additional comments: Retroperitoneal hemorrhage may occur from myelolipoma.

References: 92

Neuroblastoma, Ganglioneuroblastoma, Ganglioneuroma

Description: Tumors of neural crest origin ranging from benign (ganglioneuroma) to malignant (neuroblastoma).

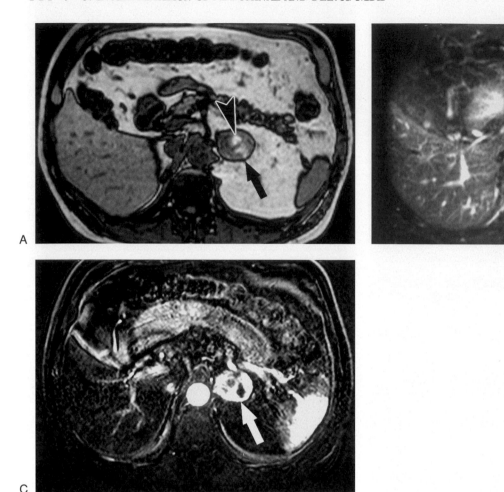

FIG. 3.65. Adrenal metastasis (renal cell carcinoma). **A:** Opposed-phase gradient echo image shows heterogeneous left adrenal mass (*arrow*) with foci of hemorrhage (*arrowhead*). Appearance not significantly different from in-phase image (not shown). **B:** Adrenal mass (*arrow*) has very high signal intensity on fat-suppressed T2-weighted image although this is nonspecific. **C:** Mass (*arrow*) demonstrates significant heterogeneous enhancement on digital subtraction gadolinium-enhanced three-dimensional gradient echo image.

Ganglioneuroblastoma has intermediate differentiation and malignant potential between neuroblastoma and ganglioneuroma.

T1: Low to intermediate signal intensity.

T2: Heterogeneous intermediate to high signal intensity. Higher signal intensity tends to correlate with myxoid stroma. Curvilinear bands of low signal intensity (Schwann cells and collagen fibers) may be seen in ganglioneuroma on T2-weighted images.

Enhancement pattern: Heterogeneous, gradually increasing enhancement.

Characteristic features: These tumors tend to be large at presentation. Ganglioneuromas are well-circumscribed masses, which may surround vessels without compromising the lumen. Neuroblastoma tends to be more irregularly shaped with areas of necrosis and hemorrhage, and may ex-

tend across midline, invade adjacent organs, or encase vessels.

Distribution: Adrenal or extraadrenal. Extraadrenal tumors occur along the paravertebral sympathetic chain. Incidence of extraadrenal tumors increases with age. Neuroblastoma tends to metastasize to bone, liver, lymph nodes, and skin.

Mimics: Adrenal cortical carcinoma.

Additional comments: Neuroblastoma and ganglioneuroblastoma are rare in adults.

References: 93, 94

Pheochromocytoma (Fig. 3.67)

Description: Paraganglioma arising from the adrenal medulla.

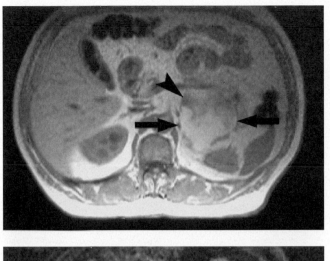

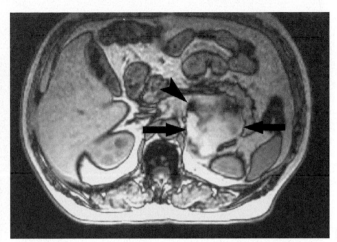

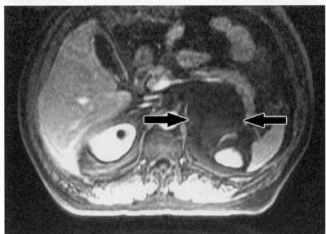

FIG. 3.66. Adrenal myelolipoma. In-phase **(A)** and opposed-phase **(B)** gradient echo images of left adrenal mass (*arrows*) show signal intensity of majority of mass to match that of subcutaneous fat. Lower signal intensity foci (*arrowheads*) within mass represent myeloid elements (note signal loss on opposed-phase image **(B)** due to myeloid elements mixed with fat). **C:** Fat-suppressed, gadolinium-enhanced T1-weighted image demonstrates uniform suppression of mass (*arrows*) with no evidence of enhancement. Note that anterior portion of images has lower signal-to-noise than posterior part. This is due to improper functioning of anterior receiver coil element during this study.

T1: Low to intermediate signal intensity.

T2: High signal intensity (best appreciated on fat-suppressed images).

Enhancement pattern: Marked enhancement that may be immediate or progressive, homogeneous or heterogeneous. Tumors larger than 3 cm typically contain nonenhancing areas of necrosis.

Characteristic features: Very high signal intensity on fat-suppressed T2-weighted images with no loss of signal on opposed-phase gradient echo images.

Distribution: Bilateral in approximately 10%. About 10% of paragangliomas are extraadrenal tumors that occur along the sympathetic chain. Typical locations include along the IVC and aorta, near the aortic bifurcation or inferior mesen-

teric artery (IMA) origin (organ of Zuckerkandl), or in the mediastinum or pelvis. Pheochromocytomas associated with MEN tend to be bilateral and intraadrenal. Metastatic disease from malignant paragangliomas occurs most commonly to the lymph nodes, bone, liver, and lung.

Atypical appearances: May be cystic or may be only mildly hyperintense on T2-weighted images.

Associations: MEN IIA, IIB, or III (see Fig. 3.128), von Hippel-Lindau disease (see Fig. 3.129), neurofibromatosis (NF-1) (see Fig. 3.131), familial pheochromocytoma, Carney triad (extraadrenal paraganglioma, gastric stromal sarcoma, pulmonary chondroma).

Mimics: Metastases, lipid-poor adenoma, adrenal cortical carcinoma.

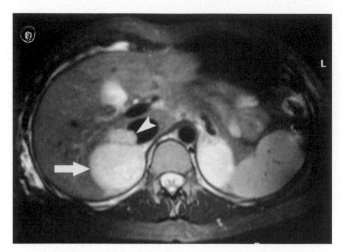

FIG. 3.67. Pheochromocytoma. Fat-suppressed T2-weighted image shows large high signal intensity mass (*arrow*) extending into inferior vena cava (*arrowhead*) in patient with hypertension and biochemical evidence of pheochromocytoma. Tumor was successfully removed surgically.

Additional comments: Pheochromocytomas are malignant in approximately 10% of cases (based on the presence of metastases). Extraadrenal paragangliomas are malignant in up to 40% of cases.

References: 95

KIDNEYS AND BLADDER

Angiomyolipoma of the Kidney (Figs. 3.68, 3.69; see Fig. 3.3)

Description: Benign tumor consisting of blood vessels, smooth muscle, and fat. Fat is often the predominant tissue element visible with imaging.

T1: May have heterogeneous signal intensity due to varying amounts of fat or the presence of hemorrhage. Many lesions may appear to consist almost entirely of fatty elements. Fat within the lesion is bright on non–fat-suppressed T1-weighted images and dark on fat-suppressed images. This pattern distinguishes angiomyolipomas from focal hemorrhage, which appears bright on both fat-suppressed and non–fat-suppressed images.

T2: Variable signal intensity depending on fat content and hemorrhage. Typically, fat within the lesion parallels fat elsewhere in the body on fat-suppressed and non–fat-suppressed images.

Enhancement pattern: Heterogeneous enhancement sparing fatty areas.

Characteristic features: A fat-containing tumor of the kidney is highly specific for angiomyolipoma, although very rare exceptions exist. Hemorrhage may be present.

Distribution: Sporadic tumors are usually solitary and unilateral. Multiple bilateral tumors are often associated with tuberous sclerosis.

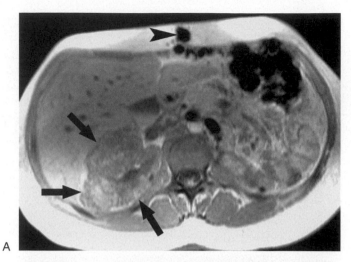

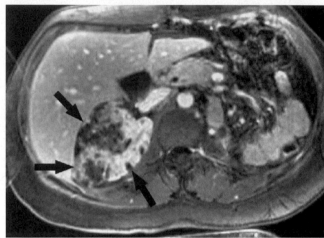

FIG. 3.68. Angiomyolipoma of kidney. In-phase **(A)** and fat-suppressed, gadolinium-enhanced **(B)** gradient echo images of right kidney demonstrate multiple heterogeneous renal masses (*arrows*). Fat within masses demonstrates high signal intensity before **(A)** and low signal intensity after fat suppression **(B)**. Note susceptibility artifact related to prior surgery on image **(A)** (*arrowhead*).

Atypical appearances: May contain only minimal fat (these lesions may appear as low signal intensity on T2-weighted images). May very rarely extend into renal vein and IVC.

Associations: Tuberous sclerosis.

Mimics: Renal cell carcinoma encompassing renal sinus fat. Liposarcoma or lipoma may very rarely mimic renal angiomyolipoma, although the vast majority of predominately fatty tumors of the kidney represent angiomyolipoma.

Additional comments: Angiomyolipomas and renal cell carcinomas (of the clear cell type) may both show significant signal loss on opposed-phase relative to in-phase gradient echo images. Therefore, T1-weighted images with and without fat suppression should be used to confirm the diagnosis of angiomyolipoma.

References: 96

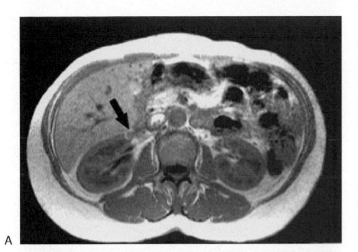

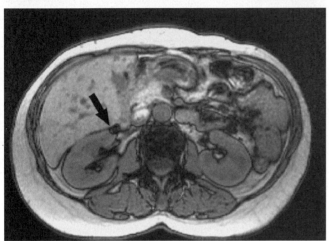

FIG. 3.69. Small angiomyolipoma of kidney. In-phase **(A)** and opposed-phase **(B)** images through kidneys show small lesion (*arrows*) of anterior lip of right kidney that demonstrates increased signal intensity on in-phase image and signal dropout on opposed-phase image (due to small size of lesion). On these sequences alone, this lesion could be mistaken for lipid-containing renal cell carcinoma.

Collecting Duct Carcinoma

Description: Aggressive malignant tumor of renal medullary origin.

T1: Isointense to renal parenchyma.

T2: Solid components hypointense to renal parenchyma.

Enhancement pattern: Enhances less than renal parenchyma.

Characteristic features: Infiltrative component with poorly defined tumor margins. Involvement of the renal medulla with extension into the renal pelvis and cortex is common.

Distribution: Unilateral and unifocal.

Atypical appearances: May appear cystic.

Mimics: Renal medullary carcinoma (associated with sickle cell trait), cortical renal cell carcinoma, transitional cell carcinoma, infection.

Additional comments: Imaging features are not specific for the diagnosis of collecting duct carcinoma.

References: 97

Cyst, Benign (Fig. 3.70)

Description: Common fluid-filled lesion of the kidney.

T1: Simple cysts are of low signal intensity. Hemorrhagic cysts have variable signal intensity from hypointense to hyperintense to renal parenchyma.

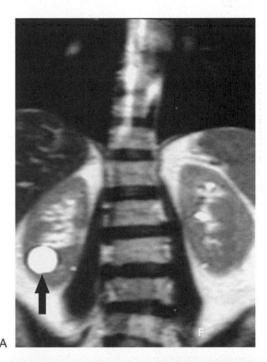

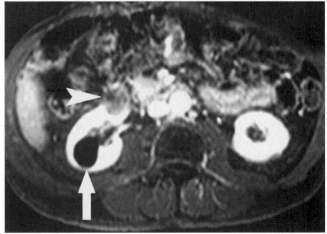

FIG. 3.70. Simple renal cyst. Simple cyst in lower pole right kidney (*arrows*) demonstrates typical high signal intensity on T2-weighted coronal image **(A)** and lack of enhancement on axial post-gadolinium, fat-suppressed T1-weighted image **(B)**. Note enhancing lesion (*arrowhead*) in anterior right kidney for comparison.

T2: Simple cysts are of very high signal intensity (equal to urine). Hemorrhagic cysts range from very dark to hyperintense to renal parenchyma.

Enhancement pattern: Nonenhancing.

Characteristic features: The appearance of a round, nonenhancing lesion with no discernible wall that parallels water on all pulse sequences is diagnostic. Hemorrhagic cysts must have no enhancing features to be considered benign. Cyst size varies greatly from a few millimeters to many centimeters in diameter.

Distribution: Frequently multiple and bilateral. May occur throughout the renal parenchyma and in the parapelvic region. May be exophytic or surrounded completely by renal parenchyma.

Atypical appearances: Thin, uniform, nonenhancing septations may be present.

Associations: Autosomal dominant polycystic kidney disease, von Hippel-Lindau disease, tuberous sclerosis, hemodialysis.

Mimics: Cystic renal cell carcinoma (suggested by mural irregularity and intense mural enhancement).

Additional comments: Signal intensity on unenhanced T1- and T2-weighted images is unreliable for distinguishing benign cysts from cystic or solid neoplasms. Therefore, enhancement characteristics are the single most important feature of a renal lesion. Parapelvic cysts may be distinguished from hydronephrosis with either a small (e.g., 2 mL) dose of intravenous gadolinium or by imaging early in the excretory phase after a standard (0.1 mmol/kg) dose of gadolinium chelate.

References: 98

Infarction, Renal (Fig. 3.71)

Description: Focal or diffuse ischemic injury to the kidney.

T1: Variable, depending on the age of the infarction and presence of hemorrhage.

T2: Variable depending on the age of the infarction and presence of hemorrhage.

Enhancement pattern: Absent enhancement of affected area, which is often peripheral and wedge-shaped with enhancement of the overlying renal capsule due to the presence of collaterals.

Characteristic features: Infarction is characterized by a wedge-shaped nonenhancing area with thin curvilinear enhancement peripherally (representing the renal capsule). Chronic infarction results in parenchymal loss, which may appear as a peripheral wedge-shaped contour defect.

Distribution: May be solitary, but often multiple and bilateral depending on the etiology. Renal infarcts from emboli often manifest between calyces, whereas renal scarring from reflux nephropathy or collecting system disease tends to involve the parenchyma overlying calyces.

Associations: Embolic source in the heart or great vessels, vasculitis or other renovascular disorder, intravenous drug use, trauma, renal interventions.

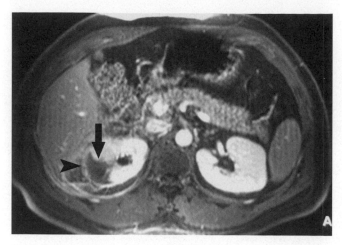

FIG. 3.71. Renal infarct. Fat-suppressed, gadolinium-enhanced T1-weighted gradient echo image demonstrates wedge-shaped, nonenhancing area (*arrow*) involving lateral right kidney. Capsular enhancement is present (*arrowhead*).

Mimics: Hypovascular neoplasm, infection.
References: 99, 100

Leiomyoma of the Bladder (Fig. 3.72)

Description: Most common benign mesenchymal tumor of the bladder.

T1: Similar signal intensity to bladder wall.

T2: Hypointense to isointense to bladder wall.

Enhancement pattern: Variable but typically modest enhancement.

Characteristic features: Well-circumscribed round or oval mass arising from bladder wall.

Distribution: Solitary. Growth may be predominantly intravesical, intramural, or extravesical. Most commonly arise from bladder base.

Atypical appearances: May have increased signal intensity or cystic areas on T2-weighted images.

Mimics: Neurofibroma (high signal intensity on T2-weighted images), low-grade leiomyosarcoma, nonmesenchymal tumors of the bladder.

References: 101

Lymphoma, Renal

Description: Lymphomatous involvement of the kidney is most often secondary. Primary renal lymphoma is extremely rare. Non-Hodgkin lymphoma is most common.

T1: Mildly hypointense to renal parenchyma.

T2: Hypointense to isointense to renal parenchyma.

Enhancement pattern: Enhancement may be minimal or absent, but when present, occurs relatively diffusely and less than renal cortex.

Characteristic features: A retroperitoneal mass extending into the renal hilum without evidence of necrosis and with

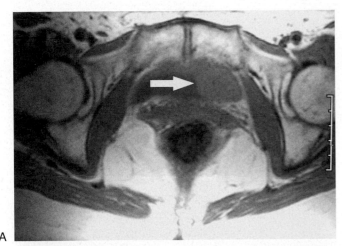

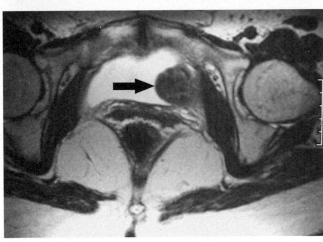

FIG. 3.72. Leiomyoma of bladder. Intramural bladder leiomyoma (*arrows*) demonstrates intermediate signal intensity on T1-weighted (**A**) and low signal intensity on T2-weighted (**B**) images of bladder.

diminished enhancement compared to the normal renal cortex is suggestive of lymphoma.

Distribution: Renal lymphoma commonly results from secondary extension of retroperitoneal disease, often into the renal hilum. However, infiltration of the perirenal space, solitary or multiple focal parenchymal masses, and diffuse infiltration of the kidney may occur.

Atypical appearances: IVC involvement is extremely rare.
Mimics: Other solid renal neoplasms.
References: 102

Multilocular Cystic Nephroma

Description: Benign cystic lesion of the kidney consisting of multiple cysts of variable size separated and surrounded by thick fibrous septa.

T1: Cysts are low in signal intensity unless they contain blood products or protein (relatively common).

T2: High signal intensity cysts with lower signal intensity septa.

Enhancement pattern: Septations enhance but cyst contents do not.

Characteristic features: Well-demarcated from normal kidney, multiple cysts with enhancing intervening septations.

Distribution: Usually unilateral. Tumor often borders or bulges into renal sinus.

Mimics: Complex cyst, cystic renal cell carcinoma, cystic Wilms tumor.

Additional comments: May be difficult to distinguish from cystic renal cell carcinoma preoperatively. Occurs most commonly in young boys and middle-aged women. Can harbor rests of Wilms' tumor and, therefore, is usually removed upon diagnosis.

References: 103, 104

Oncocytoma

Description: Benign solid tumor (oxyphilic adenoma) of the kidney.

T1: Hypointense to isointense to renal parenchyma.

T2: Variable.

Enhancement pattern: Central scar, if present, enhances to a lesser extent than remainder of tumor. Enhancement pattern may be similar to that of renal cell carcinoma.

Characteristic features: Round, well-demarcated solid mass, which may contain a central stellate scar.

Distribution: Solitary, unilateral.

Mimics: Renal cell carcinoma.

Additional comments: Cannot be reliably distinguished from renal cell carcinoma based on imaging criteria.

References: 105, 106

Pyelonephritis, Acute (Fig. 3.73)

Description: Acute bacterial infection of the kidney, usually the result of ascending urinary tract infection.

T1: Often normal, but may see loss of corticomedullary differentiation or increased signal intensity of renal medulla.

T2: High signal intensity perinephric fluid. Renal abscess may appear as focal area of high signal intensity.

Enhancement pattern: Heterogeneous enhancement with striated nephrogram. May progress to renal abscess, which appears as a focal nonenhancing area.

Characteristic features: Renal enlargement, high signal intensity perinephric fluid and fascial thickening, and striated enhancement (may appear wedge-shaped) are typical. Pyonephrosis may manifest as a debris-fluid level within a dilated collecting system.

Distribution: Multifocal abnormalities often present. Unilateral or bilateral.

Atypical appearances: Focal pyelonephritis may simulate a renal neoplasm.

Associations: Urinary tract infection.

Mimics: Embolic infarcts.

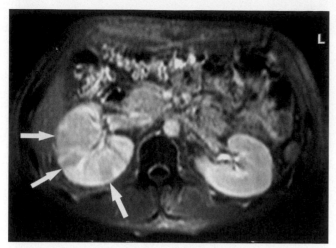

FIG. 3.73. Acute pyelonephritis. Fat-suppressed, gadolinium-enhanced T1-weighted image demonstrates low signal intensity striations (*arrows*) in right kidney secondary to acute pyelonephritis.

Additional comments: Gadolinium-enhanced inversion recovery MRI has been shown to be very sensitive for the diagnosis of pyelonephritis in children.

References: 107, 108

Renal Cell Carcinoma (Figs. 3.74, 3.75)

Description: Most common renal malignant tumor consisting of various cell types. Clear cell, papillary, granular cell, chromophobic cell, oncocytic cell, and collecting duct carcinoma are examples.

T1: Similar or slightly hypointense to renal cortex, unless complicated by hemorrhage (high signal intensity) or necrosis (low signal intensity).

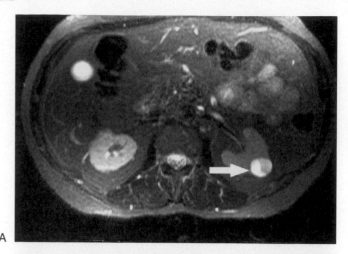

A

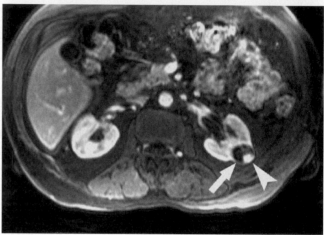

B

FIG. 3.75. Cystic renal cell carcinoma. Fat-suppressed T2-weighted **(A)** and gadolinium-enhanced T1-weighted **(B)** images show complex cystic left renal mass (*arrows*) with enhancing mural nodule (*arrowhead*).

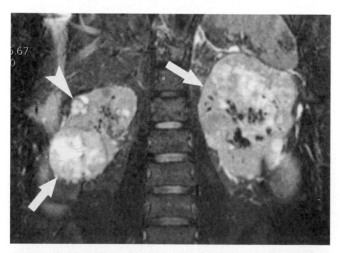

FIG. 3.74. Renal cell carcinoma. Coronal fat-suppressed T2-weighted image of the kidneys shows bilateral clear cell carcinomas (*arrows*) and right upper pole papillary renal cell carcinoma (*arrowhead*).

T2: Usually mildly hyperintense relative to renal parenchyma, although cystic or necrotic areas appear significantly more intense. Papillary type may appear hypointense to renal parenchyma.

Enhancement pattern: Large masses enhance heterogeneously with early peripheral enhancement and nonenhancing areas of tumor necrosis. Small lesions may enhance early and homogeneously, making differentiation from renal cortex difficult on the cortical phase of enhancement.

Characteristic features: Heterogeneous enhancing mass without fatty elements. Renal vein and IVC invasion may be present.

Distribution: Usually solitary and unilateral. May be multiple and bilateral, particularly in patients with von Hippel-Lindau disease (in which case they may be cystic). Most common sites of metastasis from renal cell carcinoma include lung, regional lymph nodes, liver, bone, adrenal glands, and contralateral kidney.

Atypical appearances: Renal cell carcinoma may appear predominately cystic (see Fig. 3.170). Enhancing mural nodules or thick enhancing wall or septations are clues to malignancy. Cystic components do not communicate with collecting system. Some renal cell carcinomas are relatively hypovascular (usually papillary type). Clear cell carcinoma may contain intracytoplasmic lipid (see Fig. 3.124). This can cause signal dropout on opposed-phase images, similar to that seen in some angiomyolipomas. To avoid confusion, angiomyolipomas should be diagnosed using T1-weighted images with and without fat suppression. Very rarely, renal cell carcinoma may envelop a small amount of fat that appears intratumoral. This appearance can also mimic angiomyolipoma, although being aware of this pitfall and using multiplanar reconstructions help avoid confusion.

Associations: von Hippel-Lindau disease, acquired cystic disease with chronic renal insufficiency.

Mimics: Oncocytoma, multilocular cystic nephroma, complex renal cyst, metastatic disease to kidney, xanthogranulomatous pyelonephritis.

Additional comments: To improve diagnostic confidence in the presence of renal vein and IVC invasion, we recommend the veins be evaluated with at least two different MR techniques (e.g., black blood and contrast-enhanced gradient echo). Metastases from clear cell carcinoma may contain intracellular lipid that can be demonstrated with chemical shift (in-phase and opposed-phase) imaging.

References: 109

Transitional Cell Carcinoma (Figs. 3.76, 377; see Figs. 1.51, 2.52 to 2.54)

Description: Most common malignant urothelial tumor. Most common primary malignant bladder tumor.

T1: Intermediate signal intensity.

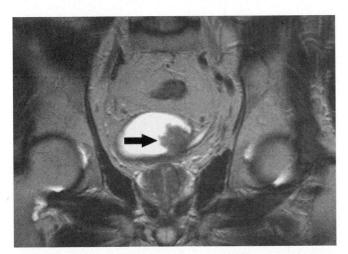

FIG. 3.76. Transitional cell carcinoma of bladder. Coronal T2-weighted image shows polypoid carcinoma (*arrow*) outlined by high signal intensity urine. This is same patient as in Figure 1.51.

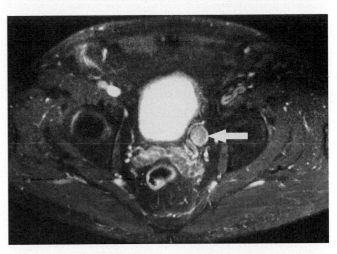

FIG. 3.77. Transitional cell carcinoma of ureter. Fat-suppressed, gadolinium-enhanced T1-weighted image of pelvis shows enhancing tumor expanding left distal ureter (*arrow*). This is same patient as in Figure 2.58.

T2: Intermediate to high signal intensity compared to bladder wall, although lower signal intensity than surrounding urine.

Enhancement pattern: Bladder transitional cell carcinoma (TCC) enhances relatively soon after arterial enhancement and earlier than bladder wall on dynamic contrast-enhanced images.

Characteristic features: Sessile enhancing filling defect in collecting system. Ureteral TCC may demonstrate classic "goblet sign" (focal ureteral dilatation around tumor) on MR urographic images. TCC of the renal pelvis may result in "faceless" kidney, resulting from obliteration of normal renal sinus anatomy.

Distribution: Often solitary, but TCC has a propensity to be multiple or bilateral. Patients are at risk for metachronous lesions. Relatively common in the bladder. Isolated ureteral tumors are uncommon. Spread by local invasion, regional lymph nodes, or distant metastases (e.g., bone).

Atypical appearances: May rarely invade renal vein and IVC.

Associations: Smoking, aniline dyes.

Mimics: Papilloma, metastasis, prostatic enlargement, endometriosis, malacoplakia, adenocarcinoma, squamous cell carcinoma, sarcoma.

Additional comments: When imaging TCC, it is important to obtain postcontrast images during the first minute after injection before a significant amount of gadolinium enters the collecting system.

References: 110 to 113

Xanthogranulomatous Pyelonephritis

Description: Chronic suppurative bacterial infection associated with obstruction of the collecting system.

T1: Hypointense cystic areas.

T2: Hyperintense cystic areas. Fluid-fluid level may be appreciated in some cases.

Enhancement pattern: Delayed but significant parenchymal enhancement due to diminished perfusion and inflammation. Poor or absent excretion of gadolinium into the involved portions of the collecting system.

Characteristic features: Renal enlargement, perinephric inflammation or extension, and dilated collecting system with thickened renal pelvic walls. Obstructing stone may be seen as signal void.

Distribution: May be focal or diffuse.

Atypical appearances: Focal disease may simulate a solid renal neoplasm.

Associations: Renal stones, staghorn calculi, proteus infection.

Mimics: Cystic renal neoplasms.

References: 114, 115

MISCELLANEOUS PERITONEUM AND RETROPERITONEUM

Abscess (Fig. 3.78)

Description: Confined collection of pus.

T1: Variable but often low, mildly heterogeneous signal intensity.

T2: Variable but often high, heterogeneous signal intensity. Layering debris may be present.

Enhancement: Enhancing wall, no enhancement of internal contents.

Characteristic features: Debris may be seen layering dependently, whereas air may appear in the nondependent portion of the cavity or interspersed throughout the collection. Air may be correctly identified by changing patient position or by the associated susceptibility artifact on a long TE gradient echo sequence.

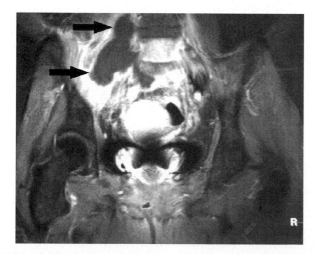

FIG. 3.78. Psoas abscess. Coronal fat-suppressed, gadolinium-enhanced T1-weighted image of pelvis shows low signal intensity fluid collection in right psoas muscle (*arrows*) with enhancing rim.

Distribution: Occurs virtually anywhere.

Associations: Recent surgery, urinary tract infection, discitis, other focus of infection.

Mimics: Complex cyst or pseudocyst, necrotic tumor, biloma, urinoma, bowel.

References: 116

Castleman Disease (Angiofollicular Lymph Node Hyperplasia)

Description: Benign proliferation of lymphocytes categorized into hyaline-vascular (most common) and plasma cell histologic subtypes.

T1: Low to intermediate signal intensity compared to liver.

T2: Hyperintense.

Enhancement pattern: Considerable early homogeneous or heterogeneous enhancement with intravenous gadolinium.

Characteristic features: Hypervascular mass that demonstrates high signal intensity on T2-weighted images.

Distribution: Occurs anywhere lymph node tissue is found. May be localized or disseminated.

Atypical appearances: Disseminated disease may be associated with diffuse lymphadenopathy, hepatosplenomegaly, ascites, or thickening of the retroperitoneal fascia.

Mimics: Lymphoma, lymph node metastases, inflammatory lymphadenopathy, granulomatous lymphadenopathy.

Additional comments: Castleman disease may mimic a variety of benign and malignant processes, including tumors of the solid organs, and should be considered in the differential diagnosis of hypervascular mass.

References: 117 to 119

Desmoid Tumor

Description: Histologically benign fibrous tumor arising from fascial or musculoaponeurotic structures. Despite the benign histology, these tumors may demonstrate an aggressive growth pattern with a high rate of recurrence after incomplete resection. Also known as aggressive fibromatosis.

T1: Low to intermediate signal intensity, although most tumors are low signal intensity.

T2: Variable, from low to high signal intensity.

Enhancement: Variable, often heterogeneous. Intense contrast enhancement may occur.

Characteristic features: Infiltrative fibrous lesion.

Distribution: May arise in the mesentery, abdominal wall, or pelvis. Usually solitary.

Associations: Familial adenomatous polyposis (Gardner syndrome).

Mimics: Soft tissue sarcoma, neurofibroma, lymphoma, carcinoid tumor.

Additional comments: High signal intensity on T2-weighted images may be associated with more rapid growth of these masses.

References: 120, 121

Mesenteric Cyst

Description: Benign, well-defined, thin-walled fluid-filled structure of the mesentery. A variety of classification systems reflects various etiologies, including lymphangiomatous or mesothelial cysts, or pseudocysts that lack an epithelial or mesothelial lining. Symptoms result from mass effect.

T1: Most commonly low signal intensity similar to simple fluid. Cysts containing sufficient protein or blood products may appear bright.

T2: Most commonly high signal intensity. Cysts complicated by hemorrhage may have lower, heterogeneous signal intensity. Fine septations may be present.

Enhancement: Nonenhancing contents. Wall and septations (if present) may enhance.

Characteristic features: Large unilocular cyst with thin walls. Signal intensity of cyst contents follows simple fluid.

Distribution: Most commonly arises from the small bowel (ileal) mesentery. Usually solitary.

Mimics: Pancreatic pseudocyst, enteric duplication cyst, cystic ovarian lesions, cystic mesothelioma.

Peritoneal Metastases (Fig. 3.79)

Description: Metastatic involvement of the peritoneal cavity by malignant tumor, most commonly arising from the ovary, colon, pancreas, or stomach. Metastatic involvement of the peritoneum is often referred to as peritoneal seeding or peritoneal implants.

T1: Low to intermediate signal intensity.

T2: Intermediate to high signal intensity.

Enhancement: Metastases typically enhance with gadolinium and become more conspicuous with fat suppression. Enhancement pattern varies with type and size of metastases.

Characteristic features: Enhancing soft tissue masses along peritoneal surfaces. Omental involvement commonly manifests as enhancing, nodular soft tissue infiltration of the omentum (omental caking).

Distribution: Common locations for peritoneal metastases include the rectouterine or rectovesical recesses, sigmoid mesocolon, perihepatic region, and omentum.

Atypical appearances: Pseudomyxoma peritonei (mucinous ascites resulting from mucinous adenocarcinoma metastases) may resemble simple ascites except mass effect on the bowel and solid organs (scalloping) is present with the former entity. Small bowel tends to float in simple ascites, but not in mucinous ascites of pseudomyxoma peritonei.

Associations: Primary ovarian, colon, gastric, or pancreatic adenocarcinoma are most common cause of peritoneal metastases.

Mimics: Peritonitis, tuberculosis, endometriosis, peritoneal disseminated leiomyomatosis.

Additional comments: The detection of peritoneal tumors may be improved by combining intravenous contrast with orally administered dilute barium, particularly when fat-suppressed T1-weighted delayed imaging is performed after a 0.2-mmol/kg (double) dose of gadolinium chelate.

References: 122, 123

Retroperitoneal Fibrosis, Idiopathic (Fig. 3.80)

Description: Inflammatory process resulting in dense fibrosis of the retroperitoneal tissues, predominately around the aorta, IVC, and ureters.

T1: Relatively low signal intensity.

T2: Relatively high signal intensity during the inflammatory stage with decreasing signal intensity as fibrosis matures. Heterogeneous high signal intensity is more common with malignant retroperitoneal processes.

Enhancement pattern: Active inflammation shows considerable enhancement. As disease progresses and mature fibrosis prevails, enhancement becomes progressively more delayed and less impressive.

Characteristic features: Fibrotic process that encases, rather than displaces, midline retroperitoneal structures. Tends not to displace aorta away from spine. Ureters may be medially deviated. May compress or obliterate inferior vena cava and iliac veins.

Distribution: May appear as a focal area of fibrosis or a diffuse process encasing the major retroperitoneal vessels and ureters. Disease may extend along the iliac vessels.

Atypical appearances: Perirenal or peripancreatic distribution may occur and simulate neoplastic processes such as lymphoma or pancreatic carcinoma.

Associations: Orbital pseudotumor, Riedel thyroiditis, sclerosing cholangitis, mediastinal fibrosis.

Mimics: Inflammatory aneurysm, lymphoma, desmoplastic metastases. Unlike lymphoma, retroperitoneal fibrosis tends not to displace the aorta away from the spine.

Additional comments: Additional secondary causes of retroperitoneal fibrosis include certain medications (e.g.,

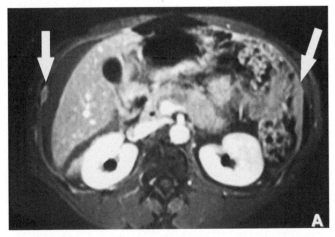

FIG. 3.79. Peritoneal metastases (ovarian primary). Fat-suppressed, gadolinium-enhanced T1-weighted image of the abdomen shows enhancing peritoneal tumor (*arrows*) in patient with metastatic ovarian carcinoma.

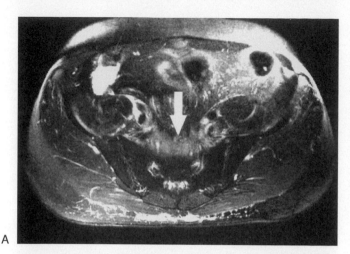

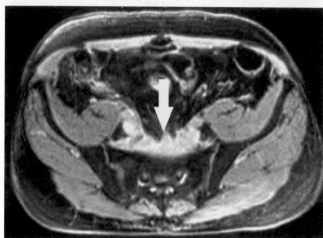

FIG. 3.80. Retroperitoneal fibrosis. Fat-suppressed T2-weighted **(A)** and delayed gadolinium-enhanced T1-weighted **(B)** images of pelvis demonstrate abnormal presacral soft tissue (*arrows*) that demonstrates mildly increased signal intensity on T2-weighted image **(A)** and homogeneous delayed enhancement **(B)**.

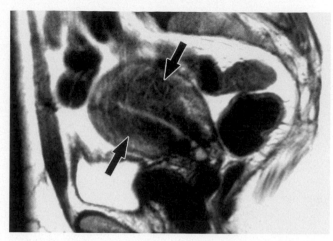

FIG. 3.81. Diffuse adenomyosis. Sagittal T2-weighted image through uterus demonstrates thickened, indistinct junctional zone (*arrows*).

dometrium on T2-weighted images) is thickened (>12 mm). The border between the junctional zone and the myometrium is often indistinct. Small bright foci are often present within the thickened junctional zone or myometrium but are not necessary for establishing the diagnosis.

Enhancement pattern: Areas of adenomyosis appear slightly hypointense to myometrium on post-gadolinium images.

Characteristic features: Thickening of the junctional zone, which may contain small bright foci on T2-weighted imaging.

Distribution: Focal or diffuse (more common). Smooth muscle hypertrophy can cause a focal masslike region of adenomyosis sometimes referred to as an adenomyoma.

methysergide), radiation treatment, prior trauma or infection, and surgery.

References: 124 to 126

FEMALE PELVIS

Adenomyosis (Figs. 3.81, 3.82)

Description: Ectopic endometrial glands within the myometrium associated with smooth muscle hypertrophy. The endometrial glands in adenomyosis are relatively unaffected by hormonal stimulation, in that the basal layer of the endometrium is involved.

T1: Usually isointense to myometrium. Occasionally, small foci of high signal may be present, corresponding to areas of hemorrhage.

T2: The junctional zone (inner layer of myometrium that normally appears as a dark band surrounding the en-

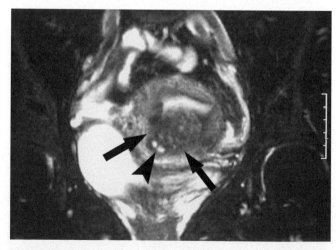

FIG. 3.82. Focal adenomyosis. Coronal fat-suppressed T2-weighted image through uterus shows focal thickening of junctional zone (*arrows*) containing small high signal foci (*arrowhead*). Note minimal distortion of endometrial stripe and serosal surface of uterus.

Atypical appearances: Adenomyoma may have a relatively well-defined margin and mimic a fibroid. Large cystic regions within adenomyosis may rarely occur.

Associations: May be associated with other gynecologic abnormalities, such as leiomyoma or endometriosis.

Mimics: Transient myometrial contractions or fibroids may occasionally mimic an adenomyoma. Adenomyosis tends to have ill-defined borders and minimal mass effect. Fibroids tend to be more clearly demarcated and exhibit greater mass effect on the endometrium or distort the serosal contour of the uterus.

Additional comments: MRI evidence of adenomyosis is common and may be incidental or asymptomatic, or associated with pain or abnormal uterine bleeding. Many centers use 12 mm as the threshold for diagnosing adenomyosis with MRI. However, not all cases of adenomyosis demonstrate this degree of junctional zone thickening. Therefore, a junctional zone that measures approximately 8 to 12 mm might be considered uncertain for the diagnosis of adenomyosis, and additional evidence of abnormality, such as focality or high signal intensity foci, should be sought.

References: 127, 128

Bartholin Gland Cyst (Fig. 3.83)

Description: Cystic lesion arising from a Bartholin (vulvovaginal) gland, possibly secondary to inflammation with retention of secretions.

T1: Intermediate to high signal intensity.

T2: High signal intensity.

Enhancement pattern: Nonenhancing. Rim enhancement may occur if infected.

Characteristic features: Cystic lesion in the classic location.

Distribution: Solitary. Involves the posterolateral lower third of the vagina (vaginal vestibule).

Atypical appearances: Infected cysts may contain air or demonstrate rim enhancement.

Mimics: Usually not a diagnostic dilemma. Urethral diverticula and Gartner duct cysts can be differentiated from Bartholin gland cysts by their characteristic locations.

References: 129

Brenner Tumor

Description: Uncommon, usually benign, epithelial ovarian neoplasm

T1: Low to intermediate signal intensity.

T2: Low signal intensity, unless cystic elements are present.

Enhancement pattern: Mild enhancement may occur.

Characteristic features: Predominantly solid mass with low signal intensity on T2-weighted sequences. CT may demonstrate calcification.

Distribution: Often unilateral and solitary, but may be bilateral.

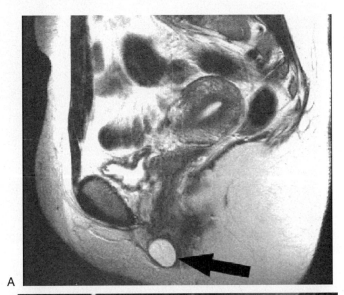

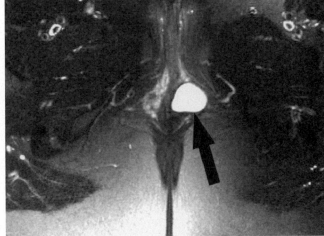

FIG. 3.83. Bartholin gland cyst. Sagittal **(A)** and axial **(B)** T2-weighted images of female pelvis show a small simple cyst (*arrows*) near vaginal vestibule.

Atypical appearances: May contain cystic elements.

Associations: May be associated with other ovarian neoplasms, particularly mucinous cystadenomas.

Mimics: Ovarian fibroma or fibrothecoma.

References: 130, 131

Cervical Carcinoma (Fig. 3.84, 3.85; see Fig. 3.209)

Description: Malignant tumor arising from the cervix. Cervical cancer is most commonly of squamous cell type.

T1: Low to intermediate signal intensity, similar to uterus and normal cervical tissue.

T2: Increased signal intensity relative to the cervical stroma.

Enhancement pattern: Early enhancement of cervical carcinoma relative to surrounding structures may be appreciated on dynamic gadolinium-enhanced images.

Characteristic features: Expansion of the cervix and disruption of the normal zonal anatomy on T2-weighted images.

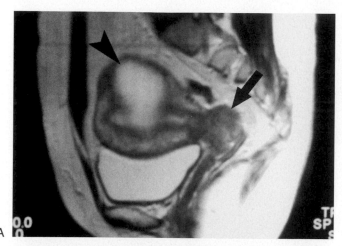

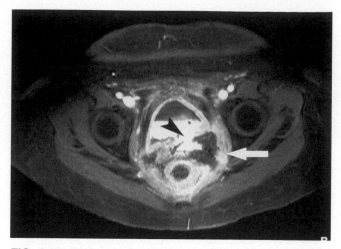

FIG. 3.85. Recurrent cervical carcinoma with vesicovaginal fistula. Fat-suppressed, gadolinium-enhanced T1-weighted image of pelvis demonstrates enhancing infiltrating pelvic tumor (*arrow*) and wide communication between bladder and vagina (*arrowhead*) allowing passage of high signal intensity gadolinium.

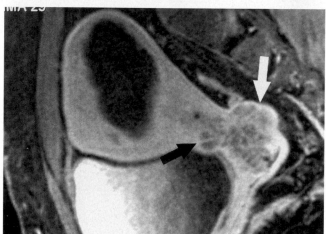

FIG. 3.84. Cervical carcinoma. **A:** Sagittal T2-weighted image shows cervical mass (*arrow*) that disrupts normally low signal intensity fibrous stroma. Note cystic fibroid (*arrowhead*). **B:** Sagittal fat-suppressed, gadolinium-enhanced T1-weighted image clearly demonstrates margins of mass (*arrows*).

Distribution: Begins in the cervix with spread predominately via local invasion of surrounding structures. Nodal metastases most commonly involve obturator, iliac, and paraaortic lymph nodes. Associated necrotic lymph nodes are likely to contain metastatic disease.

Atypical appearances: Very rarely, malignant primary cervical neoplasms other than squamous cell carcinoma may have a cystic component.

Associations: Human papillomavirus infection.

Mimics: Secondary involvement of the cervix by other malignant tumor (e.g., uterine cancer, metastasis), primary cervical lymphoma. Radiation-induced changes in the pelvis may be difficult to distinguish from recurrent cervical carcinoma. Signs of recurrent tumor include asymmetric tissue in the pelvis, an identifiable mass, lymphadenopathy, and ureteral obstruction. Increased signal intensity on T2-weighted images may be present in areas of radiation fibrosis in the absence of tumor for up to a year after radiation treatment.

Additional comments: An intact dark cervical stroma surrounding relatively bright tumor on T2-weighted images sig-

nifies absence of parametrial invasion (FIGO [International Federation of Gynecology and Obstetrics] stage I or IIa). Disruption of cervical stroma due to tumor extension indicates parametrial invasion (FIGO IIb).

References: 132 to 134

Endometrial Carcinoma (Fig. 3.86)

Description: Malignant tumor, most commonly adenocarcinoma, arising from the endometrium.

T1: Nearly isointense to uterus.

T2: Tumor is often similar in signal intensity to endometrium, but may be hypointense or hyperintense.

Enhancement pattern: Enhances less than myometrium, although the difference between tumor and myometrium decreases with time. Some evidence suggests the use of contrast-enhanced dynamic imaging improves the accuracy of assessing the depth of myometrial invasion.

Characteristic features: Widening of the endometrium (>5 mm in a postmenopausal woman). Disruption of the junctional zone implies deep myometrial invasion.

Distribution: Originates within the endometrium. Usually spreads first to pelvic lymph nodes followed by paraaortic lymph nodes. The likelihood of lymph node metastases increases markedly in the presence of deep myometrial invasion. The location of lymph node metastases is related in part to which portion of the uterus is involved. The most frequent site of hematogenous metastasis is lung. Direct invasion of the bladder or rectum should be suspected when there is loss of the normal low signal intensity wall of these structures.

Associations: Obesity, nulliparity, unopposed estrogen replacement, tamoxifen therapy, adenomatous endometrial hyperplasia.

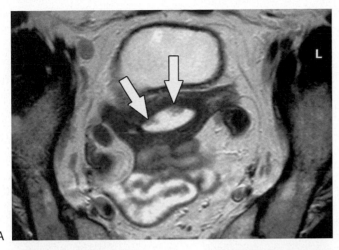

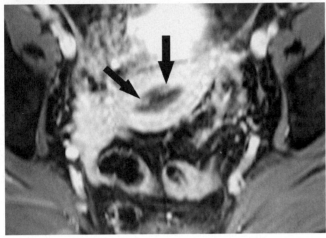

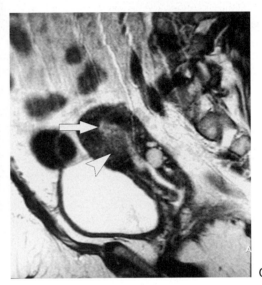

FIG. 3.86. Endometrial carcinoma. **A:** T2-weighted image oriented perpendicular to the long axis of the uterus shows thickening of the endometrium with foci of lower signal intensity (*arrows*). **B:** Fat-suppressed, gadolinium-enhanced T1-weighted image shows foci to represent enhancing tumor (*arrows*). **C:** Endometrial carcinoma in a second patient. Sagittal T2-weighted image demonstrates abnormal thickening of the endometrium (*arrow*) with lower signal intensity mass (relative to endometrium) extending slightly into myometrium (*arrowhead*). Less than 50% myometrial invasion confirmed at surgery.

Mimics: Endometrial polyp, endometrial hyperplasia, uterine sarcoma.

Additional comments: Using a 5-mm threshold for normal endometrial thickness in postmenopausal women results in high sensitivity but only moderate specificity for endometrial carcinoma. Disruption of the junctional zone on T2-weighted images or of the subendometrial enhancing line on early post-contrast T1-weighted images implies myometrial invasion. If myometrial invasion is suspected, orthogonal views should be obtained to confirm.

References: 135 to 137

Endometrial Hyperplasia

Description: Proliferation of endometrial tissue without or with cytologic atypia.

T1: Similar in signal intensity to rest of uterus.

T2: Similar in signal intensity to normal endometrium.

Enhancement pattern: Similar to normal endometrium.

Characteristic features: Diffuse thickening of the endometrium. Normal postmenopausal endometrium should not exceed 5 mm in thickness.

Distribution: Typically diffuse.

Atypical appearances: Cystic changes or asymmetric thickening may occur.

Associations: Tamoxifen therapy.

Mimics: Endometrial carcinoma, endometrial polyp.

Additional comments: Imaging cannot reliably distinguish between endometrial hyperplasia and early stage carcinoma. Some patients treated with tamoxifen may demonstrate subendometrial cysts, cystic atrophy, or markedly heterogeneous endometria with lattice-like enhancement following

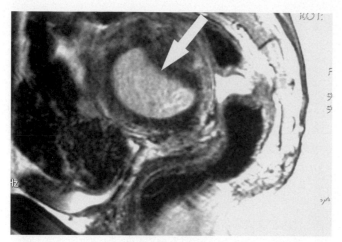

FIG. 3.87. Endometrial polyp. Sagittal T2-weighted image through uterus demonstrates nonspecific thickening of endometrium (*arrow*) representing a pathologically confirmed benign polyp.

gadolinium administration (this latter finding is often associated with polyps).

References: 138, 139

Endometrial Polyp (Fig. 3.87)

Description: Usually benign focal hyperplasia of endometrial glands and stroma projecting into uterine cavity. Although rare, malignant transformation may occur.

T1: Intermediate signal intensity, isointense to uterus.

T2: Isointense or slightly hypointense to endometrium.

Enhancement pattern: Enhances less than outer myometrium.

Characteristic features: Intratumoral cysts and low signal intensity fibrous core are more common in polyps than in carcinomas.

Distribution: Originates within the uterine cavity. May result in focal or diffuse thickening of the endometrial signal and may prolapse through endocervical canal.

Atypical appearances: Some patients treated with tamoxifen may demonstrate markedly heterogeneous endometria with lattice-like enhancement following gadolinium administration, a finding that has been associated with polyps (Fig. 3.88).

Associations: Tamoxifen therapy, endometrial hyperplasia.

Mimics: Endometrial hyperplasia and carcinoma, blood clots, early intrauterine pregnancy or retained products of conception, submucosal fibroid.

References: 138, 140, 141

Endometrioma, Endometriosis, Endometrial Implants (Figs. 3.89, 3.90)

Description: Endometriosis refers to implantation of functional endometrial glandular tissue outside of the uterus. Hor-

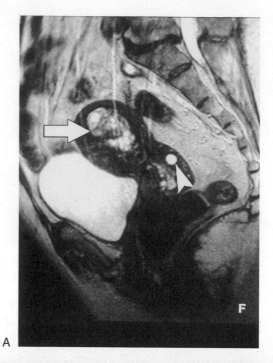

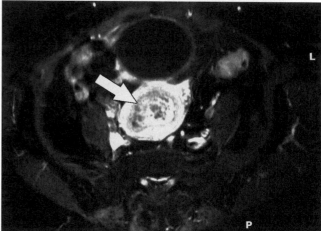

FIG. 3.88. Tamoxifen-induced changes of uterus. **A:** Sagittal T2-weighted image through uterus demonstrates thickened, heterogeneous endometrium (*arrow*) in patient being treated for breast cancer. Note nabothian cyst (*arrowhead*) in cervix. **B:** Fat-suppressed, gadolinium-enhanced T1-weighted axial image of same patient shows heterogeneous enhancement of endometrial contents (benign polyp).

monal stimulation causes cyclical hemorrhage within ectopic endometrial implants. An endometrioma consists of ectopic endometrial glands and stroma forming a cystic collection of blood products. Hemorrhage is often recurrent, resulting in blood products of varying chronicity. Endometrial implants also occur as discrete foci of ectopic endometrial tissue without formation of a cystic mass.

T1: Variable signal intensity due to wide range of chronicity of blood products. Most endometriomas and focal endometrial implants have high signal intensity resulting from

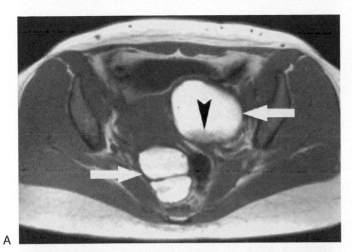

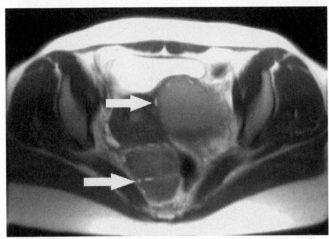

FIG. 3.89. Bilateral endometriomas. **A:** T1-weighted image through pelvis demonstrates high signal intensity adnexal fluid collections (*arrows*). Signal of collections did not suppress with fat-suppression techniques (not shown). Note debris in left adnexal lesion (*arrowhead*). **B:** Despite their cystic nature, both lesions demonstrate mild signal loss on T2-weighted image (*shading*). Note high signal follicles (*arrows*) draped around both lesions, confirming their ovarian origin. Bilateral ovarian endometriomas found at surgery.

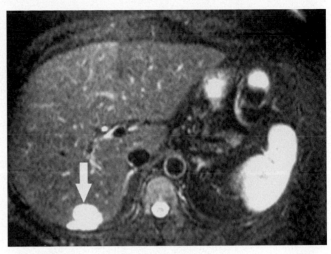

FIG. 3.90. Endometrial implant. Fat-suppressed T2-weighted image shows high signal intensity cystic lesion (*arrow*) representing perihepatic endometrial implant. At surgery, implant was seen to invaginate liver capsule.

the presence of methemoglobin. Fat-suppressed imaging increases the conspicuity of endometrial implants and helps distinguish hemorrhagic elements from fat.

T2: Variable signal intensity depending on contents, but classically endometriomas are less hyperintense than simple cysts due to the T2-shortening effect of blood products. Endometriomas commonly appear dark on T2-weighted images due to hemosiderin within the cyst contents.

Enhancement pattern: Endometrial implants enhance moderately with gadolinium, increasing their conspicuity on fat-suppressed, contrast-enhanced images. Endometriomas may show enhancement of the cyst wall, but the central contents do not enhance.

Characteristic features: Thick-walled cystic structure with increased signal intensity on T1-weighted images and variable, but typically low, signal intensity on T2-weighted im-

ages. This decreased signal intensity on T2-weighted images is often referred to as "shading." A peripheral low signal intensity rim of hemosiderin may be present. Associated adhesions are characteristic but may be difficult to appreciate with imaging. Hydrosalpinx may be present, and the dilated fallopian tubes may demonstrate increased signal intensity on T1-weighted images.

Distribution: The term endometrioma is traditionally reserved exclusively for ovarian involvement, although this distinction is of questionable value. These lesions are frequently multiple and bilateral. Other relatively common sites of involvement include rectouterine recess, uterosacral ligaments, serosal surface of the uterus, and fallopian tubes. Bowel (most commonly rectosigmoid), bladder, and ureteral involvement may occur. Bowel involvement may cause a stricture, and ureteral involvement may cause hydronephrosis or a submucosal mass. Endometriosis has a mild predilection for scar tissue and implants can occur within laparoscopy or cesarian section scars. Extraperitoneal sites are possible but rare.

Atypical appearances: Endometriosis may have a wide range of appearances and mimic a variety of benign and malignant processes. Pleural involvement has been described, resulting in catamenial pneumothorax.

Mimics: Cystic ovarian neoplasm, hemorrhagic ovarian cyst, peritoneal metastases.

Additional comments: Malignant transformation is a rare complication of endometriosis.

References: 142

Gartner Duct Cyst (Fig. 3.91)

Description: Cystic lesion of wolffian duct remnant.

T1: Typically low signal intensity, although high protein content or hemorrhage within the cyst fluid may result in high signal intensity.

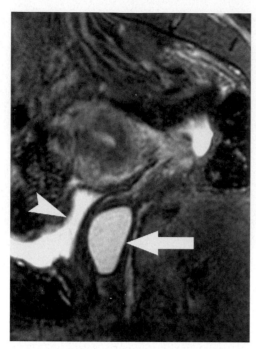

FIG. 3.91. Gartner duct cyst. Midline sagittal fat-suppressed T2-weighted image of female pelvis shows high signal intensity simple cystic lesion (*arrow*) posterior to bladder (*arrowhead*). (Courtesy of Timothy G. Sanders, M.D.)

T2: High signal intensity.

Enhancement pattern: Nonenhancing.

Characteristic features: Simple-appearing cystic lesion in typical location.

Distribution: Solitary cyst of anterolateral upper vagina.

Atypical appearances: Ectopic ureter may rarely communicate with Gartner duct cyst.

Associations: Ipsilateral renal agenesis.

Mimics: Nabothian cyst, urethral diverticulum, and Bartholin gland cyst can usually be differentiated from Gartner duct cyst by their typical location and appearance.

Additional comments: Usually asymptomatic.

References: 129

Hydrosalpinx

Description: Obstructed, dilated fallopian tube, most commonly the result of infection, inflammation, or adhesions.

T1: Low signal intensity if uncomplicated. May be high signal intensity if complicated by hemorrhage.

T2: High signal intensity.

Enhancement pattern: Nonenhancing.

Characteristic features: Typically appears as a tortuous, tubular, fluid-filled adnexal structure.

Distribution: Adnexal. Unilateral or bilateral.

Atypical appearances: Fallopian tube fluid may be lower signal intensity than simple fluid on T2-weighted images, a finding that does not necessarily imply endometriosis.

Associations: Pelvic inflammatory disease, endometriosis, adhesions.

Mimics: Adnexal cysts of various causes, tuboovarian abscess (pyosalpinx).

Additional comments: High signal intensity of fallopian tube fluid on T1-weighted images may be associated with endometriosis.

References: 143

Mature Cystic Teratoma (Dermoid Cyst) (3.92, 3.93)

Description: Slow-growing tumor of the ovary consisting of variable amounts of endodermal, mesodermal, and ectodermal tissue. This most common of ovarian neoplasms is often filled with sebaceous material.

T1: Highly variable, heterogeneous signal intensity. Fat within the lesion appears as areas of high signal intensity that suppress with fat-suppression techniques. Calcifications (such as teeth) appear as low signal intensity.

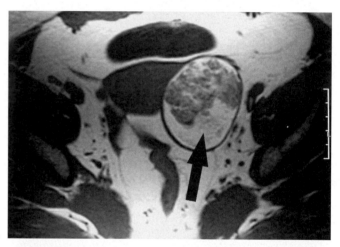

A

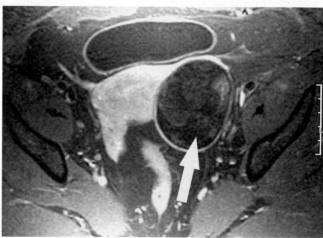

B

FIG. 3.92. Mature cystic teratoma. **A:** T1-weighted axial image through pelvis shows left adnexal mass with high signal intensity components (*arrow*). **B:** Application of fat suppression demonstrates loss of signal intensity of fatty components (*arrow*) of cystic teratoma.

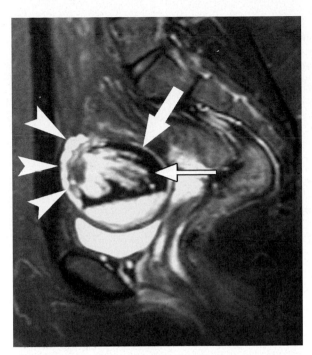

FIG. 3.93. Mature cystic teratoma. Sagittal fat-suppressed T2-weighted image of female pelvis demonstrates heterogeneous mass (*arrow*) with high signal intensity follicles (*arrowheads*) draped around it, confirming ovarian origin of mass. Low signal component of mass (*thin arrow*) represents fatty component on this fat-suppressed sequence.

T2: Variable signal intensity. Fat appears similar in intensity to subcutaneous fat.

Enhancement pattern: May demonstrate mural enhancement. The solid components of struma ovarii enhance with gadolinium.

Characteristic features: Layers of different signal intensity (e.g., fat-fluid level), dependently layering debris, or a Rokitansky nodule or protuberance (dermoid plug) may be present. The Rokitansky nodule often contains hair, bone, or teeth. Fat-water interfaces show chemical shift artifact along the frequency encoding direction. Regions of fat appear dark on fat-suppressed images. Small amounts of lipid may be detected with in-phase and opposed-phase gradient echo images.

Distribution: Adnexal. Usually unilateral, but approximately 10% are bilateral.

Atypical appearances: Some cystic teratomas may contain only minimal fat, appearing predominately cystic. In-phase and opposed-phase imaging may be helpful in revealing small amounts of fat in such lesions. Infected teratoma may contain air. Struma ovarii composed predominantly of thyroid tissue may appear as a complex cystic and solid mass. Malignant transformation should be considered when a solid, enhancing component is present, particularly when associated with transmural extension or invasion of adjacent tissues. However, enhancement of a solid component alone does not guarantee malignancy.

Mimics: Endometriomas may simulate mature cystic teratomas on non–fat-suppressed T1-weighted images. Other fat-containing masses of the female pelvis (e.g., lipoleiomyoma, liposarcoma) are much less common.

Additional comments: Although benign, these tumors are usually surgically removed as a result of the potential for complications, including torsion, intraperitoneal rupture, infection, and malignant transformation (<3%).

References: 144 to 147

Nabothian Cyst (Fig. 3.94)

Description: Cystic distention of endocervical gland.

T1: Low to intermediate signal intensity.

T2: Very high signal intensity.

Enhancement pattern: Nonenhancing.

Characteristic features: Appear as simple cysts, usually a centimeter or less in size, in the cervix.

Distribution: Located in cervix. Often multiple.

Atypical appearances: May become several centimeters in diameter.

Mimics: Gartner duct cyst, adenoma malignum.

Additional comments: Extremely common.

References: 148, 149

Ovarian Carcinoma (Fig. 3.95)

Description: Primary ovarian malignant tumor, most commonly of epithelial, germ cell, or stromal origin. Epithelial

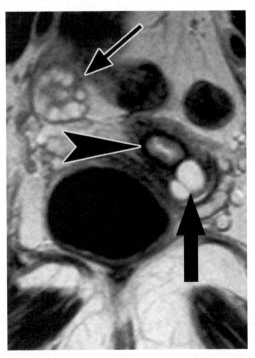

FIG. 3.94. Nabothian cyst. High resolution T2-weighted image performed axial with respect to cervix shows two small nabothian cysts (*arrow*). Note zonal anatomy of cervix (*arrowhead*) and normal right ovary with follicles (*thin arrow*).

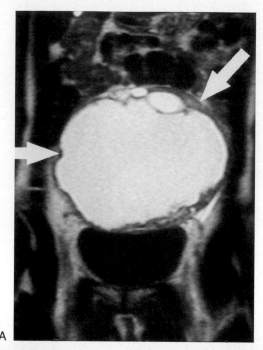

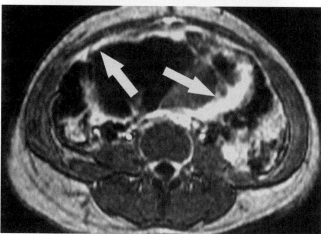

FIG. 3.95. Ovarian carcinoma. **A:** Coronal T2-weighted image demonstrates large complex cystic mass (*arrows*) with thick irregular walls occupying pelvis and lower abdomen. **B:** Following gadolinium administration, mass demonstrates thick enhancing walls and septations (*arrows*) consistent with malignant process. Mucinous cystadenocarcinoma diagnosed at surgery.

tumors are most common and include serous, mucinous, endometroid, and clear cell varieties. Germ cell tumors include dysgerminoma, immature teratoma, and endodermal sinus tumor, among other less common cell types, and tend to occur in younger patients. Of the malignant stromal tumors, the granulosa cell type is most common. Undifferentiated or other rare types of ovarian malignant tumors may occur.

T1: Variable signal intensity.

T2: Variable signal intensity. Epithelial tumors tend to have more cystic elements than other varieties. Papillary projections are also more typical of epithelial neoplasms.

Enhancement pattern: Solid soft tissue elements demonstrate enhancement. Peritoneal implants may be depicted on fat-suppressed post-gadolinium T1-weighted images.

Characteristic features: Features that suggest a malignant ovarian mass include large size, enhancing soft tissue components, thick (>3 mm) walls or septations, invasion of adjacent structures, ascites, peritoneal or omental implants (Fig. 3.79), and lymphadenopathy.

Distribution: Ovarian cancer is often unilateral, although bilateral tumors (either synchronous or metastatic) are not uncommon. Tumor spreads via direct invasion, peritoneal seeding, and lymphatic or hematogenous metastasis. Hematogenous metastases are most common in the liver and lungs. Peritoneal spread most commonly involves the pouch of Douglas, paracolic gutters, serosal surface of the bowel, omentum, and perihepatic space, although implants may occur anywhere within the peritoneum.

Mimics: Metastases to the ovaries may be difficult to distinguish from primary cancer of the ovary. Features of metastatic foci include bilaterality, sharp margins, preservation of the oval configuration of the ovary, and hypointense solid components on T2-weighted images. Peritoneal tuberculosis may mimic ovarian cancer with peritoneal metastases. Endometrial implants may simulate malignant peritoneal implants.

Additional comments: CA-125 may be elevated but is not entirely specific for ovarian cancer. Estrogen-producing tumors (e.g., granulosa cell) may result in uterine enlargement and endometrial hyperplasia.

References: 150, 151

Ovarian Cyst (Fig. 3.96)

Description: Functional cyst of the ovary including follicular, corpus luteum, and corpus albicans cysts.

T1: Isointense to simple fluid (low signal intensity).

T2: Isointense to simple fluid (very high signal intensity).

Enhancement pattern: Significant mural enhancement may occur with corpus luteum cyst.

Characteristic features: Parallels simple fluid when uncomplicated. Ovarian origin may be determined by the presence of normal follicles draped around the cyst. Functional cysts should never contain enhancing nodules or septations.

Distribution: Adnexal. Solitary or multiple. Unilateral or bilateral.

Atypical appearances: Hemorrhagic cyst may demonstrate increased signal intensity on T1-weighted images and variable signal intensity on T2-weighted images. Enlarged ovaries with multiple, complex cysts may be present in ovarian hyperstimulation syndrome.

Associations: Multiple theca lutein cysts may occur in setting of gestational trophoblastic disease or multiple gestations.

Mimics: Paraovarian cyst, peritoneal inclusion cyst. Thick enhancing wall, septations, and mural nodularity suggest

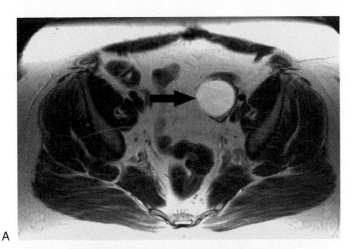

A

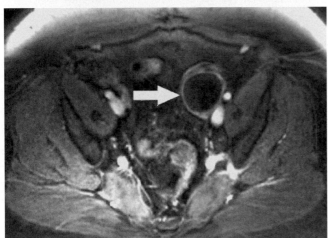

B

FIG. 3.96. Functional ovarian cyst. **A:** Axial T2-weighted image of female pelvis shows simple-appearing left ovarian cyst (*arrow*). **B:** No internal enhancement of cyst (*arrow*) is present on fat-suppressed T1-weighted image.

cystic ovarian neoplasm. Endometrioma may mimic a hemorrhagic corpus luteum cyst.

References: 152

Ovarian Fibroma/Thecoma/Fibrothecoma (see Fig. 3.187)

Description: Benign ovarian stromal tumor with variable fibrous and thecal elements. More common in perimenopausal or postmenopausal women.

T1: Low signal intensity.

T2: Low signal intensity.

Enhancement pattern: Variable.

Characteristic features: Well-defined ovarian mass with low signal intensity on all pulse sequences.

Distribution: Ovarian origin may be confirmed by the presence of normal follicles draped around mass. Bilateral tumors are rare.

Atypical appearances: High signal intensity on T2-weighted images due to myxomatous or cystic change.

Associations: Ascites may be present. Meigs syndrome refers to association of ovarian fibroma with ascites and a right pleural effusion (rare).

Mimics: Subserosal or extrauterine leiomyoma, Brenner tumor.

References: 153, 154

Ovarian Mucinous Cystadenoma

Description: Benign mucinous epithelial neoplasm of the ovary with malignant potential. Less common than serous cystadenoma.

T1: Variable signal intensity due to the presence of protein or hemorrhage.

T2: Variable signal intensity due to the presence of protein or hemorrhage.

Enhancement pattern: Septations and other soft tissue elements enhance after gadolinium administration.

Characteristic features: Multilocular cystic lesion with locules of differing signal intensity. Thick septations and soft tissue nodules or papillary projections are suggestive of carcinoma (see Fig. 3.95), but it may be difficult to distinguish between benign and malignant varieties of mucinous ovarian tumor.

Distribution: Ovarian in origin. Usually unilateral but may be bilateral.

Associations: Patients with mucinous ovarian tumors and pseudomyxoma peritonei may have a mucinous tumor of the appendix, making site of origin of the peritoneal process difficult to discern.

Mimics: Other complex cystic ovarian masses.

Additional comments: Mucinous ovarian neoplasms are benign in 80% of cases.

References: 155, 156

Ovarian Serous Cystadenoma (Fig. 3.97)

Description: Benign epithelial neoplasm of the ovary with malignant potential.

T1: Low signal intensity. The presence of hemorrhage may increase signal intensity.

T2: Very high signal intensity unless complicated by hemorrhage. Thin septations may be present. Papillary projections may be seen with benign cystadenoma but are more indicative of carcinoma.

Enhancement pattern: The use of gadolinium is most beneficial in demonstrating enhancing papillary projections, which, when present, help distinguish this neoplasm from simple functional ovarian cyst.

Characteristic features: Cystadenoma is typically thin walled and unilocular. Thin septations may be present, although solid components are typically minimal. Signal intensity usually parallels simple fluid. Cystadenocarcinoma demonstrates papillary excrescences within the cyst. Ascites, peritoneal implants, and lymphadenopathy also favor carcinoma.

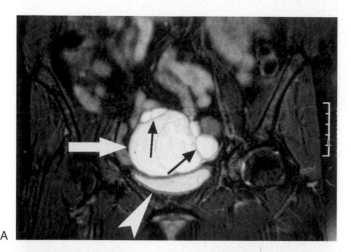

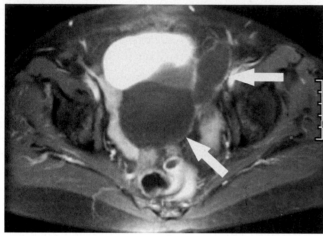

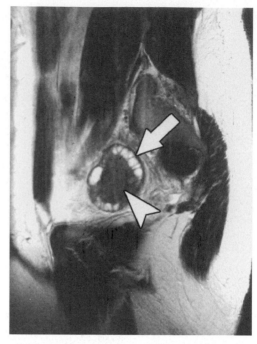

FIG. 3.98. Polycystic ovaries. Sagittal T2-weighted image through the ovary demonstrates multiple, peripherally arranged, similarly sized ovarian follicles (*arrow*). Note prominent low signal intensity ovarian stroma (*arrowhead*).

FIG. 3.97. Serous ovarian cystadenoma. A: Coronal fat-suppressed T2-weighted image shows cystic mass (*arrow*) superior to bladder (*arrowhead*). A few septa are present (*thin arrows*). B: Axial fat-suppressed, gadolinium-enhanced T1-weighted image demonstrates walls of mass (*arrows*) to be thin and without enhancing nodules. Mass was benign at surgery.

Distribution: Unilateral or bilateral. Ovarian origin of large cystic mass may be determined by the presence of normal follicles draped around the cyst.

Atypical appearances: May appear multilocular or hemorrhagic.

Mimics: Mucinous cystadenoma, hydrosalpinx, functional cyst, paraovarian cyst.

Additional comments: Approximately 60% of serous ovarian neoplasms are benign.

References: 156, 157

Polycystic Ovary Syndrome (Fig. 3.98)

Description: Hormonally mediated abnormality resulting in stimulation of ovarian follicle development without follicular maturation.

T1: Follicles not well visualized on T1-weighted images.

T2: Follicles are of high signal intensity. Central stroma is of low signal intensity.

Enhancement pattern: No specific enhancement pattern.

Characteristic features: Characterized by multiple similarly sized follicles arranged peripherally around the low signal intensity central ovarian stroma on a T2-weighted image. Ovaries commonly enlarged.

Distribution: Ovarian follicles tend to be subcapsular.

Atypical appearances: Ovaries may be near normal in size.

Associations: Stein-Leventhal syndrome (hirsutism, amenorrhea, anovulation or infertility, obesity), diabetes, endometrial hyperplasia or carcinoma.

Mimics: Normal ovaries with multiple follicles.

Additional comments: The finding of multiple peripheral ovarian cysts alone is not specific for polycystic ovaries. Correlation with clinical and laboratory data is essential.

References: 158

Urethral Diverticulum (Figs. 3.99, 3.100)

Description: Urethral outpouching presumably resulting from rupture of an infected periurethral gland into the urethral lumen.

T1: Low signal intensity.

T2: High signal intensity. Stones within a diverticulum appear as low signal intensity foci.

Enhancement pattern: Granulation tissue associated with diverticulum may enhance, although diverticulum contents should not enhance. Gadolinium-enhanced images

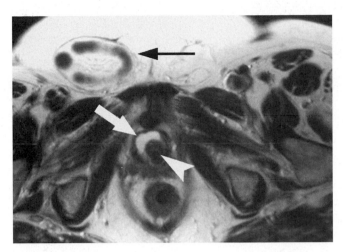

FIG. 3.99. Urethral diverticulum. Axial T2-weighted image through the lower pelvis demonstrates crescent-shaped fluid collection (*arrow*) around urethra (*arrowhead*). Note inguinal hernia containing small bowel (*thin arrow*).

performed with an endovaginal coil may also be helpful in more clearly defining the diverticulum neck.

Characteristic features: Cystic structure wrapped around the urethra is typical.

Distribution: Periurethral.

Atypical appearances: Diverticulum may completely surround urethra. High signal intensity may be present on T1-weighted images suggesting proteinaceous material within the diverticulum. Diverticulum may contain stones. Enhancing soft tissue mass associated with a urethral diverticulum should raise suspicion of associated carcinoma.

Associations: Carcinoma may arise in diverticulum. (Fig. 3.101)

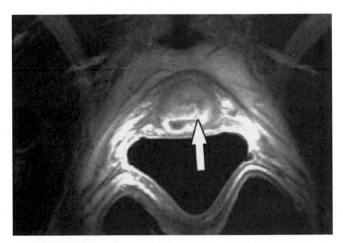

FIG. 3.100. Urethral diverticulum. Axial gadolinium-enhanced high-resolution T1-weighted image through urethra using endovaginal coil (inverted triangular signal void) demonstrates diverticulum neck (*arrow*).

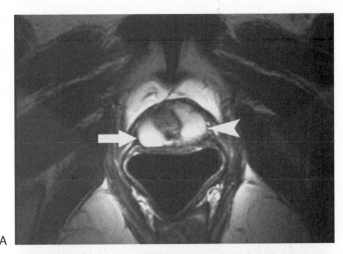

A

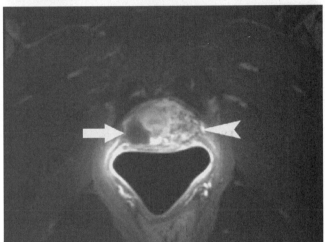

B

FIG. 3.101. Carcinoma within urethral diverticulum. **A:** Axial T2-weighted image through urethra performed with endovaginal coil shows high signal intensity urethral diverticulum (*arrow*). A high signal intensity mass (*arrowhead*) is present to the left of the urethra. **B:** Axial gadolinium-enhanced T1-weighted image at same level as **(A)** demonstrates low signal intensity urine (*arrow*) and enhancement of the mass (*arrowhead*).

Mimics: Ectopic ureterocele, Bartholin gland cyst, Gartner duct cyst.

References: 159, 160

Uterine Leiomyoma (Fibroid) (Figs. 3.102 to 3.106)

Description: Benign smooth muscle tumor commonly occurring in the uterus.

T1: Low to intermediate signal intensity relative to myometrium unless hemorrhage or fat are present. Calcifications appear as signal voids.

T2: Low signal intensity relative to the myometrium when uncomplicated by degeneration. A high signal intensity rim may be present.

Enhancement pattern: Variable. Tumors often enhance slightly less than or similar to myometrium, although brisk enhancement may also occur. Some degenerative

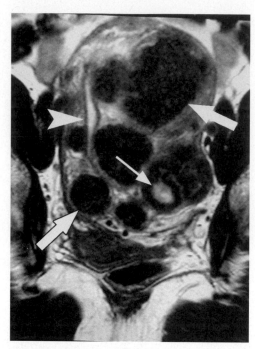

FIG. 3.102. Uterine leiomyomas. Coronal T2-weighted image through the pelvis demonstrates multiple low signal intensity intramural uterine leiomyomas (*arrows*) distorting the endometrium (*arrowhead*). One mass has undergone cystic degeneration (*thin arrow*).

leiomyomas show little or no enhancement after gadolinium injection.

Characteristic features: Clearly demarcated uterine mass of low or intermediate signal intensity on T1-weighted images and low signal intensity on T2-weighted images suggests leiomyoma. Leiomyomas greater than 3 cm in diameter commonly contain scattered foci of high signal intensity on T2-weighted images secondary to degeneration.

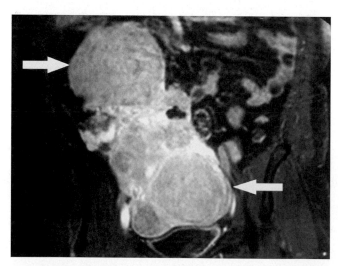

FIG. 3.103. Uterine leiomyomas. Coronal fat-suppressed, gadolinium-enhanced T1-weighted image shows significant enhancement of multiple leiomyomas (*arrows*).

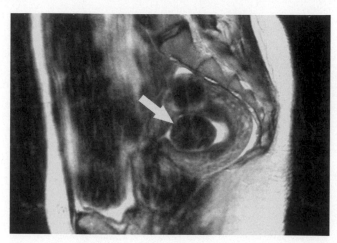

FIG. 3.104. Submucosal leiomyoma. Sagittal T2-weighted image shows submucosal fibroid (*arrow*) centered in the endometrial cavity.

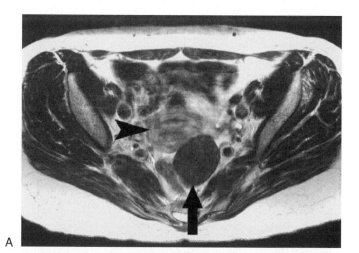

A

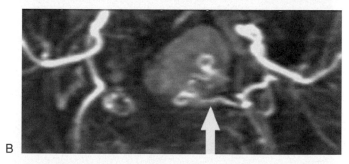

B

FIG. 3.105. Extrauterine leiomyoma. **A:** Axial T2-weighted image shows low-signal intensity mass (*arrow*) posterior to uterus (*arrowhead*). Differential diagnosis for lesion includes ovarian fibrothecoma. **B:** Maximum intensity projection reconstruction of arterial phase, three-dimensional, gadolinium-enhanced gradient echo sequence shows blood supply (*arrow*) to mass from uterine artery. At surgery, extrauterine fibroid arising from mesovarian soft tissues was found.

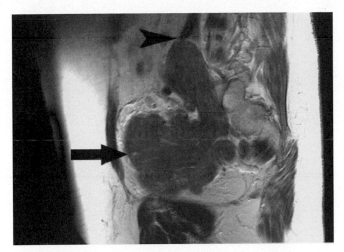

FIG. 3.106. Vascular invasive leiomyoma. Sagittal T2-weighted image demonstrates large low signal intensity mass (*arrow*) growing into inferior vena cava (*arrowhead*).

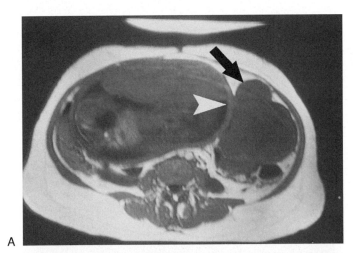

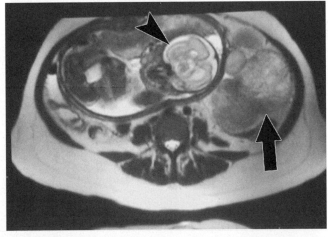

FIG. 3.107. Myxoid leiomyosarcoma. **A:** T1-weighted axial image of pregnant patient with size greater than dates shows a lobulated intermediate signal intensity mass (*arrow*) adjacent to the uterus (*arrowhead*). **B:** T2-weighted axial image shows mass (*arrow*) to have areas of high signal intensity. Arrowhead denotes fetal head. Resected specimen demonstrated invasion of surrounding fat by tumor.

Distribution: Frequently multiple. Tumor locations categorized as submucosal, intramural, subserosal, or cervical in location. May be pedunculated. Rarely, leiomyomas may occur outside of the uterus within the pelvis. Benign metastasizing leiomyoma may spread to remote areas of the body. Invasion of the pelvic veins occurs rarely.

Atypical appearances: Areas of hemorrhagic degeneration appear as high signal intensity on T1-weighted images. Areas of cystic, hyaline or myxoid degeneration appear as increased signal intensity on T2-weighted images. Pedunculated subserosal leiomyoma may simulate an ovarian mass, while submucosal leiomyoma may prolapse into the vagina. Subserosal leiomyomas may also undergo torsion. Lipoleiomyoma (very rare) contains fat that parallels fat elsewhere on all pulse sequences. Leiomyomas may very rarely demonstrate venous invasion. Sarcomatous transformation is rare but difficult to specifically detect with imaging unless tumor becomes invasive (tumor enlargement alone is nonspecific) (Fig. 3.107).

Mimics: Ovarian fibroma or fibrothecoma, focal adenomyosis, myometrial contraction.

Additional comments: Leiomyomas may enlarge during pregnancy (although growth is unpredictable) or with oral contraceptive use. They may regress after menopause. Well-vascularized, enhancing leiomyomas are more likely to respond to embolotherapy. Following successful embolization therapy, uterine leiomyomas should appear smaller and show reduced or absent enhancement on follow-up imaging. Subserosal fibroids may respond poorly to embolization in some cases because of parasitized or alternate blood supply.

References: 161, 162

MALE PELVIS

Benign Prostatic Hypertrophy (Fig. 3.108)

Description: Common proliferative disorder of the glandular and stromal elements of the transitional zone of the prostate.

T1: Low to intermediate signal intensity similar to normal prostatic tissue.

T2: Heterogeneous, intermediate to high signal intensity when hyperplasia of glandular elements predominates. Stromal hyperplasia may result in intermediate or decreased signal intensity on T2-weighted images. Cystic changes may be present in glandular benign prostatic hypertrophy (BPH).

Enhancement pattern: Gadolinium enhancement of BPH tends to be slower and more heterogeneous than prostate carcinoma.

Characteristic features: Heterogeneous high signal intensity nodules with peripheral hypointense rims on T2-weighted images are typical of glandular BPH. Small cystic component is common. When large, BPH compresses the peripheral zone or protrudes into the bladder base.

Distribution: Occurs in transitional and periurethral glandular zones.

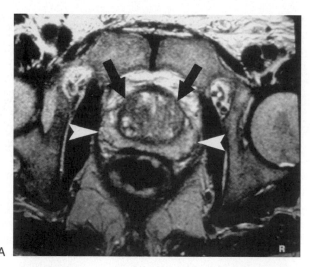

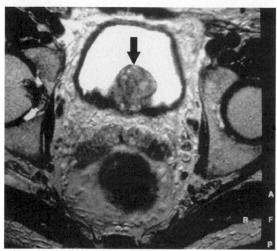

FIG. 3.108. Benign prostatic hypertrophy. **A:** High-resolution axial T2-weighted image through the lower pelvis demonstrates rounded, heterogeneous enlargement of the central gland of the prostate (*arrows*). Peripheral zone marked by arrowheads. **B:** More cephalad slice from same sequence as **(A)** shows hypertrophic central gland (*arrow*) protruding into bladder, an appearance that may be mistaken for primary bladder mass.

Atypical appearances: BPH may infiltrate the peripheral zone, mimicking prostate cancer.

Mimics: Centrally occurring prostate carcinoma.

References: 163 to 166

Cryptorchid Testis (Figs. 3.109, 3.110)

Description: Incomplete testicular descent into the scrotum resulting in an ectopic location of the testis.

T1: Parallels normal testis (intermediate signal intensity).

T2: Parallels normal testis (bright signal intensity).

Enhancement pattern: MR venography may demonstrate enhancing spermatic vessels, providing a clue as to the location of the testis.

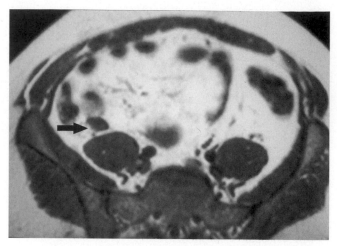

FIG. 3.109. Cryptorchid testis. Axial T1-weighted image at level of iliac wings demonstrates olive-shaped low signal intensity testis (*arrow*) anterior to right psoas muscle. (Courtesy of Neal Dalrymple, M.D.)

Characteristic features: The cryptorchid testis resembles a normal testis in signal intensity and morphology. Identification of the mediastinum testis may assist in correctly characterizing a cryptorchid testis.

Distribution: Most commonly located in the inguinal canal, but can be located anywhere along the normal route of descent from the retroperitoneum to the scrotum.

Atypical appearances: Undescended testis may be atrophic, with low signal intensity on T1- and T2-weighted sequences.

Associations: Abnormal spermatogenesis. Increased risk of testicular carcinoma. Patent processus vaginalis may result in hernia.

Mimics: Lymph node.

References: 167, 168

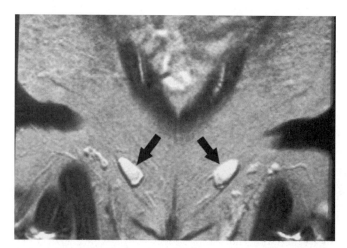

FIG. 3.110. Bilateral undescended testes. Coronal T2-weighted image through the inguinal canals show both testes (*arrows*) as high signal intensity ovoid structures.

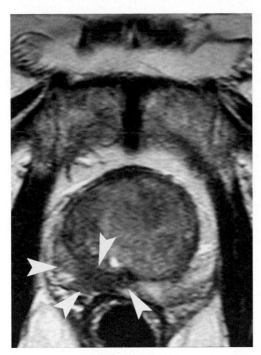

FIG. 3.111. Prostate carcinoma. Axial T2-weighted image demonstrates low signal intensity carcinoma (*arrowheads*) arising in normally high signal intensity peripheral zone of prostate.

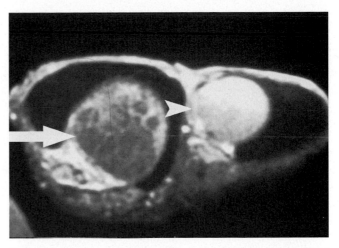

FIG. 3.112. Testicular cancer. Axial gadolinium-enhanced T1-weighted image through scrotum demonstrates enlargement of right testis containing mass (*arrow*), which enhances weakly compared with normal left testis (*arrowhead*). Bilateral hydroceles are present. (Courtesy of Neal Dalrymple, M.D.)

Prostate Carcinoma (Fig. 3.111; see Figs. 3.205, 3.206)

Description: Most common malignant tumor of the prostate.

T1: Isointense to peripheral zone.

T2: Hypointense to surrounding high signal intensity peripheral zone.

Enhancement pattern: Early, rapid enhancement. Increased enhancement relative to surrounding peripheral zone.

Characteristic features: Appears as a low signal intensity focus in the otherwise high signal intensity peripheral zone on T2-weighted images.

Distribution: The majority of prostate carcinomas arise in the peripheral zones (>70%), with significantly fewer arising in the transitional and central zones.

Atypical appearances: Tumors arising from the transitional or central zones may mimic BPH. Prostate carcinoma may rarely be increased in signal intensity or isointense to the peripheral zone on T2-weighted images. Cystic prostate carcinoma may occur, but is rare. Mucinous carcinoma of the prostate may appear as high signal intensity on T1-weighted images but is also quite rare.

Mimics: Chronic or granulomatous prostatitis, or postbiopsy hemorrhage may mimic prostate cancer (high signal intensity on T1-weighted images is common with hemorrhage but rare with prostate carcinoma). Amyloid deposits in the seminal vesicles may cause a decrease in signal intensity of the seminal vesicles on T2-weighted images, mimicking infiltration with carcinoma.

Additional comments: High signal intensity may be seen in the peripheral zone on T1- and T2-weighted images after prostate biopsy. Therefore, a waiting period of at least 3 weeks after biopsy is recommended before prostate MRI. MR spectroscopy will likely become routine for the evaluation of prostate cancer with MRI.

References: 169 to 171

Testicular Cancer (Figs. 3.112 to 3.114)

Description: Malignant tumor of the testis of either germ cell or stromal cell origin. Germ cell tumors include seminoma and nonseminomatous tumors such as embryonal cell

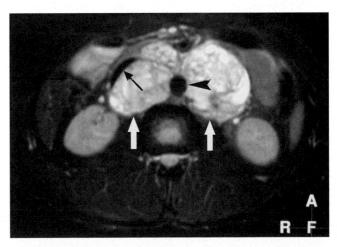

FIG. 3.113. Testicular cancer metastases, germ cell primary. Axial fat-suppressed T2-weighted image through the kidneys demonstrates multiple bulky, cystic-appearing lymph node metastases (*arrows*) surrounding the aorta (*arrowhead*) and displacing the inferior vena cava (*thin arrow*).

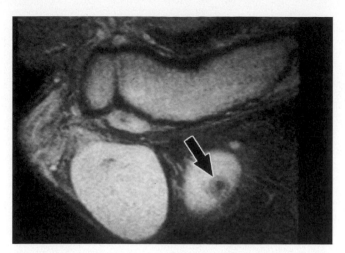

FIG. 3.114. Burned out testicular tumor. T2-weighted image through the scrotum demonstrates low signal intensity focus (*arrow*) within the left testis representing the nonviable remnant of a small testicular tumor.

carcinoma, yolk sac tumor, teratocarcinoma, and choriocarcinoma. Pure germ cell tumors are most commonly seminoma. However, germ cell tumors are commonly of mixed histology, especially when nonseminomatous. Stromal cell tumors include Leydig and Sertoli cell tumors.

T1: Tumor is most commonly isointense to testis. Nonseminomatous germ cell tumors may have high signal intensity foci related to hemorrhage.

T2: Tumor is most commonly hypointense to testis. Seminomas tend to be homogeneously hypointense and well defined. Nonseminomatous germ cell tumors tend to be more heterogeneous with high signal intensity foci related to necrosis or cystic areas.

Enhancement pattern: Cancers usually enhance less than normal testis after gadolinium administration.

Characteristic features: Most seminomas are well-defined, relatively homogeneous testicular masses. Nonseminomatous germ cell tumors tend to be more heterogeneous in signal intensity. Testicular cancer may enlarge the testis. Metastases to retroperitoneal nodes may have a multicystic appearance.

Distribution: Usually unilateral. Synchronous contralateral tumor may occur but is rare. The majority of bilateral tumors occur asynchronously. Tumor may invade spermatic cord or metastasize to lymph nodes, lung, brain, bone, and liver. The lymph node drainage pattern parallels the course of the gonadal veins, often resulting in nodal metastases to the left renal hilar region and right paracaval region before pelvic nodal metastases. Pelvic nodes become involved when local invasion is present. Invasion of gonadal and renal vein may occur.

Atypical appearances: A malignant testicular mass may rarely be isointense to normal testis. Seminoma very rarely appears as high signal intensity on T2-weighted images. Metastases from testicular cancer may be present with only

a small area of scar within the testis representing the primary tumor ("burned-out" or regressed tumor).

Associations: Cryptorchid testis, intersex syndromes, testicular microlithiasis (the extent of the association between microlithiasis and testicular carcinoma is controversial).

Mimics: Lymphoma (lymphoma usually manifests as homogeneous diffuse involvement of the testis), metastasis, orchitis, sarcoidosis, adrenal rests.

Additional comments: Seminomas tend to occur in older patients than nonseminomatous tumors. Approximately 20% of patients have retroperitoneal lymphadenopathy at presentation. Seminomas are radiosensitive and prognosis is generally good.

References: 172

REFERENCES

1. Elizondo G, Weissleder R, Stark DD, et al. Amebic liver abscess: diagnosis and treatment evaluation with MR imaging. *Radiology* 1987;165:795–800.
2. Ralls PW, Henley DS, Colletti PM, et al. Amebic liver abscess: MR imaging. *Radiology* 1987;165:801–804.
3. Semelka RC, Kelekis NL, Sallah S, et al. Hepatosplenic fungal disease: diagnostic accuracy and spectrum of appearances on MR imaging. *AJR* 1997;169:1311–1316.
4. Mendez RJ, Schiebler ML, Outwater EK, et al. Hepatic abscesses: MR imaging findings. *Radiology* 1994;190:431–436.
5. Balci NC, Semelka RC, Noone TC, et al. Pyogenic hepatic abscesses: MRI findings on T1- and T2-weighted and serial gadolinium-enhanced gradient-echo images. *J Magn Reson Imaging* 1999;9:285–290.
6. Chung KY, Mayo-Smith WW, Saini S, et al. Hepatocellular adenoma: MR imaging features with pathologic correlation. *AJR* 1995;165:303–308.
7. Grazioli L, Federle MP, Ichikawa T, et al. Liver adenomatosis: clinical, histopathologic, and imaging findings in 15 patients. *Radiology* 2000;216:395–402.
8. Koyama T, Fletcher JG, Johnson CD, et al. Primary hepatic angiosarcoma: findings at CT and MR imaging. *Radiology* 2002;222:667–673.
9. Mortele B, Mortele K, Seynaeve P, et al. Hepatic bile duct hamartomas (von Meyenburg complexes): MR and MR cholangiography findings. *J Comput Assist Tomogr* 2002;26:438–443.
10. Mortelé KJ, Ros PR. Cystic focal liver lesions in the adult: differential CT and MR imaging features. *Radiographics* 2001;21:895–910.
11. Worawattanakul S, Semelka RC, Noone TC, et al. Cholangiocarcinoma: spectrum of appearances on MR images using current techniques. *J Magn Reson Imaging* 1998;16:993–1003.
12. Maetani Y, Itoh K, Watanabe C, et al. MR imaging of intrahepatic cholangiocarcinoma with pathologic correlation. *AJR* 2001;176:1499–1507.
13. Matos C, Nicaise N, Deviere J, et al. Choledochal cysts: comparison of findings at MR cholangiopancreatography and endoscopic retrograde cholangiopancreatography in eight patients. *Radiology* 1998;209:443–448.
14. Kim SH, Lim JH, Yoon HK, et al. Choledochal cyst: comparison of MR and conventional cholangiography. *Clin Radiol* 2000;55:378–383.
15. Govil S, Justus A, Korah I, et al. Choledochal cysts: evaluation with MR cholangiography. *Abdom Imaging* 1998;23:616–619.
16. Ohtomo K, Baron RL, Dodd GD III, et al. Confluent hepatic fibrosis in advanced cirrhosis: evaluation with MR imaging. *Radiology* 1993;189:871–874.
17. Vitellas KM, Tzalonikou MT, Bennett WF, et al. Cirrhosis: spectrum of findings on unenhanced and dynamic gadolinium-enhanced MR imaging. *Abdom Imaging* 2001;26:601–615.
18. Krinsky GA, Lee VS. MR imaging of cirrhotic nodules. *Abdom Imaging* 2000;25:471–482.
19. Krinsky GA, Lee VS, Nguyen MT, et al. Siderotic nodules at MR imaging: regenerative or dysplastic? *J Comput Assist Tomogr* 2000;24:773–776.

20. Buetow PC, Buck JL, Pantongrag-Brown L, et al. Undifferentiated (embryonal) sarcoma of the liver: pathologic basis of imaging findings in 28 cases. *Radiology* 1997;203:779–783.

21. Siegelman ES, Rosen MA. Imaging of hepatic steatosis. *Semin Liver Dis* 2001;21:71–80.

22. Ichikawa T, Federle MP, Grazioli L, et al. Fibrolamellar hepatocellular carcinoma: imaging and pathologic findings in 31 recent cases. *Radiology* 1999;213:352–361.

23. Ba-Ssalamah A, Schima W, Schmook MT, et al. Atypical focal nodular hyperplasia of the liver: imaging features of nonspecific and liver-specific MR contrast agents. *AJR* 2002;179:1447–1456.

24. Paley MR, Mergo PJ, Torres GM, et al. Characterization of focal hepatic lesions with ferumoxides-enhanced T2-weighted MR imaging. *AJR* 2000;175:159–163.

25. Vilgrain V, Boulos L, Vullierme MP, et al. Imaging of atypical hemangiomas of the liver with pathologic correlation. *Radiographics* 2000;20:379–397.

26. Coumbaras M, Wendum D, Monnier-Cholley L, et al. CT and MR imaging features of pathologically proven atypical giant hemangiomas of the liver. *AJR* 2002;179:1457–1463.

27. Kadoya M, Matsui O, Takashima T, et al. Hepatocellular carcinoma: correlation of MR imaging and histopathologic findings. *Radiology* 1992;183:819–825.

28. Kelekis NL, Semelka RC, Worawattanakul S, et al. Hepatocellular carcinoma in North America: a multiinstitutional study of appearance on T1-weighted, T2-weighted, and serial gadolinium-enhanced gradient-echo images. *AJR* 1998;170:1005–1013.

29. Baron RL, Peterson MS. Screening the cirrhotic liver for hepatocellular carcinoma with CT and MR imaging: opportunities and pitfalls. *Radiographics* 2001;21:S117–S132.

30. Kelekis NL, Semelka RC, Siegelman ES, et al. Focal hepatic lymphoma: magnetic resonance demonstration using current techniques including gadolinium enhancement. *Magn Reson Imaging* 1997;15:625–636.

31. Sica GT, Ji H, Ros PR. CT and MR imaging of hepatic metastases. *AJR* 2000;174:691–698.

32. Ohtomo K, Itai Y, Ohtomo Y, et al. Regenerating nodules of liver cirrhosis: MR imaging with pathologic correlation. *AJR* 1990;154:505–507.

33. Murakami T, Kuroda C, Marukawa T, et al. Regenerating nodules of hepatic cirrhosis: MR findings with pathologic correlation. *AJR* 1990;155:1227–1231.

34. Kim T, Baron RL, Nalesnik MA. Infarcted regenerative nodules in cirrhosis: CT and MR imaging findings with pathologic correlation. *AJR* 2000;175:1121–1125.

35. Krinsky GA, Lee VS, Nguyen MT, et al. Siderotic nodules in the cirrhotic liver at MR imaging with explant correlation: no increased frequency of dysplastic nodules and hepatocellular carcinoma. *Radiology* 2001;218:47–53.

36. Dodd GD III, Baron RL, Oliver JH III, et al. Spectrum of imaging findings of the liver in end-stage cirrhosis: part I, gross morphology and diffuse abnormalities. *AJR* 1999;173:1031–1036.

37. Dodd GD III, Baron RL, Oliver JH III, et al. Spectrum of imaging findings of the liver in end-stage cirrhosis: part II, focal abnormalities. *AJR* 1999;173:1185–1192.

38. Jeong YY, Mitchell DG, Kamishima T. Small (<20 mm) enhancing hepatic nodules seen on arterial phase MR imaging of the cirrhotic liver: clinical implications. *AJR* 2002;178:1327–1334.

39. Siegelman ES, Rosen MA. Imaging of hepatic steatosis. *Semin Liver Dis* 2001;21:71–80.

40. Vilgrain V, Lewin M, Vons C, et al. Hepatic nodules in Budd-Chiari syndrome: imaging features. *Radiology* 1999;210:443–450.

41. Noone TC, Semelka RC, Siegelman ES, et al. Budd-Chiari syndrome: spectrum of appearances of acute, subacute, and chronic disease with magnetic resonance imaging. *J Magn Reson Imaging* 2000;11:44–50.

42. Brancatelli G, Federle MP, Grazioli L, et al. Large regenerative nodules in Budd-Chiari syndrome and other vascular disorders of the liver: CT and MR imaging findings with clinicopathologic correlation. *AJR* 2002;178:877–883.

43. Siegelman ES, Mitchell DG, Semelka RC. Abdominal iron deposition: metabolism, MR findings, and clinical importance. *Radiology* 1996;199:13–22.

44. Schlund JF, Semelka RC, Kettritz, et al. Transient increased segmental hepatic enhancement distal to portal vein obstruction on dynamic gadolinium-enhanced gradient echo MR images. *J Magn Reson Imaging* 1995;5:375–377.

45. Ito K, Mitchell DG, Outwater EK, et al. Primary sclerosing cholangitis: MR imaging features. *AJR* 1999;172:1527–1533.

46. Revelon G, Rashid A, Kawamoto S, et al. Primary sclerosing cholangitis: MR imaging findings with pathologic correlation. *AJR* 1999;173:1037–1042.

47. Dodd GD III, Baron RL, Oliver JH, et al. End-stage primary sclerosing cholangitis: CT findings of hepatic morphology in 36 patients. *Radiology* 1999;211:357–362.

48. Warshauer DM, Semelka RC, Ascher SM. Nodular sarcoidosis of the liver and spleen: appearance on MR images. *J Magn Reson Imaging* 1994;4:553–557.

49. Yoshimitsu K, Honda H, Jimi M, et al. MR diagnosis of adenomyomatosis of the gallbladder and differentiation from gallbladder carcinoma: importance of showing Rokitansky-Aschoff sinuses. *AJR* 1999;172:1535–1540.

50. Yoshimitsu K, Honda H, Aibe H, et al. Radiologic diagnosis of adenomyomatosis of the gallbladder: comparative study among MRI, helical CT, and transabdominal US. *J Comput Assist Tomogr* 2001;25:843–850.

51. Loud PA, Semelka RC, Kettritz U, et al. MRI of acute cholecystitis: comparison with the normal gallbladder and other entities. *Magn Reson Imaging* 1996;14:349–355.

52. Hakansson K, Leander P, Ekberg O, et al. MR imaging in clinically suspected acute cholecystitis. A comparison with ultrasonography. *Acta Radiol* 2000;41:322–328.

53. Ukaji M, Ebara M, Tsuchiya Y, et al. Diagnosis of gallstone composition in magnetic resonance imaging: in vitro analysis. *Eur J Radiol* 2002;41:49–56.

54. Schwartz LH, Black J, Fong Y, et al. Gallbladder carcinoma: findings at MR imaging with MR cholangiopancreatography. *J Comput Assist Tomogr* 2002;26:405–410.

55. Tseng JH, Wan YL, Hung CF, et al. Diagnosis and staging of gallbladder carcinoma. Evaluation with dynamic MR imaging. *Clin Imaging* 2002;26:177–182.

56. Urrutia M, Mergo PJ, Ros LH, et al. Cystic masses of the spleen: radiologic-pathologic correlation. *Radiographics* 1996;16:107–129.

57. Minami M, Itai Y, Ohtomo K, et al. Siderotic nodules in the spleen: MR imaging of portal hypertension. *Radiology* 1989;172:681–684.

58. Sagoh T, Itoh K, Togashi K, et al. Gamna-Gandy bodies of the spleen: evaluation with MR imaging. *Radiology* 1989;172:685–687.

59. Ramani M, Reinhold C, Semelka RC, et al. Splenic hemangiomas and hamartomas: MR imaging characteristics of 28 lesions. *Radiology* 1997;202:166–172.

60. Weissleder R, Elizondo G, Stark DD, et al. The diagnosis of splenic lymphoma by MR imaging: value of superparamagnetic iron oxide. *AJR* 1989;152:175–180.

61. Ito K, Murata T, Nakanishi T. Cystic lymphangioma of the spleen: MR findings with pathologic correlation. *Abdom Imaging* 1995;20:82–84.

62. Hahn PF, Weissleder R, Stark DD, et al. MR imaging of focal splenic tumors. *AJR* 1988;150:823–827.

63. Mirowitz SA, Brown JJ, Lee JK, et al. Dynamic gadolinium-enhanced MR imaging of the spleen: normal enhancement patterns and evaluation of splenic lesions. *Radiology* 1991;179:681–686.

64. Kaneko K, Onitsuka H, Murakami J, et al. MRI of primary spleen angiosarcoma with iron accumulation. *J Comput Assist Tomogr* 1992;16:298–300.

65. Falk S, Krishnan J, Meis JM. Primary angiosarcoma of the spleen. A clinicopathologic study of 40 cases. *Am J Surg Pathol* 1993;17:959–970.

66. Rabushka LS, Kawashima A, Fishman E. Imaging of the spleen: CT with supplemental MR examination. *Radiographics* 1994;14:307–332.

67. Ha HK, Kim HH, Kim BK, et al. Primary angiosarcoma of the spleen. CT and MR imaging. *Acta Radiol* 1994;35:455–458.

68. Piironen A. Severe acute pancreatitis: contrast-enhanced CT and MRI features. *Abdom Imaging* 2001;26:225–233.

69. Merkle EM, Gorich J. Imaging of acute pancreatitis. *Eur J Radiol* 2002;12:1979–1992.
70. Lopez Hänninen E, Amthauer H, Hosten N, et al. Prospective evaluation of pancreatic tumors: accuracy of MR imaging with MR cholangiopancreatography and MR angiography. *Radiology* 2002;224:34–41.
71. Irie H, Honda H, Baba S, et al. Autoimmune pancreatitis: CT and MR characteristics. *AJR* 1998;170:1323–1327.
72. Kim T, Murakami T, Takamura M, et al. Pancreatic mass due to chronic pancreatitis: correlation of CT and MR imaging features with pathologic findings. *AJR* 2001;177:367–371.
73. Johnson PT, Outwater EK. Pancreatic carcinoma versus chronic pancreatitis: dynamic MR imaging. *Radiology* 1999;212:213–218.
74. Usuki N, Okabe Y, Miyamoto T. Intraductal mucin-producing tumor of the pancreas: diagnosis by MR cholangiopancreatography. *J Comput Assist Tomogr* 1998;22:875–879.
75. Silas AM, Morrin MM, Raptopoulos V, et al. Intraductal papillary mucinous tumors of the pancreas. *AJR* 2001;176:179–185.
76. Maire F, Hammel P, Terris B, et al. Intraductal papillary and mucinous pancreatic tumour: a new extracolonic tumour in familial adenomatous polyposis. *Gut* 2002;51:446–449.
77. Thoeni RF, Mueller-Lisse UG, Chan R. Detection of small, functional islet cell tumors in the pancreas: selection of MR imaging sequences for optimal sensitivity. *Radiology* 2000;214:483–490.
78. Ichikawa T, Peterson MS, Federle MP, et al. Islet cell tumor of the pancreas: biphasic CT versus MR imaging in tumor detection. *Radiology* 2000;216:163–171.
79. Owen NJ, Sohaib SA, Peppercorn PD, et al. MRI of pancreatic neuroendocrine tumours. *Br J Radiol* 2001;74:968–973.
80. Buetow PC, Rao P, Thompson LD. From the archives of the AFIP. Mucinous cystic neoplasms of the pancreas: radiologic-pathologic correlation. *Radiographics* 1998;18:433–449.
81. Grogan JR, Saeian K, Taylor A, et al. Making sense of mucin-producing pancreatic tumors. *AJR* 2001;176:921–929.
82. Compton CC. Serous cystic tumors of the pancreas. *Semin Diagn Pathol* 2000;17:43–55.
83. Buetow PC, Buck JL, Pantongrag-Brown L, et al. Solid and papillary epithelial neoplasm of the pancreas: imaging-pathologic correlation on 56 cases. *Radiology* 1996;199:707–711.
84. Mitchell DG, Crovello M, Matteucci T, et al. Benign adrenocortical masses: diagnosis with chemical shift MR imaging. *Radiology* 1992;185:345–351.
85. Heinz-Peer G, Honigschnabl S, Schneider B, et al. Characterization of adrenal masses using MR imaging with histopathologic correlation. *AJR* 1999;173:15–22.
86. Mayo-Smith WW, Boland GW, Noto RB, et al. State-of-the-art adrenal imaging. *Radiographics* 2001;21:995–1012.
87. Chung JJ, Semelka RC, Martin DR. Adrenal adenomas: characteristic postgadolinium capillary blush on dynamic MR imaging. *J Magn Reson Imaging* 2001;13:242–248.
88. Schlund JF, Kenney PJ, Brown ED, et al. Adrenocortical carcinoma: MR imaging appearance with current techniques. *J Magn Reson Imaging* 1995;5:171–174.
89. Otal P, Escourrou G, Mazerolles C, et al. Imaging features of uncommon adrenal masses with histopathologic correlation. *Radiographics* 1999;19:569–581.
90. Hamrick-Turner JE, Cranston PE, Shipkey FH. Cavernous hemangiomas of the adrenal glands: MR findings. *Magn Reson Imaging* 1994;12:1263–1267.
91. Ichikawa T, Ohtomo K, Uchiyama G, et al. Contrast-enhanced dynamic MRI of adrenal masses: classification of characteristic enhancement patterns. *Clin Radiol* 1995;50:295–300.
92. Rao P, Kenney PJ, Wagner BJ, et al. Imaging and pathologic features of myelolipoma. *Radiographics* 1997;17:1373–1385.
93. Radin R, David CL, Goldfarb H, et al. Adrenal and extra-adrenal retroperitoneal ganglioneuroma: imaging findings in 13 adults. *Radiology* 1997;202:703–707.
94. Rha SE, Byun JY, Jung SE, et al. Neurogenic tumors in the abdomen: tumor types and imaging characteristics. *Radiographics* 2003;23:29–43.
95. Krebs TL, Wagner BJ. MR imaging of the adrenal gland: radiologic-pathologic correlation. *Radiographics* 1998;18:1425–1440.
96. Jinzaki M, Tanimoto A, Narimatsu Y, et al. Angiomyolipoma: imaging findings in lesions with minimal fat. *Radiology* 1997;205:497–502.
97. Pickhardt PJ, Siegel CL, McLarney JK. Collecting duct carcinoma of the kidney: are imaging findings suggestive of the diagnosis? *AJR* 2001;176:627–633.
98. Balci NC, Semelka RC, Patt RH, et al. Complex renal cysts: findings on MR imaging. *AJR* 1999;172:1495–1500.
99. Kim SH, Park JH, Han JK, et al. Infarction of the kidney: role of contrast enhanced MRI. *J Comput Assist Tomogr* 1992;16:924–928.
100. Choo SW, Kim SH, Jeong YG, et al. MR imaging of segmental renal infarction: an experimental study. *Clin Radiol* 1997;52:65–68.
101. Chen M, Lipson SA, Hricak H. MR imaging evaluation of benign mesenchymal tumors of the urinary bladder. *AJR* 1997;168:399–403.
102. Semelka RC, Kelekis NL, Burdeny DA, et al. Renal lymphoma: demonstration by MR imaging. *AJR* 1996;166:823–827.
103. Dikengil A, Benson M, Sanders L, et al. MRI of multilocular cystic nephroma. *Urol Radiol* 1988;10:95–99.
104. Kettritz U, Semelka RC, Siegelman ES, et al. Multilocular cystic nephroma: MR imaging appearance with current techniques, including gadolinium enhancement. *J Magn Reson Imaging* 1996;6:145–148.
105. Harmon WJ, King BF, Lieber MM. Renal oncocytoma: magnetic resonance imaging characteristics. *J Urol* 1996;155:863–867.
106. Newhouse JH, Wagner BJ. Renal oncocytomas. *Abdom Imaging* 1998;23:249–255.
107. Poustchi-Amin M, Leonidas JC, Palestro C, et al. Magnetic resonance imaging in acute pyelonephritis. *Pediatr Nephrol* 1998;12:579–580.
108. Lonergan GJ, Pennington DJ, Morrison JC, et al. Childhood pyelonephritis: comparison of gadolinium-enhanced MR imaging and renal cortical scintigraphy for diagnosis. *Radiology* 1998;207:377–384.
109. Outwater EK, Bhatia M, Siegelman ES, et al. Lipid in renal clear cell carcinoma: detection on opposed phase gradient-echo MR images. *Radiology* 1997;205:103–107.
110. Barentsz JO, Ruijs SH, Strijk SP. The role of MR imaging in carcinoma of the urinary bladder. *AJR* 1993;160:937–947.
111. Weeks SM, Brown ED, Brown JJ, et al. Transitional cell carcinoma of the upper urinary tract: staging by MRI. *Abdom Imaging* 1995;20:365–367.
112. Barentsz JO, Jager GJ, van Vierzen PB, et al. Staging urinary bladder cancer after transurethral biopsy: value of fast dynamic contrast-enhanced MR imaging. *Radiology* 1996;201:185–193.
113. Tekes A, Kamel IR, Imam K, et al. MR imaging features of transitional cell carcinoma of the urinary bladder. *AJR* 2003;180:771–777.
114. Mulopulos GP, Patel SK, Pessis D. MR imaging of xanthogranulomatous pyelonephritis. *J Comput Assist Tomogr* 1986;10:154–156.
115. Verswijvel G, Oyen R, Van Poppel H. Xanthogranulomatous pyelonephritis: MRI findings in the diffuse and focal type. *Eur Radiol* 2000;10:586–589.
116. Cohen JM, Weinreb JC, Maravilla KR. Fluid collections in the intraperitoneal and extraperitoneal spaces: comparison of MR and CT. *Radiology* 1985;155:705–708.
117. Irsutti M, Paul JL, Selves J, et al. Castleman disease: CT and MR imaging features of a retroperitoneal location in association with paraneoplastic pemphigus. *Eur Radiol* 1999;9:1219–1221.
118. Aygun C, Tekin MI, Demirhan B, et al. A case of incidentally detected Castleman's disease with retroperitoneal paravertebral localization. *Int J Urol* 2000;7:22–25.
119. Kim TJ, Han JK, Kim YH, et al. Castleman disease of the abdomen: imaging spectrum and clinicopathologic correlations. *J Comput Assist Tomogr* 2001;25:207–214.
120. Healy JC, Reznek RH, Clark SK, et al. MR appearances of desmoid tumors in familial adenomatous polyposis. *AJR* 1997;169:465–472.
121. Shields CJ, Winter DC, Kirwan WO, et al. Desmoid tumors. *Eur J Surg Oncol* 2001;27:701–706.
122. Chou CK, Liu GC, Chen LT, et al. MRI demonstration of peritoneal implants. *Abdom Imaging* 1994;19:95–101.
123. Low RN, Barone RM, Lacey C, et al. Peritoneal tumor: MR imaging with dilute oral barium and intravenous gadolinium-containing contrast agents compared with unenhanced MR imaging and CT. *Radiology* 1997;204:513–520.
124. Mulligan SA, Holley HC, Koehler RE, et al. CT and MR imaging in the evaluation of retroperitoneal fibrosis. *J Comput Assist Tomogr* 1989;13:277–281.
125. Arrive L, Hricak H, Tavares NJ, et al. Malignant versus nonmalignant

retroperitoneal fibrosis: differentiation with MR imaging. *Radiology* 1989;172:139–143.

126. Vivas I, Nicolas AI, Velazquez P, et al. Retroperitoneal fibrosis: typical and atypical manifestations. *Br J Radiol* 2000;73:214–222.

127. Reinhold C, Tafazoli F, Mehio A, et al. Uterine adenomyosis: endovaginal US and MR imaging features with histopathologic correlation. *Radiographics* 1999;19:S147–S160.

128. Byun JY, Kim SE, Choi BG, et al. Diffuse and focal adenomyosis: MR imaging findings. *Radiographics* 1999;19:S161–S170.

129. Siegelman ES, Outwater EK, Banner MP, et al. High-resolution MR imaging of the vagina. *Radiographics* 1997;17:1183–1203.

130. Outwater EK, Siegelman ES, Kim B, et al. Ovarian Brenner tumors: MR imaging characteristics. *J Magn Reson Imaging* 1998;16:1147–1153.

131. Moon WJ, Koh BH, Kim SK, et al. Brenner tumor of the ovary: CT and MR findings. *J Comput Assist Tomogr* 2000;24:72–76.

132. Hricak H, Lacey CG, Sandles LG, et al. Invasive cervical carcinoma: comparison of MR imaging and surgical findings. *Radiology* 1988;166:623–631.

133. Weber TM, Sostman HD, Spritzer CE, et al. Cervical carcinoma: determination of recurrent tumor extent versus radiation changes with MR imaging. *Radiology* 1995;194:135–139.

134. Nicolet V, Carignan L, Bourdon F, et al. MR imaging of cervical carcinoma: a practical staging approach. *Radiographics* 2000;20:1539–1549.

135. Hricak H, Stern JL, Fisher MR, et al. Endometrial carcinoma staging by MR imaging *Radiology* 1987;162:297–305.

136. Frei KA, Kinkel K. Staging endometrial cancer: role of magnetic resonance imaging. *J Magn Reson Imaging* 2001;13:850–855.

137. Ascher SM, Reinhold C. Imaging of cancer of the endometrium. *Radiol Clin North Am* 2002;40:563–576.

138. Ascher SM, Johnson JC, Barnes WA, et al. MR imaging appearance of the uterus in postmenopausal women receiving tamoxifen therapy for breast cancer: histopathologic correlation. *Radiology* 1996;200:105–110.

139. Nalaboff KM, Pellerito JS, Ben-Levi E. Imaging the endometrium: disease and normal variants. *Radiographics* 2001;21:1409–1424.

140. Brown JJ, Thurnher S, Hricak H. MR imaging of the uterus: low-signal-intensity abnormalities of the endometrium and endometrial cavity. *J Magn Reson Imaging* 1990;8:309–313.

141. Grasel RP, Outwater EK, Siegelman ES, et al. Endometrial polyps: MR imaging features and distinction from endometrial carcinoma. *Radiology* 2000;214:47–52.

142. Gougoutas CA, Siegelman ES, Hunt J, et al. Pelvic endometriosis: various manifestations and MR imaging findings. *AJR* 2000;175:353–358.

143. Outwater EK, Siegelman ES, Chiowanich P, et al. Dilated fallopian tubes: MR imaging characteristics. *Radiology* 1998;208:463–469.

144. Yamashita Y, Hatanaka Y, Torashima M, et al. Mature cystic teratomas of the ovary without fat in the cystic cavity. *AJR* 1994;163:613–616.

145. Yamashita Y, Hatanaka Y, Takahashi M, et al. Struma ovarii: MR appearances. *Abdom Imaging* 1997;22:100–102.

146. Kido A, Togashi K, Konishi I, et al. Dermoid cysts of the ovary with malignant transformation. *AJR* 1999;172:445–449.

147. Outwater EK, Siegelman ES, Hunt JL. Ovarian teratomas: tumor types and imaging characteristics. *Radiographics* 2001;21:475–490.

148. Li H, Sugimura K, Yoshida M, et al. Markedly high signal intensity lesions in the uterine cervix on T2-weighted imaging: differentiation between mucin-producing carcinomas and nabothian cysts. *Radiat Med* 1999;17:137–143.

149. Yamashita Y, Takahashi M, Katabuchi H, et al. Adenoma malignum: MR appearances mimicking nabothian cysts. *AJR* 1994;162:649–650.

150. Ha HK, Baek SY, Kim SH, et al. Krukenberg's tumor of the ovary: MR imaging features. *AJR* 1995;164:1435–1439.

151. Yamashita Y, Hatanaka Y, Torashima M, et al. Characterization of sonographically indeterminate ovarian tumors with MR imaging—a logistic regression analysis. *Acta Radiol* 1997;38:572–577.

152. Outwater EK, Mitchell DG. Normal ovaries and functional cysts: MR appearance. *Radiology* 1996;198:397–402.

153. Troiano RN, Lazzarini KM, Scoutt LM, et al. Fibroma and fibrothecoma of the ovary: MR imaging findings. *Radiology* 1997;204:795–798.

154. Ueda J, Furukawa T, Higashino K, et al. Ovarian fibroma of high signal intensity on T2-weighted MR image. *Abdom Imaging* 1998;23:657–658.

155. Kinoshita T, Ishii K, Naganuma H, et al. MR findings of ovarian tumours with cystic components. *Br J Radiol* 2000;73:333–339.

156. Jung SE, Lee JM, Rha SE, et al. CT and MR imaging of ovarian tumors with emphasis on differential diagnosis. *Radiographics* 2002;22:1305–1325.

157. Ghossain MA, Buy JN, Ligneres C, et al. Epithelial tumors of the ovary: comparison of MR and CT findings. *Radiology* 1991;181:863–870.

158. Kimura I, Togashi K, Kawakami S, et al. Polycystic ovaries: implications of diagnosis with MR imaging. *Radiology* 1996;201:549–552.

159. Kim B, Hricak H, Tanagho EA. Diagnosis of urethral diverticula in women: value of MR imaging. *AJR* 1993;161:809–815.

160. Blander DS, Rovner ES, Schnall MD, et al. Endoluminal magnetic resonance imaging in the evaluation of urethral diverticula in women. *Urology* 2001;57:660–665.

161. Murase E, Siegelman ES, Outwater EK, et al. Uterine leiomyomas: histopathologic features, MR imaging findings, differential diagnosis, and treatment. *Radiographics* 1999;19:1179–1197.

162. Ueda H, Togashi K, Konishi I, et al. Unusual appearances of uterine leiomyomas: MR imaging findings and their histopathologic backgrounds. *Radiographics* 1999;19:S131–S145.

163. Schiebler ML, Tomaszewski JE, Bezzi M, et al. Prostate carcinoma and benign prostatic hyperplasia: correlation of high-resolution MR and histopathologic findings. *Radiology* 1989;172:131–137.

164. Way WG, Brown JJ, Lee JK, et al. MR imaging of benign prostatic hypertrophy using a Helmholtz-type surface coil. *Magn Reson Imaging* 1992;10:341–349.

165. Lovett K, Rifkin MD, McCue PA, et al. MR imaging characteristics of noncancerous lesions of the prostate. *Magn Reson Imaging* 1992;2:35–39.

166. Ishida J, Sugimura K, Okizuka H, et al. Benign prostatic hyperplasia: value of MR imaging for determining histologic type. *Radiology* 1994;190:329–331.

167. Nguyen HT, Coakley F, Hricak H. Cryptorchidism: strategies in detection. *Eur Radiol* 1999;9:336–343.

168. Lam WW, Tam PK, Ai VH, et al. Using gadolinium-infusion venography to show the impalpable testis in pediatric patients. *AJR* 2001;176:1221–1226.

169. Mirowitz SA, Brown JJ, Heiken JP. Evaluation of the prostate and prostatic carcinoma with gadolinium-enhanced endorectal coil MR imaging. *Radiology* 1993;186:153–157.

170. Jager GJ, Ruijter ET, van de Kaa CA, et al. Dynamic TurboFLASH subtraction technique for contrast-enhanced MR imaging of the prostate: correlation with histopathologic results. *Radiology* 1997;203:645–652.

171. Bartolozzi C, Crocetti L, Menchi I, et al. Endorectal magnetic resonance imaging in local staging of prostate carcinoma. *Abdom Imaging* 2001;26:111–122.

172. Woodward PJ, Sohaey R, O'Donohue MJ, et al. From the archives of the AFIP: tumors and tumorlike lesions of the testis: radiologic-pathologic correlation. *Radiographics* 2002;22:189–216.

SECTION 3.3

Differential Diagnoses for Abdominal and Pelvic Magnetic Resonance Imaging

Successful implementation of abdominal and pelvic magnetic resonance imaging (MRI) consists of the following steps: creation of high-quality images, detection of significant abnormalities, and development of a meaningful differential diagnosis. This section concentrates on the third step–development of a meaningful differential diagnosis. The lists of differential diagnoses that follow reflect commonly encountered or particularly challenging clinical scenarios. With each entity listed, one or more brief differentiating features are provided to assist in narrowing the differential diagnosis. Also included are lists that are not differential diagnoses per se, but rather provide concise information on related clinical entities (e.g., syndromes). Not listed are some very rare entities and highly unusual manifestations of more common diseases. Therefore, the information presented here cannot be considered a substitute for a thorough search of the imaging literature.

PSEUDOTUMORS OF THE ABDOMEN AND PELVIS

Focal fat and fatty sparing—Focal fatty infiltration is common in the liver and may mimic a focal mass (see Fig. 3.18). Multifocal fatty infiltration may simulate hepatic metastases. Focal fatty sparing in an otherwise diffusely fatty infiltrated liver may also appear round and masslike (Fig. 3.115). Focal fat may also mimic a mass in the pancreas (Fig. 3.116). These entities are readily characterized on in-phase and opposed-phase imaging (the fatty areas lose signal on opposed-phase images). Contrast enhancement of infiltrated areas usually parallels that of normal parenchyma. Some tumors also contain intracellular lipid and may simulate focal fat.

Transient hepatic intensity difference (THID)—Increased enhancement of a hepatic segment or lobe during the arterial phase of enhancement. This enhancement usually fades to approach that of normal liver on portal venous and equilibrium phase images. THID is caused by a regional reduction of portal flow with compensatory increased arterial flow to the involved segment or lobe. THID is often seen in the absence of any identifiable cause but should prompt careful scrutiny of the images for associated tumor or vascular abnormality.

Duodenal diverticulum (Fig 3.117)—Common cause of pancreatic head pseudotumor. The presence of air or an air-fluid level within the lesion and continuity with the duodenal lumen are helpful differentiating features.

Gastric diverticulum (Fig 3.118)—Common cause of adrenal pseudotumor. The presence of air within the lesion or continuity with the gastric fundus should suggest this entity.

Varices (Fig. 3.119)—Common cause of adrenal, gastric, or esophageal pseudotumor. Varices occur in the setting of portal hypertension, are tubular, and parallel the veins in signal intensity after intravenous gadolinium administration.

Plane-dependent adrenal pseudotumor (Fig. 3.120)—Imaging through the broad, flat portion of a normal adrenal gland may create the appearance of a mass lesion.

Accessory spleen (Fig. 3.121)—Accessory spleens, or splenules, may mimic adrenal, pancreatic, or peritoneal tumors. Accessory splenic tissue parallels normal spleen on unenhanced and contrast-enhanced MR images. Splenules show decreased signal on T2- and T2*-weighted images after ferumoxides administration due to the presence of reticuloendothelial system cells.

Phase ghost (Figs. 3.122, 3.123)—Common cause of liver (usually left lateral lobe), pancreatic, and vertebral pseudotumor. Occurs in the phase-encoding direction of the image and lines up with offending structure (e.g., aorta). Multiple ghosts of alternating high and low signal intensity should be sought. The appearance of phase ghosts is usually sufficiently typical to exclude a true lesion. Rarely, a true lesion of the left hepatic lobe may appear similar to a phase ghost from the aorta (see Fig. 3.123). The absence of additional ghosts elsewhere in the plane of the aorta should arouse suspicion. Swapping the phase and frequency directions on a repeat scan confirms the nature of the lesion (a true lesion persists in the same location).

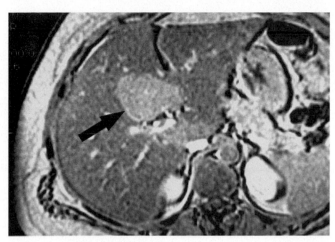

FIG. 3.115. Focal fatty sparing. Gadolinium-enhanced opposed-phase gradient echo image demonstrates masslike area of focal fatty sparing (*arrow*) in central portion of liver. Liver was homogeneous on all other sequences (not shown).

FAT- OR LIPID-CONTAINING LESIONS OF THE ABDOMEN AND PELVIS

Adrenal adenoma (see Fig. 3.63)—Intracellular lipid is best demonstrated on in-phase and opposed-phase images.

Adrenal cortical carcinoma—Lipid-rich cells may be present, but the large and often necrotic appearance of the majority of these tumors makes confusion with benign adenoma unlikely.

Adrenal myelolipoma (see Fig. 3.66)—Usually a predominantly fatty mass with areas of myeloid elements. Predominantly fatty tumors are well demonstrated with fat saturation,

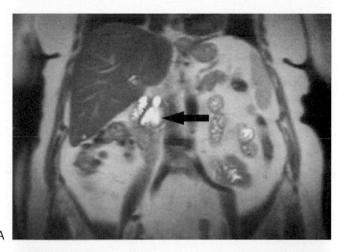

A

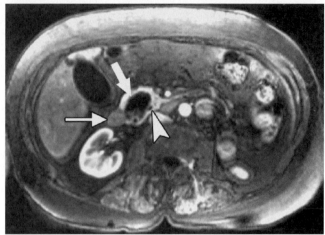

B

FIG. 3.117. Duodenal diverticulum simulating pancreatic mass. **A:** Coronal HASTE image shows apparent cystic mass (*arrow*) in region of pancreatic head. **B:** Fat-suppressed, gadolinium-enhanced gradient echo image shows duodenal diverticulum in same patient as **(A)** simulating cystic pancreatic head mass between duodenum (*thin arrow*) and pancreatic duct (*arrowhead*).

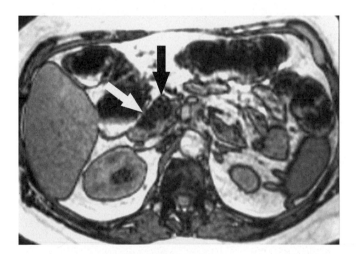

FIG. 3.116. Focal fatty infiltration of pancreas. T1-weighted opposed-phase gradient echo image shows focal area of low signal intensity (*arrows*) in region of pancreatic head caused by focal fat infiltration. This area was normal on all other sequences, including the in-phase image (not shown). Bile duct and pancreatic duct were normal.

whereas opposed-phase imaging may be useful when similar amounts of fat and myeloid elements are intermixed.

Renal angiomyolipoma (see Figs. 3.3, 3.68)—Small lesions are well demonstrated on in-phase and opposed-phase images, whereas larger lesions with prominent areas of fat are best demonstrated with standard fat suppression techniques (e.g., fat saturation, short tau inversion recovery [STIR], spectral presaturation inversion recovery [SPIR]).

Benign cystic teratoma (see Figs. 3.92, 3.93)—This adnexal mass is best characterized with standard fat suppression techniques (fat saturation, STIR, SPIR).

Clear cell carcinoma of kidney (Fig 3.124)—A small percentage of these tumors contain significant concentrations of intracellular lipid, which can be demonstrated on in-phase and opposed-phase images. Care should be taken not to confuse these lesions with angiomyolipomas. Although macroscopic fatty elements are exceedingly uncommon in

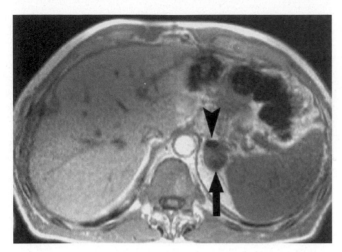

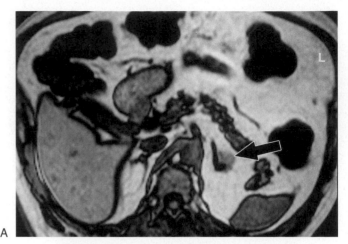

FIG. 3.118. Gastric diverticulum simulating adrenal mass. T1-weighted spoiled gradient echo image shows mass (*arrow*) in expected location of left adrenal gland. Clue to correct diagnosis of gastric diverticulum is susceptibility artifact caused by air (*arrowhead*) in nondependent portion of mass.

renal cell carcinoma, tumors may rarely engulf renal sinus fat.

Focal nodular hyperplasia (FNH) (Fig. 3.125)—A rare manifestation of FNH, intracellular lipid is best demonstrated with in-phase and opposed-phase imaging.

Hepatic adenoma (see Fig. 3.6)—Intracellular lipid is common within this entity and best demonstrated with in-phase and opposed-phase imaging.

Hepatocellular carcinoma (Fig 3.126)—Intracellular lipid is best demonstrated with in-phase and opposed-phase imaging.

Lipoma—Occurs throughout the body, most often in or adjacent to muscles or normal fatty deposits. Can also occur within bones and solid parenchymal organs such as the liver

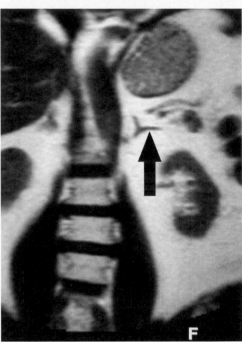

FIG. 3.120. Plane-dependent pseudotumor of adrenal gland. **A:** Axial opposed-phase gradient echo image through abdomen shows apparent mass (*arrow*) of left adrenal gland caused by partial volume effect. **B:** Coronal image through left adrenal gland shows no evidence of mass.

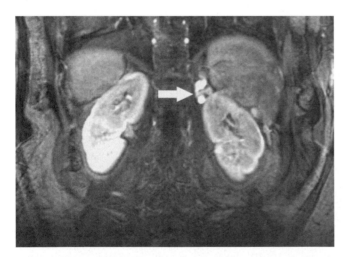

FIG. 3.119. Varices simulating adrenal mass. Coronal fat-suppressed, gadolinium-enhanced T1-weighted image shows enhancing suprarenal varices (*arrow*) that might be mistaken for adrenal mass on other sequences.

and pancreas. Composed almost entirely of fat, lipomas are best characterized by acquiring a T1-weighted sequence of the area of interest with and without frequency-selective fat saturation.

Lipoleiomyoma—Rare benign tumor that may occur in the uterus or ovary. Uterine lipoleiomyoma may be associated with ordinary leiomyomas.

Liposarcoma—Well-differentiated liposarcoma may be difficult to distinguish from benign lipoma. Alternatively, liposarcoma may contain relatively little fat. Larger areas of fat are well demonstrated by scanning with and without standard fat suppression techniques. Enhancing soft tissue elements within a fatty mass favor liposarcoma over lipoma.

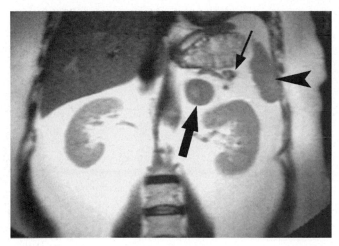

FIG. 3.121. Accessory spleen simulating adrenal mass. Left suprarenal mass (*arrow*) followed signal intensity of spleen (*arrowhead*) on all sequences. Diagnosis of accessory spleen was suggested by MRI, but biopsy was performed, revealing only blood and lymphocytes. Question mark (*thin arrow*) was coincidental but appropriate.

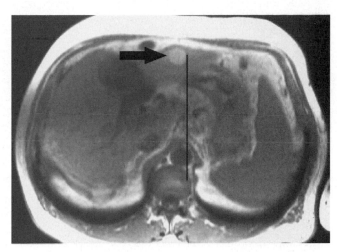

FIG. 3.123. Liver nodule simulating phase ghost. T1-weighted spoiled gradient echo image shows high signal intensity cirrhotic nodule (*arrow*) in left hepatic lobe that resembles a phase ghost from aorta. Note, however, that nodule does not exactly align with aorta (*black line*).

Malignant ovarian teratoma—Enhancing soft tissue elements and invasion of adjacent structures suggests malignant nature of this mass.

References: 1, 2

SELECTED SYNDROMES AND MULTISYSTEM ABNORMALITIES AFFECTING THE ABDOMEN AND PELVIS

Multiple endocrine neoplasia (MEN)—Autosomal dominant neoplastic abnormality predominantly affecting the endocrine system.

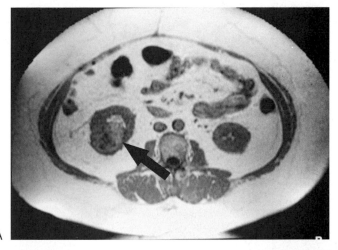

A

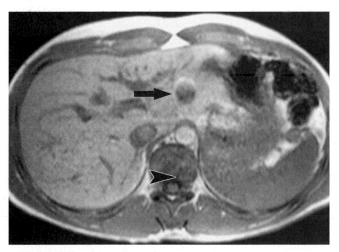

FIG. 3.122. Phase ghost simulating hepatic mass. Round, low signal intensity lesion (*arrow*) in left hepatic lobe is actually ghost produced by aorta. A similar but fainter ghost is seen over spine (*arrowhead*).

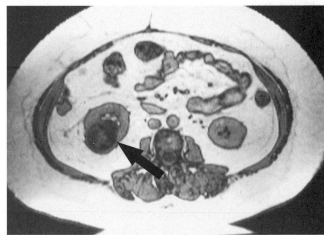

B

FIG. 3.124. Lipid-containing clear cell carcinoma of kidney. Axial in-phase gradient echo image **(A)** shows mass of right kidney to contain high signal intensity elements (*arrow*) that lose signal intensity on opposed-phase image **(B)**.

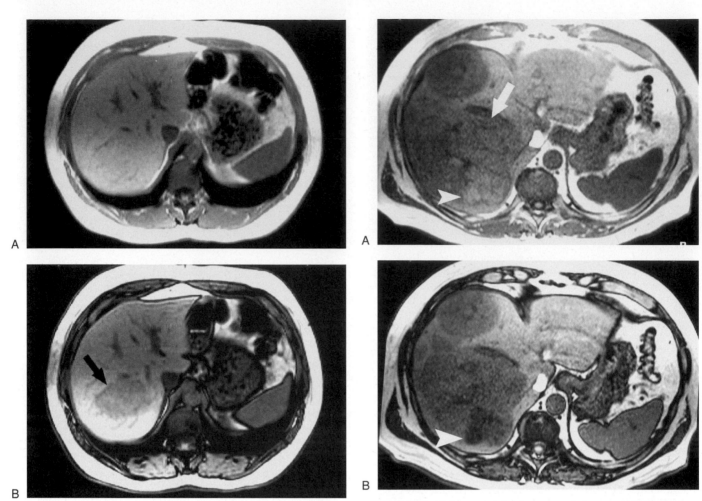

FIG. 3.125. Lipid-containing focal nodular hyperplasia (FNH). **A:** In-phase T1-weighted gradient echo image of liver shows homogeneous signal intensity of liver. **B:** Opposed-phase image performed as part of same sequence as **(A)** shows area of signal loss (*arrow*) in right hepatic lobe corresponding to surgically confirmed FNH.

FIG. 3.126. Lipid-containing hepatocellular carcinoma. **A:** In-phase T1-weighted gradient echo image of large hepatic mass (*arrow*) shows area of slightly higher signal intensity (*arrowhead*) posteriorly. **B:** Opposed-phase image performed as part of same sequence as **(A)** shows focal area of signal loss (*arrowhead*) consistent with intracytoplasmic lipid.

MEN I (Wermer)—Abdominal manifestations include pancreatic islet cell tumors, which are more likely to be malignant and multiple than sporadic cases. Gastrinoma is a common tumor type in the setting of MEN (Fig. 3.127). Other abnormalities include pituitary and parathyroid adenoma.

MEN IIa (Sipple)—Primary abdominal manifestation is pheochromocytoma (Fig. 3.128), which has a high incidence of bilaterality in these patients. Other manifestations include parathyroid adenoma and medullary carcinoma of the thyroid.

MEN IIb (III, mucosal neuroma syndrome)—Also associated with pheochromocytoma. The other primary abdominal manifestation of MEN IIb is intestinal neuromas. Also associated with mucosal neuromas elsewhere and medullary carcinoma of the thyroid.

Von Hippel-Lindau disease (VHL) (Fig. 3.129)—Autosomal dominant neurocutaneous syndrome. Abdominal and

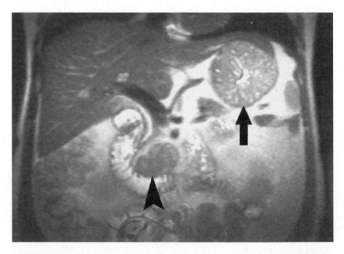

FIG. 3.127. Gastrinoma in multiple endocrine neoplasia I syndrome. Coronal HASTE image demonstrates marked rugal fold thickening in the stomach (*arrow*) due to gastrinoma near pancreatic head (*arrowhead*).

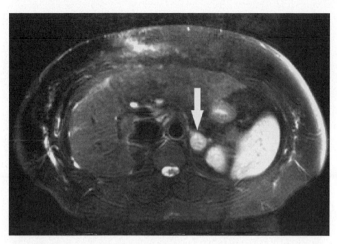

FIG. 3.128. Pheochromocytoma in multiple endocrine neoplasia IIa syndrome. Axial fat-suppressed T2-weighted image shows high signal intensity left adrenal pheochromocytoma (*arrow*).

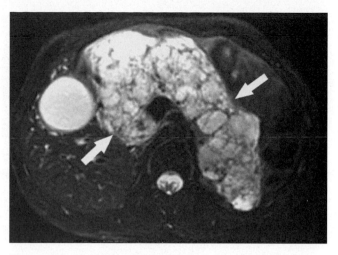

FIG. 3.130. Von Hippel-Lindau disease. Axial fat-suppressed T2-weighted image of pancreas (*arrows*) demonstrates extensive pancreatic cysts.

pelvic manifestations include pheochromocytomas, pancreatic islet cell tumors, pancreatic cysts, pancreatic serous cystadenomas, renal cysts, renal cell carcinomas, papillary cystadenoma of the epididymis, and ovarian cysts. Pancreatic and renal cysts tend to be multiple and may be extensive. VHL can be distinguished from autosomal dominant polycystic kidney disease by the extensive pancreatic involvement (Fig. 3.130). Renal cell carcinoma is common in patients with VHL and bilateral or multiple tumors are often present. These malignant renal tumors may appear cystic and be difficult to differentiate from the multiple other benign renal cysts. Other manifestations include

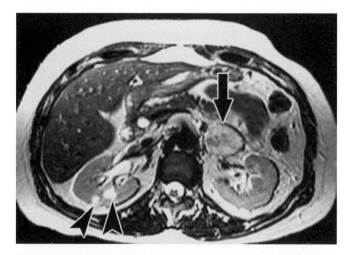

FIG. 3.129. Von Hippel-Lindau disease. Axial T2-weighted image of the abdomen shows large high signal intensity left adrenal mass (*arrow*) and small right renal cysts (*arrowheads*). At surgery, bilateral pheochromocytomas and islet cell tumor of pancreas were removed. Bilateral cystic renal cell carcinomas were also present, but could not be identified as malignant by imaging.

central nervous system (CNS) hemangioblastoma and retinal angioma.

Tuberous sclerosis (Bourneville disease)—Autosomal dominant neurocutaneous syndrome characterized by some combination of adenoma sebaceum, seizures, and mental retardation. Abdominal manifestations include multiple renal cysts and angiomyolipomas (see Fig. 3.68). Renal involvement with cysts may be extensive. Angiomyolipomas are often multiple, may grow over time, and are prone to hemorrhage. Angiomyolipomas may also occur in the liver. Extraabdominal manifestations include cardiac rhabdomyomas.

Neurofibromatosis type 1 (Von Recklinghausen disease)—Autosomal dominant disorder characterized by peripheral neurofibromas and café-au-lait spots. Abdominal manifestations include neurofibromas, neurofibrosarcoma, and pheochromocytoma (Fig. 3.131). Neurofibromas tend to have very high signal intensity on T2-weighted images. Neurofibromatosis type 1 has also been associated with gastrointestinal (GI) stromal tumors and somatostatinomas. Neurofibromas may also occur within the GI tract.

Autosomal dominant polycystic kidney disease—A genetic disorder of very high penetrance but variable expression. Named for the typical extensive renal cystic involvement (Fig. 3.132), this disorder is also associated with cysts of the liver and other viscera such as the spleen and pancreas. Liver involvement may exceed that of the kidneys. Pancreatic cysts are rare and involvement is typically not as extensive as may be seen with VHL disease. Cysts are often of variable signal intensity on T1- and T2-weighted images due to hemorrhage. Also associated are saccular cerebral aneurysms.

Hereditary hemorrhagic telangiectasia (Osler-Weber-Rendu syndrome) (Figs. 3.133, 3.134)—Hereditary vascular disorder resulting in multiple telangiectasias and arteriovenous malformations in various organs, including the GI tract, liver, lungs, skin, and CNS. Vascular malformations of the bowel are often not visible with MRI. However, involvement

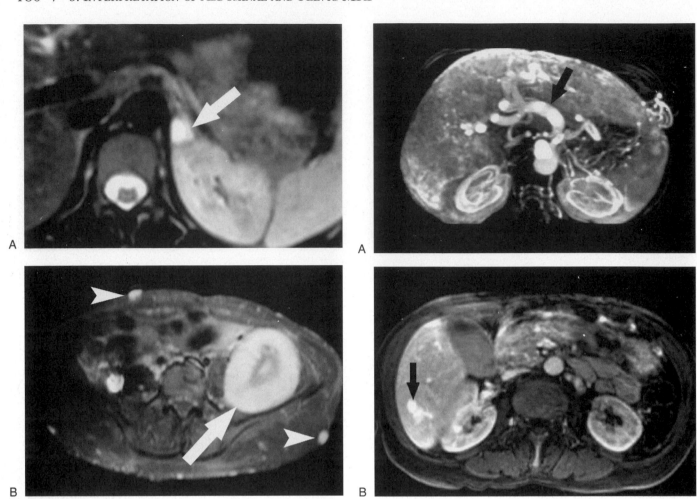

FIG. 3.131. Neurofibromatosis. **A:** Fat-suppressed T2-weighted image shows small high signal intensity left adrenal pheochromocytoma (*arrow*) in patient with NF-1. **B:** Lower image from same patient demonstrates a large plexiform neurofibroma (*arrow*) and multiple cutaneous neuromas (*arrowheads*).

FIG. 3.133. Hereditary hemorrhagic telangiectasia (HHT). **A:** Maximum intensity projection of arterial phase three-dimensional gradient echo sequence shows massively enlarged hepatic artery (*arrow*) in patient with HHT. **B:** Vascular malformation is present in right hepatic lobe of different patient with HHT (*arrow*).

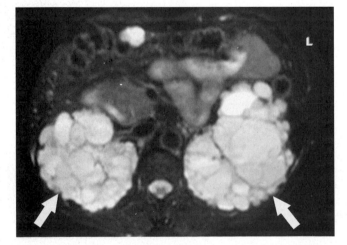

FIG. 3.132. Autosomal dominant polycystic kidney disease. Fat-suppressed T2-weighted image demonstrates extensive bilateral renal involvement with cysts (*arrows*).

of the liver by multiple arteriovenous malformations (AVMs) may be well demonstrated. As a result of the arteriovenous shunting in the liver, the hepatic artery may become quite large.

Mayer-Rokitansky-Küster-Hauser syndrome (Fig. 3.135) —This syndrome occurs when the müllerian ducts fail to develop, resulting in variable degrees of agenesis or hypoplasia of the uterus and vagina. The diagnosis is readily made with MRI when an absent or rudimentary uterus is noted in the presence of intact ovaries in a patient with no surgical history. Skeletal and renal anomalies (renal agenesis or malposition) may be present.

References: 3 to 8

DISORDERS OF IRON METABOLISM AND DEPOSITION

Primary (idiopathic) hemochromatosis—Autosomal recessive disorder resulting in increased intestinal absorption of

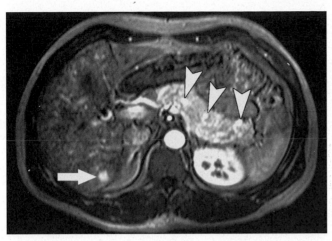

FIG. 3.134. Hereditary hemorrhagic telangiectasia (HHT). Axial gadolinium-enhanced three-dimensional gradient echo image through abdomen of patient with HHT shows multiple pancreatic (*arrowheads*) and hepatic (*arrow*) vascular malformations.

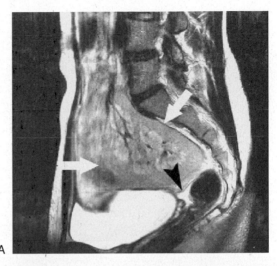

A

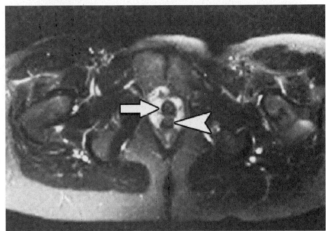

B

FIG. 3.135. Mayer-Rokitansky-Küster-Hauser syndrome. **A:** Sagittal T2-weighted image through pelvis of female patient with amenorrhea reveals absence of uterus with only small amount of fluid occupying space between bladder and rectum (*arrowhead*). Solitary pelvic kidney (*arrows*) is noted. **B:** Axial fat-suppressed T2-weighted image through lower pelvis in same patient as **(A)** shows normal urethra (*arrow*) surrounded by high signal intensity periurethral veins. Vagina (*arrowhead*) lacks normal "H" shape.

iron. Excess iron accumulates, not in the reticuloendothelial system, but in the hepatocytes and parenchymal cells of a variety of other organs such as the pancreas, pituitary gland, heart, joints, and skin (Fig. 3.136). Excess iron is well demonstrated on T2- and T2*-weighted images. Hepatic iron eventually leads to cirrhosis, and patients are at markedly increased risk for hepatocellular carcinoma. Pancreatic involvement may lead to diabetes. It is important to distinguish primary hemochromatosis from transfusional hemochromatosis, because the former condition is potentially lethal and can be treated with phlebotomy or chelation if detected at an early stage. An abnormally dark liver on T2- or T2*-weighted images associated with normal splenic signal intensity should arouse suspicion for primary hemochromatosis. Abnormal darkening of the pancreas further supports this diagnosis, although histologic confirmation via liver biopsy is usually necessary. Rarely, reduced myocardial signal intensity is also seen in patients with primary hemochromatosis.

Paroxysmal nocturnal hemoglobinuria (PNH)—Rare acquired hemolytic disorder resulting from an abnormal clone of hematopoietic stem cells susceptible to complement-mediated lysis. Intravascular hemolysis requiring multiple transfusions results in hemosiderosis. Iron is also deposited in the renal cortex, giving a characteristic appearance of decreased signal intensity on T2- and T2*-weighted images (Fig. 3.137). Because these patients are predisposed to vascular thromboses, a search should be performed for evidence of occlusion of the visualized abdominal and pelvic veins including the hepatic and portal veins.

Hemolytic anemias and transfusional iron overload—Iron overload resulting from multiple blood transfusions can usually be distinguished from primary hemochromatosis, because in the case of multiple transfusions, the iron accumulates within the reticuloendothelial system. Therefore, the T2* effect of the excess iron is manifested initially in the

liver and spleen, but not the pancreas. T2- and T2*-weighted images are more sensitive than T1-weighted images for detecting excess iron. With in-phase and opposed-phase imaging, excess iron usually creates the opposite effect from fatty infiltration of the liver, causing signal loss on the in-phase image. (The longer echo time [TE] of the in-phase image results in greater T2*-weighting). Once the excess iron exceeds the storage capacity of the reticuloendothelial system, parenchymal deposition of iron occurs. This may result in pancreatic signal loss similar to that seen with primary hemochromatosis.

The signal abnormalities in patients with hemolytic anemia are more complex and are influenced by the transfusional history and rate of intestinal iron absorption. Some patients

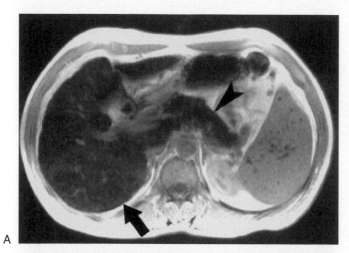

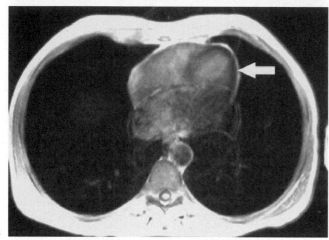

FIG. 3.136. Primary hemochromatosis. A: Axial in-phase T1-weighted gradient echo image demonstrates markedly diminished signal intensity in liver (*arrow*) and pancreas (*arrowhead*) due to parenchymal iron deposition. Liver is cirrhotic. B: Axial in-phase gradient echo image through lower chest of same patient as in (A) reveals decreased signal in left ventricular myocardium (*arrow*) consistent with iron deposition.

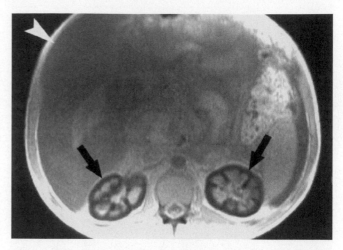

FIG. 3.137. Paroxysmal nocturnal hemoglobinuria (PNH). Axial in-phase T1-weighted gradient echo sequence demonstrates markedly diminished signal intensity in renal cortices (*arrows*) in patient with PNH. Patient also had hepatic and portal vein thrombosis. Note ascites (*arrowhead*).

the diaphragm in paraesophageal type and moves above the esophageal hiatus with the sliding variety. Sliding hiatal hernia is very common.

Inguinal (see Fig. 3.99)—Herniation of peritoneal contents in the inguinal region. Indirect hernia occurs through internal inguinal ring into inguinal canal, coursing along the spermatic cord. Direct hernia (much less common) occurs medial to the deep (inferior) epigastric artery.

Incisional—Herniation of peritoneal contents through a surgically created abdominal wall defect.

Lumbar (Petit's triangle hernia)—Protrusion of hernia sac in the region between the lowest rib and the iliac crest. Hernia

with hemolytic anemia have increased iron absorption without the need for blood transfusion. This may result in MRI findings similar to primary hemochromatosis. Patients with sickle cell disease or intravascular hemolysis from a prosthetic heart valve may demonstrate iron-related renal cortical signal loss identical to that seen with PNH (Fig. 3.138).

References: 9

COMMON HERNIAS

Bochdalek (Fig. 3.139)—Relatively common dorsolateral diaphragmatic hernia.

Femoral—Herniation of peritoneal contents through the femoral ring into the femoral canal. Hernia sac may extend through saphenous opening. It is more common in women.

Hiatal (Fig. 3.140)—Gastric herniation through the esophageal hiatus. Gastroesophageal junction remains below

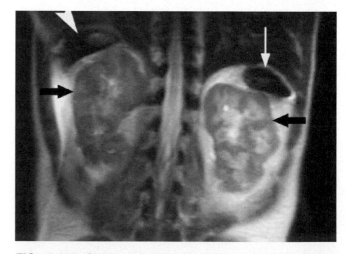

FIG. 3.138. Sickle cell anemia. Coronal HASTE image demonstrates decreased signal intensity of renal cortices bilaterally (*arrows*). Note decreased signal intensity of liver (*arrowhead*) and spleen (*thin arrow*).

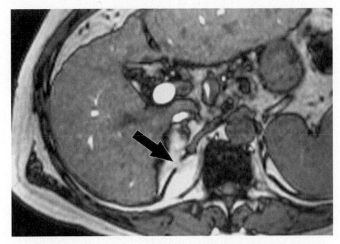

FIG. 3.139. Bochdalek hernia. Small posterior diaphragmatic defect is noted on right (*arrow*). Note nodular liver contour and hypertrophy of lateral segment of left hepatic lobe in patient with cirrhosis.

contents can include mesenteric or omental fat, bowel, and rarely kidney or spleen.

Parastomal—Protrusion of peritoneal contents through a defect created for an ostomy.

Spigelian—Lateral ventral hernia through a defect in the aponeurosis between the transversus abdominis and rectus abdominis muscles.

Richter—Protrusion of the antimesenteric wall of a bowel loop through a hernia ring resulting in focal strangulation.

Traumatic (Fig. 3.141)—History of significant blunt abdominal trauma. Associated hemorrhage may appear as high signal intensity on T1-weighted images.

Umbilical (paraumbilical)—Protrusion of peritoneal contents through the anterior abdominal wall at the umbilicus.

References: 10

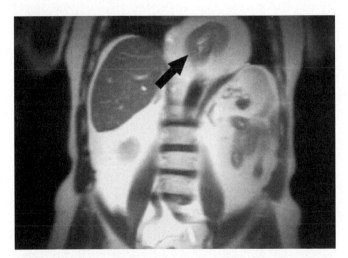

FIG. 3.140. Hiatal hernia. Coronal HASTE image shows herniation of stomach (*arrow*) and surrounding fat into mediastinum.

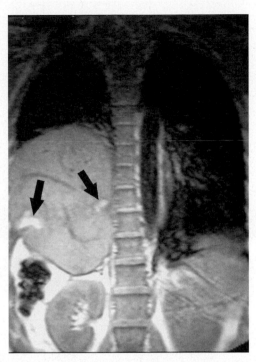

FIG. 3.141. Traumatic diaphragmatic hernia. Coronal T1-weighted gradient echo image shows cephalad displacement of liver into thorax through diaphragmatic defect. High signal intensity hemorrhage is present along rent in diaphragm (*arrows*).

CYSTIC-APPEARING LIVER LESION

Abscess (Fig. 3.142; see Figs. 3.2, 3.5)—Nonenhancing fluid collection with enhancing rim. Internal debris or gas may be present. Abscesses are often multiple.

Bile duct hamartoma (Fig. 3.143; see Fig 3.8)—Small (usually < 1 cm), multiple, nonenhancing lesions. Often mistaken for simple cysts.

Biloma—Communication with biliary tree may be visible. May accumulate mangafodipir in the setting of an active bile leak.

Biliary cystadenoma or carcinoma (see Fig. 3.9)—Multilocular cyst with enhancing wall, septa, and mural nodules.

Choledochal cyst—Communicates with biliary tree. Central dot sign (portal triad vessels partially surrounded by dilated duct) often present with Caroli disease (see Fig. 3.13).

Cystic metastasis (ovarian, gastric, sarcoma, others) (Fig. 3.144)—Multiple, often with thick enhancing walls. Primary tumor or other evidence of metastatic disease may be visible.

Embryonal sarcoma (see Fig. 3.17)—Occurs predominantly in older children and adolescents, although young adults may develop embryonal sarcoma. Myxoid stroma makes these solid tumors appear cystic with areas of high signal intensity on T2-weighted images. Embryonal sarcoma typically exhibits heterogeneous enhancement of the periphery and septa on contrast-enhanced images.

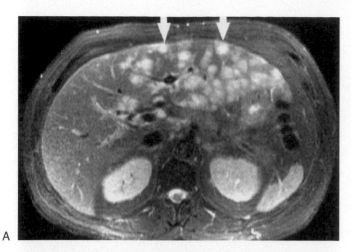

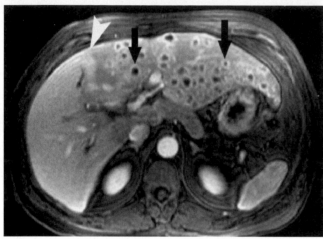

FIG. 3.142. Hepatic abscesses. **A:** Axial fat-suppressed T2-weighted image through liver shows multiple high signal intensity lesions throughout left lobe (*arrows*). **B:** Lesions demonstrate ring enhancement (*arrows*) on fat-suppressed, gadolinium-enhanced three-dimensional gradient echo images. Lesions resolved after antibiotic therapy. Right lobe was free of lesions, and right portal vein was absent, suggesting enteric source for abscesses. Note increased enhancement of right hepatic lobe (*arrowhead*).

Hematoma—Often heterogeneous with areas of increased signal intensity on T1-weighted images due to methemoglobin. History of trauma, recent biopsy, or other predisposing factor (e.g., liver tumor, thrombocytopenia, coagulopathy) is usually present.

Hydatid disease—Parasitic infection caused by *Echinococcus granulosus*. Endemic in sheep-raising regions, because domesticated livestock serve as intermediate hosts. Multiple, peripherally arranged daughter cysts are often visible on T2-weighted images.

Necrotic primary hepatic tumor—Irregular, thick enhancing rim usually present.

Simple cyst (see Fig. 3.15)—Nonenhancing fluid collection with no discernible wall.

References: 11

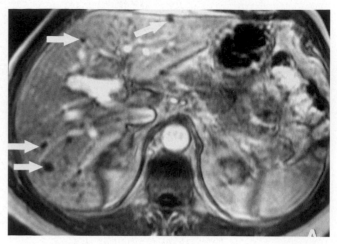

FIG. 3.143. Bile duct hamartomas. Gadolinium-enhanced T1-weighted gradient echo image shows multiple tiny, nonenhancing lesions throughout liver (*arrows*). This is same patient as in Figure 3.8.

LIVER LESION WITH A CENTRAL "SCAR"

Cavernous hemangioma (Fig 3.145)—Demonstrates nodular peripheral enhancement with nonenhancement of central scar.

Fibrolamellar hepatocellular carcinoma—Central scar, when present, is dark on T1- and T2-weighted images. Central scar typically does not enhance unless very delayed images are obtained.

Focal nodular hyperplasia (FNH) (Fig. 3.146)—FNH tends to be inconspicuous on all but arterial phase contrast-enhanced MR images ("stealth tumor"). Typically abuts the liver capsule and demonstrates marked enhancement on arterial phase images. Central scar is dark on T1-weighted images, is bright on T2-weighted images, and exhibits delayed (equilibrium phase) enhancement.

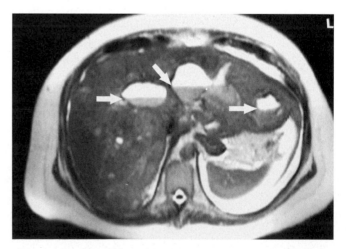

FIG. 3.144. Cystic metastases. Multiple cystic liver lesions demonstrating fluid-fluid levels (*arrows*) in patient with metastatic squamous cell carcinoma.

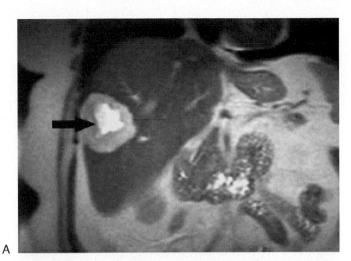

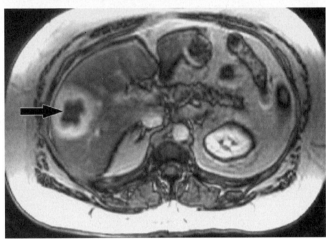

FIG. 3.145. Atypical hemangioma. Appearance of hemangioma in right hepatic lobe is atypical due to differing signal characteristics of center (*arrow*) and periphery of lesion on coronal HASTE image (**A**) and lack of central enhancement (*arrow*) on delayed gadolinium-enhanced T1-weighted image (**B**).

Hepatocellular adenoma—Central scars are uncommon but may occur as a consequence of intratumoral hemorrhage.

Peripheral cholangiocarcinoma (Fig 3.147)—Nonenhancement of central portions of tumor due to fibrosis or necrosis. Peripheral portions of tumor demonstrate gradual progressive enhancement.

TRANSIENT HEPATIC INTENSITY DIFFERENCE

Aberrant venous drainage—Anatomic variations in venous drainage (e.g., capsular veins, accessory cystic vein, or aberrant right gastric vein) may result in areas of transiently increased signal intensity on arterial phase images. Common locations for this phenomenon include the subcapsular liver and areas adjacent to the falciform ligament and gallbladder fossa.

Cirrhosis—Arterial-portal shunting is common in cirrhosis and may be confused for hepatocellular carcinoma on dynamic contrast-enhanced images.

Hemangioma—Mass associated with THID demonstrates typical imaging characteristics of hemangioma.

Hepatic vein thrombosis, obstruction, or occlusion—Abnormal signal intensity or abnormal/absent enhancement of hepatic veins is present. Intrahepatic venous collaterals may be visible in chronic cases.

Idiopathic—Occasionally, peripheral, wedge-shaped THID occurs without associated mass or discernible hepatic vascular abnormality.

Inflammation—THID may occur adjacent to an inflammatory process such as acute cholecystitis.

Portal vein thrombosis, obstruction, or occlusion (see Fig. 3.38)—Thrombosis is suggested by abnormal signal intensity or abnormal/absent enhancement of portal veins. A primary or metastatic liver tumor may also invade or obstruct portal vein branches.

Vena cava obstruction—Medial segment of left lobe often affected. Enlarged collateral thoracic veins often present with superior vena cava obstruction. Images through the thorax may demonstrate a mass, thrombus, or stenosis obstructing the superior vena cava.

Tumor—Tumors with increased arterial blood supply may cause increased enhancement of the surrounding hepatic parenchyma. Transient intensity difference is occasionally seen with hilar cholangiocarcinoma related to vascular compromise or biliary obstruction (Fig. 3.148). Any tumor that compresses or obstructs a portal vein branch may cause THID.

References: 12

POSTTREATMENT APPEARANCE OF THE LIVER AND MALIGNANT LIVER TUMORS

Ablative Therapies

A variety of local ablative therapies are performed for focal malignant hepatic tumors, including cryotherapy, laser thermal ablation, microwave coagulation therapy, percutaneous ethanol ablation, and radiofrequency ablation. MRI is useful to follow response to treatment. Most of these techniques induce a thermal injury (freeze or burn) in the tumor and surrounding liver. The exception is ethanol ablation, which creates tumor death through cellular dehydration and vascular thrombosis. Regardless of mechanism, these techniques all produce a focal area of tissue necrosis. This necrotic area appears avascular on contrast-enhanced MR images, although a thin enhancing rim of granulation tissue may persist for several months after treatment. The appearance of the ablated tissue is variable on precontrast T1- and T2-weighted images. Most lesions demonstrate diminished signal intensity on T2-weighted images, presumably resulting from tissue dehydration and devascularization, although focal areas of markedly increased intensity may be seen corresponding

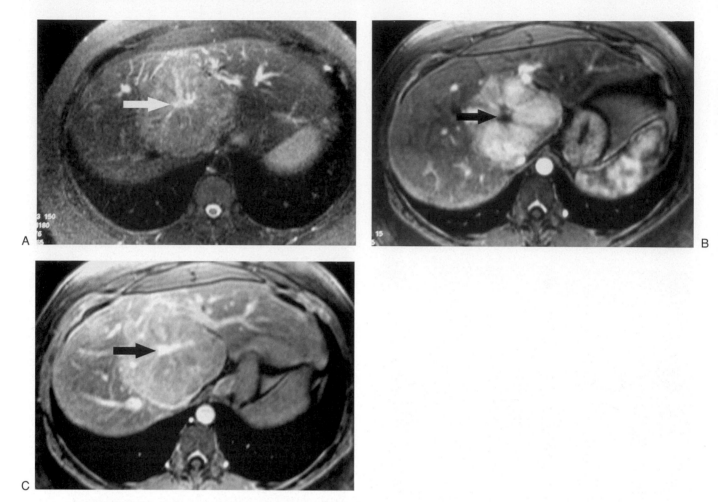

FIG. 3.146. Appearance of scar in focal nodular hyperplasia. Central scar is high signal intensity on T2-weighted image (*arrow*) **(A)**, low signal intensity on early contrast-enhanced image (*arrow*) **(B)**, and demonstrates delayed enhancement (*arrow*) **(C)**. Note brisk arterial enhancement of mass **(B)**.

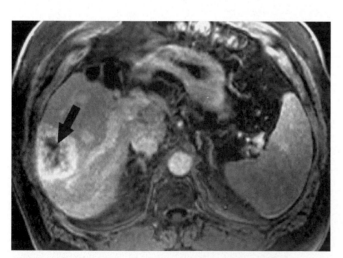

FIG. 3.147. Cholangiocarcinoma. Fat-suppressed T1-weighted image shows incomplete central enhancement of cholangiocarcinoma (*arrow*) of right hepatic lobe despite delay of 10 minutes after administration of gadolinium.

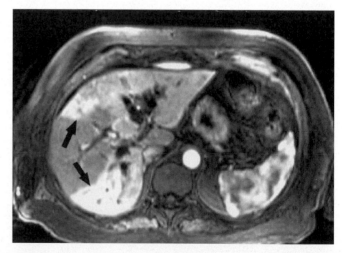

FIG. 3.148. Transient hepatic intensity difference associated with cholangiocarcinoma. Arterial phase fat-suppressed image demonstrates relative hyperperfusion of left hepatic lobe and right posterior segment (*arrows*) in patient with obstructing cholangiocarcinoma. Portal vein was patent on other images (not shown).

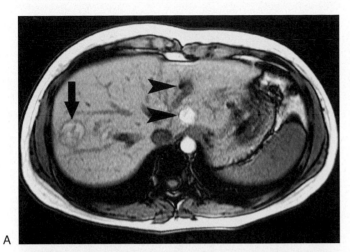

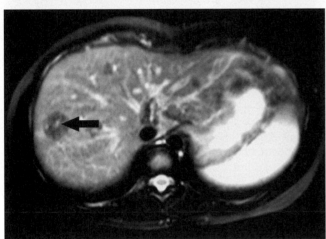

FIG. 3.149. Radiofrequency ablation lesion. **A:** T1-weighted spoiled gradient echo image demonstrates sharply defined lesion (*arrow*) of slightly heterogeneous high signal intensity near dome of liver. Lesion has thin low signal intensity capsule. Note phase ghosts (*arrowheads*) from aorta. **B:** Fat suppressed T2-weighted image of same lesion as **(A)** shows predominantly low signal intensity with the exception of tiny high signal intensity foci (*arrow*). Appearance of this lesion was stable over a period of 6 months.

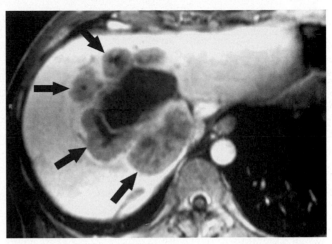

FIG. 3.150. Recurrence of tumor after radiofrequency ablation. Fat-suppressed, gadolinium-enhanced T1-weighted image of liver demonstrates enhancing tumor (*arrows*) surrounding prior ablation site for neuroendocrine metastasis.

to hemorrhage or liquefaction. Increased signal intensity is common on T1-weighted images due to hemorrhage or proteinaceous material (Fig. 3.149). Successfully treated lesions should progressively decrease in size following ablation. Areas of moderately increased signal intensity on T2-weighted images, areas of nodular or intratumoral enhancement with gadolinium, or lesion enlargement should be viewed as possible tumor recurrence or evidence of residual disease (Fig. 3.150).

Chemoembolization

Chemoembolization of the liver is a treatment option for patients who cannot undergo hepatic resection or local ablative therapy. Malignant hepatic tumors treated with transar-

terial chemoembolization undergo characteristic changes in appearance on MR images. Because transarterial chemoembolization is designed to interrupt the blood supply of the target tumor, successfully embolized tumors demonstrate minimal arterial enhancement with intravenous contrast, although arterial-portal shunting may be present. Delayed contrast-enhanced images may demonstrate peripheral enhancement related to either residual tumor or inflammation, making them potentially less useful than early images. Treated hepatocellular carcinoma may have variable signal intensity on T1- and T2-weighted images after chemoembolization. On T2-weighted images, increased signal intensity may be the result of residual tumor, liquefied necrosis, or inflammatory infiltration. Decreased signal intensity on T2-weighted images results from coagulative necrosis. Hepatocellular carcinomas that convert from hyperintense to hypointense on T2-weighted images tend not to recur.

External Irradiation

Radiation therapy that includes a portion of the liver in the treatment port may cause hepatocellular injury resulting in signal abnormalities on MR images. Typically, a sharp demarcation corresponding to the treatment port exists between normal and injured liver. Radiation-induced edema manifests as decreased hepatic signal intensity on T1-weighted images and increased hepatic signal intensity on T2-weighted images. Patients with fatty infiltration of the liver may show decreased fat deposition in the irradiated portion of the liver. Prolonged enhancement of the injured liver parenchyma following the administration of gadolinium chelates may also be present. This pattern of gadolinium enhancement may be useful to distinguish recurrent hepatocellular carcinoma from radiation-induced injury. Uptake of intravenously administered superparamagnetic iron oxide contrast material may be diminished in the irradiated portion of the liver.

Systemic Chemotherapy

MRI may demonstrate changes in the appearance of hepatic metastatic lesions treated with systemic chemotherapy. MRI findings that suggest a favorable response to treatment include an increase in lesion signal intensity on T1-weighted images and a decrease in lesion signal intensity on T2-weighted images. Treated metastases may occasionally mimic the appearance of hemangiomas on subsequent MRI examinations, demonstrating high signal intensity on T2-weighted images and peripheral nodular enhancement. Patients with infiltrating breast carcinoma metastases previously treated with chemotherapy may develop a cirrhosis-like macronodular appearance to the liver.

References: 13 to 32

BILE DUCT FILLING DEFECTS

Air and gas—Move with changes in patient position; associated with susceptibility artifact.

Blood clot—Often conforms to duct; may demonstrate high signal intensity on T1-weighted images.

Crossing vessel (see Fig. 2.46)—An artifact of MR cholangiopancreatography (MRCP). A crossing vessel should be visible on individual source images.

Flow artifact (see Fig. 2.47)—Inconsistent on multiple different pulse sequences. Common with HASTE images. Steady-state gradient echo sequences (trueFISP, balanced-FFE, FIESTA) usually eliminate artifact.

Stones (Fig. 3.151)—Characterized on T2-weighted images as one or more low signal intensity foci within the bile duct. The signal intensity of stones varies on T1-weighted images depending on their composition.

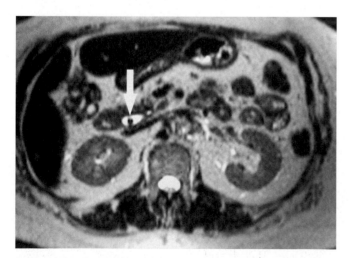

FIG. 3.151. Choledocholithiasis. Small stone is present in distal common bile duct (*arrow*) on axial HASTE image.

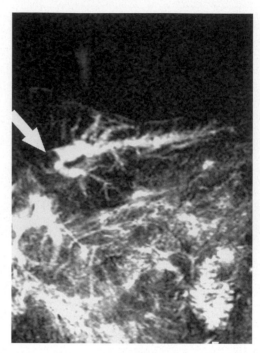

FIG. 3.152. Tumor invading bile duct. Coronal thick-slab magnetic resonance cholangiopancreatography image shows obstructing filling defect in left hepatic duct due to hepatocellular carcinoma, an unusual manifestation.

Tumor (Fig. 3.152)—May expand duct; often associated with parenchymal mass and enhances with contrast.

DILATED BILE DUCTS

Acute cholangitis—Characterized by biliary dilatation with mildly thickened, enhancing bile duct walls on fat-suppressed, post-gadolinium T1-weighted images. Liver parenchyma drained by affected biliary segments may demonstrate increased signal intensity on T2-weighted images and relative increased enhancement following gadolinium administration. Liver abscess or portal vein thrombosis may complicate infectious cholangitis.

Acquired immunodeficiency syndrome (AIDS) cholangiopathy (Fig. 3.153)—Findings of AIDS cholangiopathy may appear similar to those seen with sclerosing cholangitis. Inflammation of the bile ducts results in strictures, focal dilatations, and pruning, whereas inflammation of the gallbladder may manifest as wall thickening resembling acute acalculous cholecystitis.

Ampullary tumor (Fig. 3.154)—Dilated intrahepatic and extrahepatic bile ducts are seen to the level of the ampulla. The actual tumor mass may be difficult to visualize but, when present, appears as a filling defect protruding into the duodenum in the expected location of the ampulla. Duodenal distention with water or other oral contrast agent facilitates visualization of the mass. Fat-suppressed, contrast-enhanced T1-weighted sequences may demonstrate enhancement of the

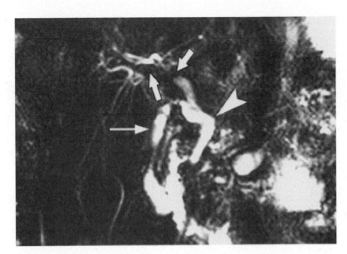

FIG. 3.153. Acquired immunodeficiency syndrome cholangiopathy. Thick-slab magnetic resonance cholangiopancreatography demonstrates multiple bile duct strictures (*arrows*) with mild segmental dilatation of intrahepatic bile ducts. *Arrowhead* denotes common bile duct; thin arrow denotes gallbladder.

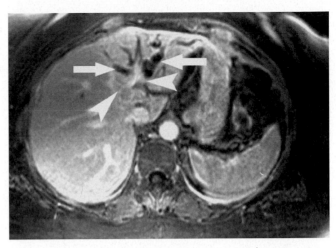

FIG. 3.155. Cholangiocarcinoma. Delayed fat-suppressed, gadolinium-enhanced T1-weighted image demonstrates dilated bile ducts (*arrows*) that converge on area of subtle abnormal enhancement (*arrowheads*) corresponding to tumor.

mass, which may invade the surrounding pancreatic head or cause pancreatic duct dilatation.

Cholangiocarcinoma (Fig. 3.155)—Typically causes bile duct thickening with delayed enhancement of the tumor mass.

Choledochal cyst (Fig. 3.156)—May be associated with anomalous union of the pancreatic and common bile ducts.

Choledocholithiasis—One or more focal filling defects within the common duct are typically present. Stones impacted at the ampulla may be difficult to detect.

Duodenal tumor—Duodenal thickening or mass may be seen. Duodenal distention with water or other oral contrast agent improves detection.

Functional obstruction (Fig. 3.157)—Suggested when no mass, stone, or other cause for obstruction is present. Repeated imaging may be necessary to demonstrate ampullary portion of common bile duct.

Lymphadenopathy—Uncommon cause of biliary obstruction, usually occurring in the setting of malignant tumor. Lymph nodes often best seen on fat-suppressed T2-weighted images or gadolinium-enhanced fat-suppressed T1-weighted images.

Metastases (Fig. 3.158)—Associated with primary malignant tumor. Colorectal metastases may mimic cholangiocarcinoma.

Mirizzi syndrome (Fig. 3.159)—Associated with acute cholecystitis. Impacted cystic duct stone may be visible.

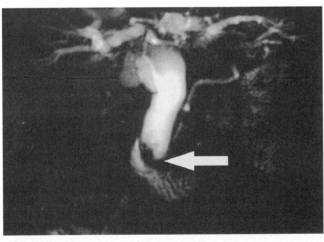

FIG. 3.154. Ampullary carcinoma. Thick-slab magnetic resonance cholangiopancreatography image shows obstruction of the distal common bile duct (*arrow*). Note abrupt transition and subtle irregularity supporting malignant nature of obstruction.

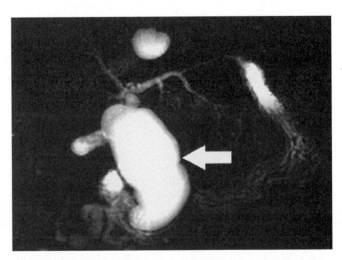

FIG. 3.156. Choledochal cyst. Thick-slab magnetic resonance cholangiopancreatography image demonstrates marked fusiform dilatation of common bile duct due to type I choledochal cyst.

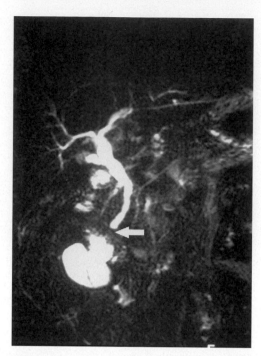

FIG. 3.157. Mild bile duct dilatation without obstructing mass or stricture. Coronal thick-slab magnetic resonance cholangiopancreatography demonstrates mild dilatation of common bile duct with abrupt termination and nonvisualization of the papillary segment (*arrow*). Percutaneous cholangiogram (not shown) revealed identical anatomic findings, but after delay of several minutes, contrast emptied into duodenum with visualization of the papillary segment.

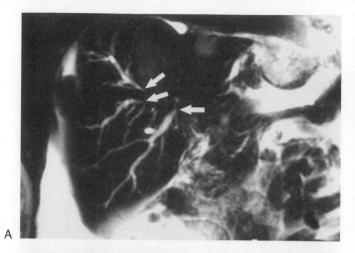

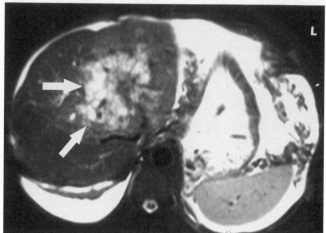

FIG. 3.158. Metastatic colon cancer obstructing bile ducts **(A)**. Coronal thick-slab magnetic resonance cholangiopancreatography shows segmental intrahepatic bile duct dilatation with obstruction (*arrows*) secondary to large colon cancer metastasis (*arrows*) **(B)** seen on axial fat-suppressed T2-weighted examination.

Pancreatic carcinoma—Often results in common bile or pancreatic duct dilatation with abrupt termination of the obstructed ducts. Pancreatic mass is usually visible. Vascular encasement may be present.

Pancreatitis, acute (Fig. 3.160)—Associated with elevation of serum amylase and lipase. C-loop of duodenum may appear widened on MRCP images. Peripancreatic edema and inflammation are visible on fat-suppressed T2-weighted images. Pancreatic duct is usually not dilated in acute pancreatitis.

Postinflammatory or iatrogenic stricture (Fig 3.161)—No associated mass; gradual tapering of duct on MRCP images. History of common duct stones, biliary intervention, or pancreatitis is often elicited.

Recurrent pyogenic cholangitis—Characterized by marked biliary dilatation associated with strictures, periductal abscesses, and biliary pigment stones. Affected segments may undergo parenchymal atrophy. Cholangitis results from an inflammatory or fibrotic response to parasitic infiltration (e.g., *Clonorchis sinensis*).

Sclerosing cholangitis—Bile duct strictures, typically multifocal. May involve intrahepatic and extrahepatic ducts. Bile duct enhancement may be seen after gadolinium administration. Abnormal ductal enhancement is usually due to inflammation, but these patients are also at increased risk for developing cholangiocarcinoma.

References: 33

CYSTIC PANCREATIC MASS

Abscess—Clinical signs of infection usually present.

Choledochal cyst– Communicates with bile duct.

Congenital cyst (Fig 3.162)—Usually simple and unilocular. Association exists with VHL disease and (rarely) with autosomal dominant polycystic kidney disease.

Cystic and papillary epithelial neoplasm (solid and papillary epithelial neoplasm) (see Fig. 3.62)—Contains cystic and solid elements. Most common in pancreatic tail. Tends to occur in young females.

Cystic islet cell tumor—Very rare. Laboratory data are helpful in cases of functioning tumors.

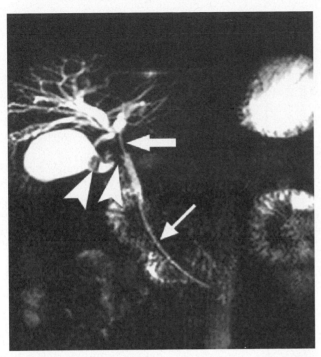

FIG. 3.159. Common hepatic duct obstruction due to acute cholecystitis. Thick-slab magnetic resonance cholangiopancreatography demonstrates stricture of common hepatic duct (*arrow*) due to inflammation caused by stones impacted in the gallbladder neck and cystic duct (*arrowheads*). Note biliary stent (*thin arrow*).

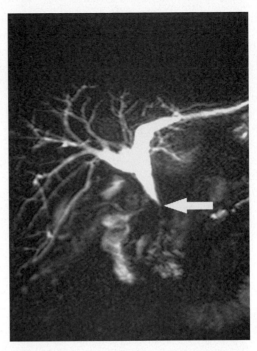

FIG. 3.161. Benign common bile duct stricture secondary to prior episode of pancreatitis. Thick-slab magnetic resonance cholangiopancreatography shows smoothly tapering stricture of common bile duct (*arrow*) in patient with prior history of pancreatitis.

Intraductal papillary mucinous tumor (IPMT) (see Fig. 3.57)—Often found incidentally. Diffuse or segmental dilatation of main pancreatic duct is often seen. Branch duct involvement may have "cluster of grapes" appearance and communication with main pancreatic duct may be visible. IPMT of the branch duct type is most common in uncinate process.

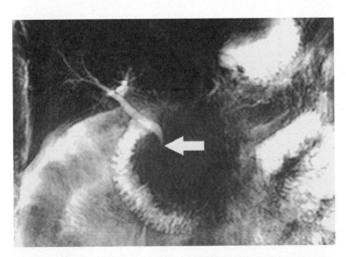

FIG. 3.160. Acute pancreatitis. Thick-slab magnetic resonance cholangiopancreatography demonstrates wide duodenal c-loop with smooth tapering of the common bile duct (*arrow*). Distal pancreatic duct not visualized due to pancreatic inflammation.

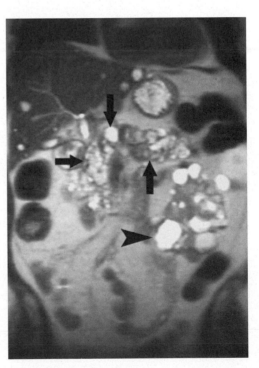

FIG. 3.162. Pancreatic cysts in Von Hippel-Lindau disease (VHL). Coronal HASTE image demonstrates numerous pancreatic cysts (*arrows*) in patient with VHL. Note also renal cysts (*arrowhead*).

Mucinous cystadenoma and cystadenocarcinoma (see Fig. 3.59)—Cysts typically greater than 2 cm in size. They do not communicate with pancreatic duct. They are most common in body and tail of pancreas. They most often occur in the 40- to 60-year age range with slight female predominance.

Necrotic ductal adenocarcinoma—Uncommon manifestation of pancreatic cancer; infiltrative, poorly marginated.

Pseudocyst (see Fig. 3.60)—Occurs as complication of pancreatitis. May communicate with pancreatic duct. Fibrous capsule may be evident.

Serous cystadenoma (Fig. 3.163; see Fig. 3.61)—Typically occurs in older (>60 years) females. Radiating septations and

central signal void may be present. Cysts are typically small (<2 cm).

References: 34

SOLID PANCREATIC MASS

Acinar cell carcinoma- Very rare exocrine tumor. May appear as a predominately solid mass or as a cystic mass. Solid portions enhance with intravenous contrast.

Ductal adenocarcinoma (see Figs. 3.55, 4.17)—Most common malignant pancreatic tumor. Most common in the pancreatic head and least common in the pancreatic tail. Pancreatic head tumors are usually associated with biliary and pancreatic duct dilatation (double duct sign). Tumor enhances in delayed manner compared with normal pancreas. Vascular encasement common.

Focal pancreatitis—Usually does not obstruct the pancreatic duct. Pancreatic duct may be seen traversing region of inflammatory mass (penetrating duct sign).

Islet cell tumor (Fig. 3.164; see Fig. 3.58)—Typically hypervascular. Often bright on fat-suppressed T2-weighted images.

Lymphoma (Fig. 3.165)—Often associated with lymphadenopathy.

Metastasis—May be multifocal. Evidence of metastatic disease is often present elsewhere.

DILATED PANCREATIC DUCT

Ampullary stone—Round signal void near ampulla. Bile duct is usually dilated.

Ampullary tumor—Mass may be visible protruding into duodenum.

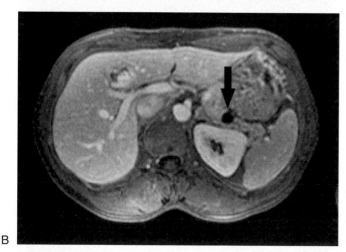

FIG. 3.163. Serous cystadenoma of pancreas. **A:** Thick-slab magnetic resonance cholangiopancreatography image demonstrates small cystic lesion (*arrow*) in tail of pancreas. **B:** Fat-suppressed, gadolinium-enhanced T1-weighted gradient echo image shows no significant enhancement of lesion (*arrow*). Serous cystadenoma was found at surgery.

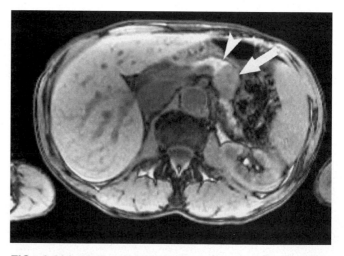

FIG. 3.164. Malignant islet cell tumor of pancreas. T1-weighted gradient echo image of abdomen demonstrates mass (*arrow*) near junction of pancreatic body and tail. Note that mass (*arrow*) is lower in signal intensity than adjacent normal pancreatic parenchyma (*arrowhead*).

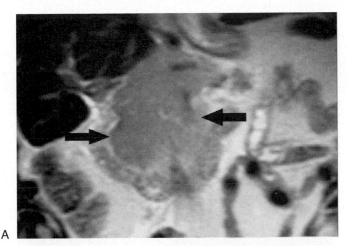

A

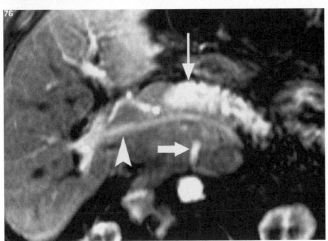

B

FIG. 3.165. Secondary involvement of pancreas with lymphoma. **A:** Coronal HASTE image demonstrates large soft tissue mass (*arrows*) in expected region of pancreatic head. **B:** Fat-suppressed, gadolinium-enhanced gradient echo image shows infiltrating mass encasing the superior mesenteric artery (*arrow*) and portal vein (*arrowhead*). Normally enhancing pancreatic body (*thin arrow*) is seen surrounded by mass. Biopsy revealed non-Hodgkin's lymphoma.

Chronic pancreatitis (Figs. 3.166, 3.167; see Figs. 2.41, 3.56)—Branch duct ectasia and multiple focal strictures and dilatations of pancreatic duct typically present ("chain of lakes" appearance). Pancreatic duct stones or pseudocysts may be visible.

Intraductal papillary mucinous tumor (Fig. 3.168; see Fig. 2.44)—Associated with ectatic branch ducts and focal or diffuse main duct dilatation, often to the level of the ampulla. One or more cystic lesions with a "cluster of grapes" appearance may be present. Bile duct is rarely dilated.

Obstructing pancreatic tumor (see Fig. 2.43)—Pancreatic duct terminates abruptly. Biliary dilatation often present when tumor occurs in pancreatic head. Vascular encasement may be present.

Reference: 35

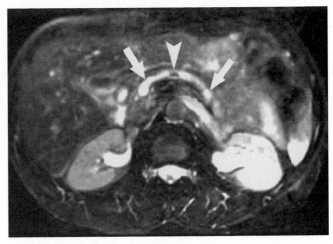

FIG. 3.166. Chronic pancreatitis. Axial fat-suppressed T2-weighted image demonstrates dilated pancreatic duct (*arrows*) with intraductal stone (*arrowhead*). Pancreas is atrophic.

ADRENAL MASS

Adenoma (see Fig. 3.63)—Signal loss on opposed-phase relative to in-phase gradient echo images is most characteristic appearance. Adenomas typically enhance early and wash out rapidly after intravenous gadolinium administration.

Adrenal cortical carcinoma—Rare and tends to be large and necrotic or hemorrhagic at time of diagnosis. May invade adjacent organs or veins. Intracytoplasmic lipid may occasionally be detected on in-phase and opposed-phase images.

Cyst (see Fig. 3.64)—Follows signal intensity of fluid. Nonenhancing. Complicated cysts may mimic other lesions.

Hemangioma—Bright on T2-weighted images. Peripheral enhancement is typical. Central portion often does not enhance.

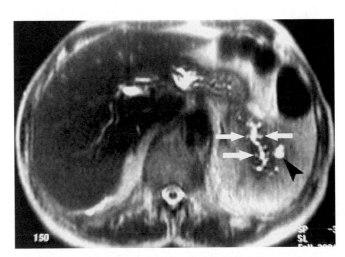

FIG. 3.167. Chronic pancreatitis. Axial HASTE image demonstrates dilated duct in pancreatic tail with multiple ectatic branch ducts (*arrows*). Note small pseudocyst (*arrowhead*).

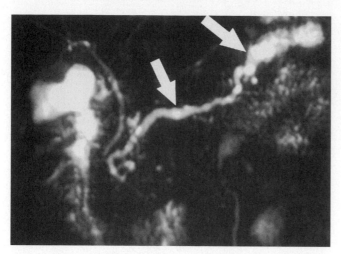

FIG. 3.168. Intraductal papillary mucinous tumor. Coronal thick-slab magnetic resonance cholangiopancreatography image shows diffuse dilatation of mucin-filled main pancreatic duct (*arrows*) and several ectatic branch ducts. (Reprinted with permission from the *American Journal of Roentgenology.* Leyendecker JR, Elsayes KM, Gratz BI, et al. MR cholangiopancreatography: spectrum of pancreatic duct abnormalities. *AJR* 2002;179:1465–1471.)

Lymphoma—Usually non-Hodgkin type. Lymphoma has nonspecific appearance similar to metastatic disease. Normal adrenal shape may be maintained. Lymphadenopathy is often present elsewhere.

Metastasis (see Fig. 3.65)—Typically does not lose signal on opposed-phase relative to in-phase gradient echo images. Presence of intracytoplasmic lipid is extremely rare in metastases. Prolonged washout after intravenous gadolinium administration is typical. Primary malignant tumor present elsewhere.

Myelolipoma (see Fig. 3.66)—Fat-containing portions of this lesion parallel signal intensity of surrounding retroperitoneal fat on all pulse sequences. Solid myeloid elements are often present.

Pheochromocytoma (see Figs. 3.67, 3.128, 3.129, 3.131)—Often very bright on fat-suppressed T2-weighted images. Pheochromocytoma often demonstrates early, intense enhancement and is associated with neurofibromatosis, VHL disease, MEN, and other less common syndromes. Elevated catecholamine levels are present.

References: 36

CYSTIC RENAL MASS

Abscess—Signs and symptoms of infection typically present.

Calyceal diverticulum (Fig. 3.169)—Pericalyceal location. Fills with contrast on delayed gadolinium-enhanced images.

Dilated collecting system—Accumulates intravenously administered gadolinium. Communication of cystic spaces is usually visible.

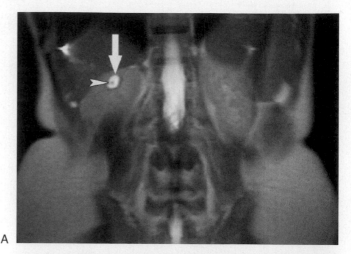

A

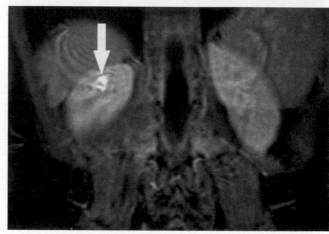

B

FIG. 3.169. Calyceal diverticulum. **A:** Coronal HASTE image shows small cystic lesion (*arrow*) containing stone (*arrowhead*) in upper pole of right kidney. **B:** Cyst filled with contrast on delayed gadolinium-enhanced images (*arrow*).

Hydatid cyst—History of exposure to endemic area is helpful. T1- and T2-weighted images may demonstrate low signal intensity rim and peripherally arranged daughter cysts.

Multilocular cystic nephroma—Multiple cysts with thick enhancing septations present. It is very difficult to distinguish from cystic renal cell carcinoma.

Renal cell carcinoma (Fig 3.170)—Mural nodules or thick enhancing walls and septations are present.

Simple cyst (see Fig. 3.70)—Imperceptible wall, no enhancement.

References: 37

SOLID RENAL MASS

Adenoma—Small, solid mass, indistinguishable from renal cell carcinoma.

Angiomyolipoma (Fig. 3.171)—Contains macroscopic fat of variable amounts. Usually hypervascular.

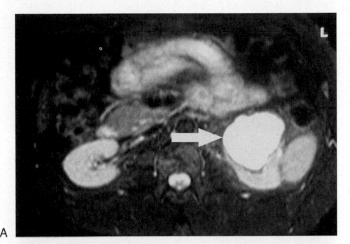

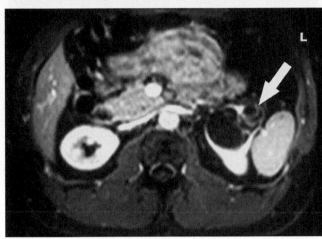

FIG. 3.170. Cystic renal cell carcinoma. A: Axial fat-suppressed T2-weighted image demonstrates high signal intensity cystic lesion (*arrow*) of left kidney. B: Following gadolinium administration, enhancing septations (*arrow*) are noted within cyst.

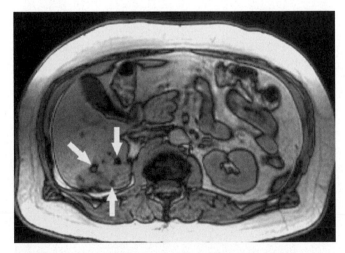

FIG. 3.171. Angiomyolipoma with small amounts of fat. Axial opposed-phase gradient echo image shows multiple foci of signal loss (*arrows*) within right renal angiomyolipoma signifying presence of small amounts of fat.

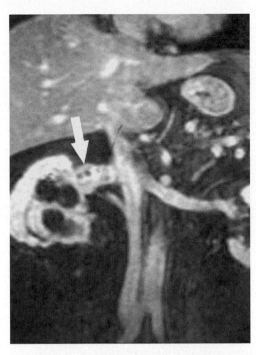

FIG. 3.172. Renal hemangioma. Coronal fat-suppressed, gadolinium-enhanced gradient echo image shows complex enhancing renal mass extending into right renal vein (*arrow*).

Focal pyelonephritis—Signs and symptoms of infection typically present.

Hemangioma (Fig 3.172)—Very rare. Hypervascular.

Infarct (see Fig. 3.71)—Wedge-shaped with nonenhancing center and thin rim of enhancement along adjacent capsule.

Lymphoma—May present as multiple bilateral renal masses, retroperitoneal mass invading kidney, diffusely infiltrating mass, perinephric mass, or solitary renal mass. Mildly enhancing after gadolinium administration.

Metastasis—Primary tumor or metastases may be visible elsewhere. Bilateral involvement is common.

Oncocytoma—Central stellate scar may be present. Cannot be reliably distinguished from renal cell carcinoma with imaging studies.

Renal cell carcinoma (see Fig. 3.74)—Commonly appears as heterogeneous, enhancing mass. Renal vein and inferior vena cava invasion may occur with other tumors but is most common with renal cell carcinoma.

Reninoma/juxtaglomerular tumor—Results in hypertension associated with elevated renin levels. MR angiography may be helpful to exclude renal artery stenosis.

Transitional cell carcinoma—May result in obliteration of renal sinus fat (faceless kidney). Filling defect may be seen in distended collecting system on T2-weighted images.

Xanthogranulomatous pyelonephritis—Delayed enhancement of renal parenchyma after gadolinium administration with poor or absent excretion of contrast material into collecting system is typical. Associated renal calculus appears as signal void.

References: 38

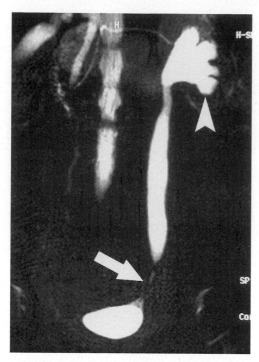

FIG. 3.173. Benign ureteral stricture. Coronal thick-slab static MR urogram image demonstrates smoothly tapered stricture (*arrow*) of distal ureter related to prior stone disease and instrumentation. Stricture has resulted in hydronephrosis (*arrowhead*).

DILATED URETER

Acute pyelonephritis—Signs and symptoms of infection are present. Striated nephrogram may be visible after intravenous gadolinium administration.

Benign stricture (Fig 3.173)—History of prior inflammation, procedure, stone, or radiation is helpful. Typically characterized by smooth gradual tapering without associated mass.

Bladder outlet obstruction (see Fig. 1.35)—Enlarged prostate, bilateral ureterectasis, bladder distention, bladder trabeculation, or bladder diverticula may be present.

Congenital megaureter—Involves distal ureter just before ureterovesical junction. Often incidental and asymptomatic. May be bilateral.

Diuresis—Bilateral (when both kidneys function) ureteral dilatation without evidence of obstructing lesion. Increased urine output. Normal renal enhancement after gadolinium administration.

Endometriosis with obstruction—Unilateral obstruction of distal ureter present in woman of childbearing age. May be associated with high signal intensity or enhancing mass on fat-suppressed T1-weighted images.

Extraureteral obstructing tumor (cervical carcinoma, fibroids, lymphoma, primary retroperitoneal tumor) (Fig 3.174)—Evidence of extraureteral mass or adenopathy adjacent to or encasing ureter.

Intraluminal obstruction (nonneoplastic)—May be caused by stone, blood clot, or sloughed papilla. Ureteral filling de-

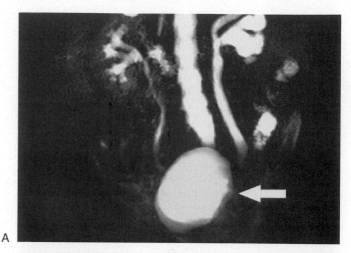

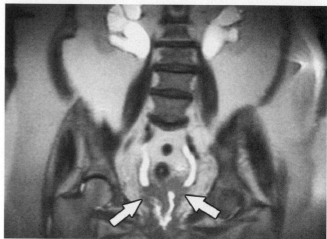

FIG. 3.174. Squamous cell carcinoma (vaginal primary) invading ureter and bladder. **A:** Oblique coronal thick-slab static MR urogram demonstrates bilateral hydroureteronephrosis with irregularity of left posterolateral bladder (*arrow*). **B:** Coronal HASTE image shows tumor (*arrows*) infiltrating around both distal ureters.

fect seen on T2-weighted images. No enhancement following intravenous gadolinium administration. Blood clot may demonstrate increased signal intensity on T1-weighted images. Hematuria is often present.

Metastasis (obstructing)—Primary malignant neoplasm present. Enhancing soft tissue mass present.

Pregnancy—Gravid uterus present without evidence of obstructing stone.

Prior obstruction (relieved)—History of recent ureteral obstruction helpful.

Prior surgery/iatrogenic obstruction—History of prior procedure or instrumentation is helpful. Susceptibility artifact may be present at level of obstruction due to surgical clips.

Retroperitoneal fibrosis—Medial deviation of mid ureters with smooth tapering at level of obstruction. Abnormal retroperitoneal signal intensity and enhancement surround aorta or iliac vessels.

Retrocaval ureter (Fig 3.175)—Abrupt medial deviation of right ureter at the approximate level of L3 vertebra.

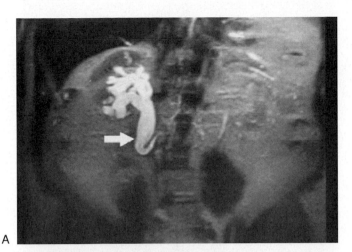

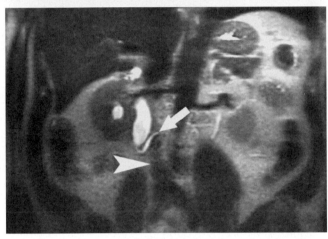

FIG. 3.175. Retrocaval ureter. **A:** Maximum intensity projection of coronal HASTE acquisition shows hydronephrosis of right kidney and proximal ureteral dilatation (*arrow*). **B:** Coronal HASTE source image shows ureter (*arrow*) passing behind inferior vena cava (*arrowhead*).

Tuberculosis—Strictures alternating with dilated segments are typical. Evidence of renal involvement may be present.

Ureterocele—Cystic dilatation of distal ureter within bladder wall protruding into bladder lumen (Cobra head sign). Duplicated collecting system is present in setting of ectopic ureteral insertion (Fig 3.176).

Uroepithelial tumor (see Fig. 2.53)—Intraluminal filling defect that enhances following gadolinium administration. Goblet sign may be present.

Vesicoureteral reflux—No evidence of obstructing lesion. Renal scarring may be present.

BLADDER MASS

Benign prostatic hypertrophy (BPH) (see Fig. 3.108)—Enlarged central zone of prostate may protrude into bladder base.

Bladder papilloma (Fig 3.177)—Enhancing, smooth, small polypoid filling defect, best demonstrated on gadolinium-enhanced T1-weighted images obtained before

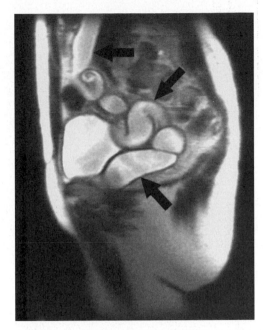

FIG. 3.176. Ectopic ureteral insertion. Sagittal HASTE image demonstrates dilated, tortuous ureter (*arrows*) due to ectopic insertion. This is same patient as in Figure 2.53.

urine enhances. May be difficult to distinguish from small transitional cell carcinoma with imaging.

Bladder stone—Nonenhancing mobile signal void in dependent portion of bladder.

Blood clot—Nonenhancing signal abnormality that may fill bladder or layer dependently. May demonstrate increased signal intensity on T1-weighted images.

Carcinoma (transitional cell, squamous cell, adenocarcinoma) (Fig. 3.178; see Fig. 3.76)—Mass typically enhances earlier than bladder wall following intravenous gadolinium administration.

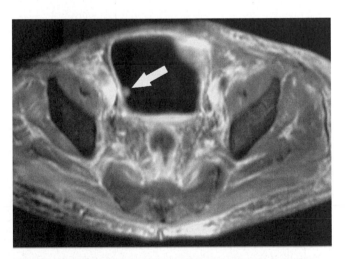

FIG. 3.177. Bladder papilloma. Fat-suppressed, gadolinium-enhanced T1-weighted gradient echo image demonstrates small enhancing papilloma (*arrow*). This lesion was difficult to detect on other sequences (not shown).

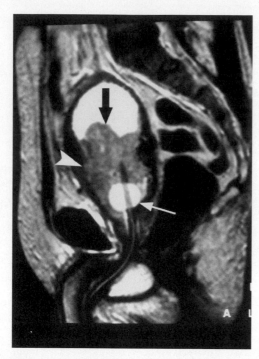

FIG. 3.178. Transitional cell carcinoma of bladder. Coronal T2-weighted image demonstrates large transitional cell carcinoma (*arrow*) occupying much of bladder lumen and invading bladder wall (*arrowhead*). Note Foley catheter balloon (*thin arrow*).

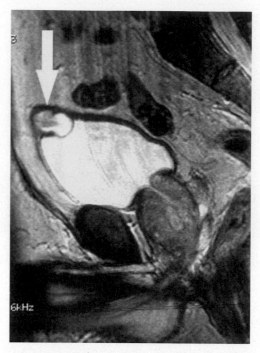

FIG. 3.179. Urachal tubulovillous neoplasm. Sagittal T2-weighted image demonstrates urachal remnant at bladder dome (*arrow*) containing small soft tissue mass.

Endometriosis—Heterogeneous mass with high signal intensity components on T1-weighted images or cystic areas on T2-weighted images. Occurs in women of childbearing age. Posterior bladder wall involvement is more common.

Leiomyoma (see Fig. 3.72)—Smoothly margined intramural mass with relatively low signal intensity on T2-weighted images.

Metastasis—Known primary malignant tumor present. Mass enhances following gadolinium administration.

Urachal tumor (Fig. 3.179)—Mass extends from anterior bladder dome near midline. May extend into space of Retzius or anterior abdominal wall. High signal intensity on T2-weighted images. May appear cystic.

Ureterocele—Cystic dilatation of intravesical ureter. May need to adjust window and level settings to appreciate thin wall.

RETROPERITONEAL MASS

Abscess (see Fig. 3.78)—High signal intensity center on T2-weighted images. Thick, enhancing wall present. May be associated with urinary tract infection or discitis.

Aneurysm/pseudoaneurysm (Fig. 3.180)—Contiguous with abdominal aorta or one of its branches. Appears round or lobulated. Associated thrombus may appear bright on fat-suppressed T1-weighted images. Arterial phase enhancement

may be present, although some pseudoaneurysms demonstrate delayed enhancement after intravenous gadolinium due to slow flow.

Castleman disease—Usually appears as noninfiltrating soft tissue mass. Low to intermediate signal intensity on T1-weighted images and hyperintense on T2-weighted images. Hypervascular. Septa may be present. Calcifications may appear as signal voids.

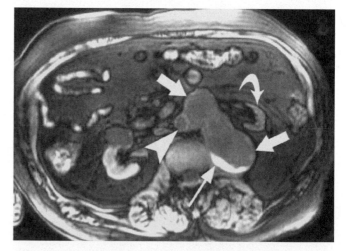

FIG. 3.180. Retroperitoneal pseudoaneurysm secondary to renal stent placement. Fat-suppressed T1-weighted gradient echo image demonstrates lobulated mass (*arrows*) in direct continuity with aorta (*arrowhead*). Crescentic area of high signal intensity (*thin arrow*) is clue to presence of blood products. Note small displaced kidney (*curved arrow*).

Extramedullary hematopoiesis—Associated with chronic anemia. Retroperitoneal sites include renal pelvis and paraspinal regions (usually lower thoracic). Typically homogeneous in appearance with increased signal intensity on T2-weighted images. Exhibits moderate homogeneous enhancement after intravenous gadolinium administration.

Hemangiopericytoma—Very hypervascular.

Hematoma—May demonstrate high signal intensity on T1-weighted images. May be associated with anticoagulation, cardiac catheterization, aortic aneurysm, or trauma.

Leiomyosarcoma—More common in females. Tumors are usually large at presentation with areas of necrosis being relatively common. Lesions tend to be hypervascular.

Lipoma or liposarcoma—Lipomas are well-defined, nonenhancing tumors that parallel fat on all sequences. A well-differentiated liposarcoma may contain considerable fat with some enhancing soft tissue elements. Poorly differentiated tumors may consist predominantly of soft tissue elements with very little fat. Myxoid liposarcoma may appear very bright on T2-weighted images.

Lymphangioma (Fig. 3.181)—Multiloculated, insinuating cystic mass. Thin septations are often present. More common in children.

Lymphoma (Fig 3.182)—Most common retroperitoneal malignant tumor. Bulky retroperitoneal and mesenteric adenopathy typical of non-Hodgkin lymphoma. Lymphadenopathy may coalesce into a large confluent mass that envelops vessels (sandwich sign). May invade kidneys, pancreas, or adrenal glands.

Lymph node metastases—History or findings of primary neoplasm are helpful (e.g., prostate, cervical, testicular, breast, colon, lung, melanoma, pancreatic, or renal primary). May be difficult to distinguish from reactive lymph nodes, although metastatic nodes tend to reach larger size. May appear necrotic. Testicular cancer metastases may appear cystic (see Fig. 3.113).

Malignant fibrous histiocytoma (Fig. 3.183)—Large, heterogeneous, enhancing mass. Calcifications may be present on computed tomography (CT) scan.

Metastasis—History of primary malignant tumor helpful.

Neuroblastoma, ganglioneuroblastoma, ganglioneuroma —Predominantly occur in young patients. Extraadrenal location increases with age. Neuroblastoma is very rare in adults. High signal intensity on T2-weighted images. Enhance with contrast. Neuroblastoma may invade organs or encase vessels.

Neurofibroma and neurofibrosarcoma (see Fig. 3.131B)— History or findings of neurofibromatosis are helpful. Usually bright on T2-weighted images (the tumor periphery may be of higher signal intensity than the center as a result of myxoid degeneration) and enhances with contrast. Differentiation between benign and malignant lesions may be difficult, although neurofibrosarcoma tends to be larger, more heterogeneous, and more infiltrative than neurofibroma.

Nonneoplastic lymphadenopathy—Associated with a large variety of infectious and inflammatory etiologies,

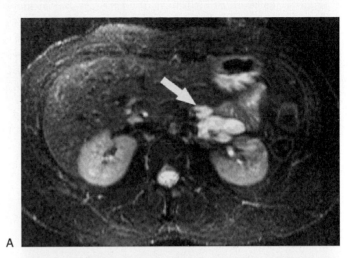

A

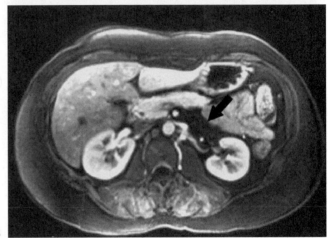

B

FIG. 3.181. Lymphangioma. Lobulated retroperitoneal fluid collection (*arrows*) demonstrating high signal intensity on fat-suppressed T2-weighted image **(A)** and no enhancement on fat-suppressed, gadolinium-enhanced T1-weighted gradient echo image **(B)**.

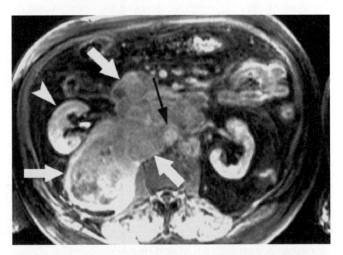

FIG. 3.182. Lymphoma. Fat-suppressed, gadolinium-enhanced gradient echo image demonstrates large heterogeneously enhancing retroperitoneal mass (*arrows*) displacing right kidney (*arrowhead*) and encasing aorta (*thin arrow*). Biopsy revealed non-Hodgkin lymphoma.

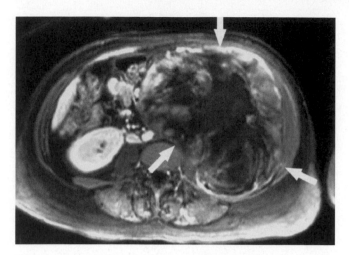

FIG. 3.183. Malignant fibrous histiocytoma. Axial fat-suppressed, gadolinium-enhanced gradient echo image shows large, heterogeneously enhancing mass (*arrows*). Despite retroperitoneal origin, mass significantly displaces peritoneal contents.

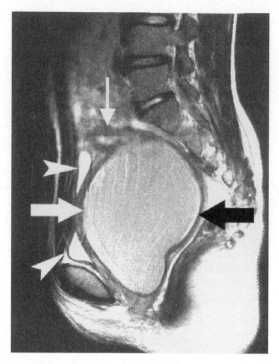

FIG. 3.184. Hematocolpos in patient with uterus didelphys. Sagittal T2-weighted image of pelvis demonstrates large fluid-filled vagina (*arrows*) compressing bladder (*arrowheads*). Note continuity of fluid with superiorly displaced uterine horn (*thin arrow*).

including human immunodeficiency virus, mycobacterial infections, sarcoidosis, and Castleman disease.

Paraganglioma—Occurs in paraspinal region or near origin of inferior mesenteric artery. Demonstrates increased signal intensity on T2-weighted images and tends to be very hypervascular. Hemorrhagic necrosis may manifest as fluid-fluid level.

Pancreatic carcinoma—Infiltrative mass encasing vessels. The mass within the pancreas may be difficult to detect, making perivascular extension the predominant finding in some patients.

Retroperitoneal fibrosis (see Fig. 3.80)—Surrounds aorta and involves ureters. Signal intensity on T2-weighted images decreases as fibrosis matures. Active inflammation enhances considerably, but enhancement becomes more delayed as fibrous tissue predominates.

References: 39, 40

CYSTIC MASS OF THE FEMALE PELVIS (NOT ADNEXAL)

Abscess—Associated with pelvic inflammatory disease, Crohn disease, appendicitis, or diverticulitis. Demonstrates rim enhancement.

Bartholin gland cyst (see Fig. 3.83)—Near vaginal vestibule. Cystic on T2-weighted images, variable signal intensity on T1-weighted images.

Degenerated fibroid—Irregular, thick-walled cavity. Arises from uterus. Other leiomyomas often present.

Ectopic ureterocele—Inserts distal to trigone. Usually associated with upper pole ureter of duplex kidney.

Endometrial implant—May demonstrate high signal intensity on T1-weighted images and variable signal intensity on T2-weighted images. Often associated with adhesions.

Gartner duct cyst (see Fig. 3.91)—Occurs along anterolateral upper vagina. Simple appearing if not complicated by hemorrhage.

Hematocolpos (Fig. 3.184)—Vagina distended with fluid that may demonstrate increased signal intensity on T1-weighted images or contain debris. Often initially detected during puberty. May be associated with other genitourinary anomalies.

Nabothian cyst (see Fig. 3.94)—Involves cervix. Often multiple, small, and round.

Obstructed uterus (Fig. 3.185)—Associated with abnormal cervix (cervical carcinoma, cervical stenosis). Uterine contents may demonstrate high signal intensity on T1-weighted images.

Urethral diverticulum (see Figs. 3.99, 3.100)—Wraps around urethra on axial images. May see neck of diverticulum with endovaginal coil. May contain calculi.

CYSTIC MASS OF THE FEMALE PELVIS (ADNEXAL)

Cystic teratoma (see Figs. 3.92, 3.93)—Also referred to as dermoid cyst. Contains fatty elements that lose signal on fat-suppressed sequences. Debris, fat-fluid level, or Rokitansky nodule may be present. Bilateral lesions not uncommon.

Ectopic pregnancy—Positive pregnancy test. Complex cystic mass, often associated with pelvic fluid. Fallopian tube

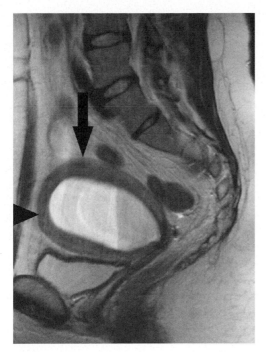

FIG. 3.185. Obstructed uterus. Sagittal T2-weighted image demonstrates distended fluid-filled uterus (*arrows*) due to obstructed outflow. Patient had prior surgical removal of cervix with subsequent scarring.

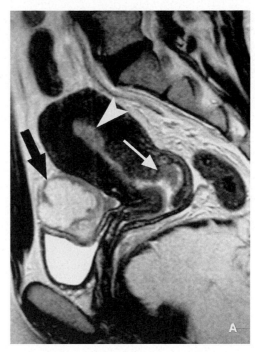

FIG. 3.186. Ovarian metastasis from endometrial carcinoma versus second primary malignant tumor. Sagittal T2-weighted image demonstrates cystic left ovarian mass with thick irregular walls (*arrow*) and abnormal endometrium (*arrowhead*) extending into upper cervix (*thin arrow*). Upon pathologic inspection, endometrioid adenocarcinoma was found in uterus and ovary. Ovarian mass was thought to be most likely metastatic from uterus based on histology.

may appear bright on T1-weighted images. Endometrium may be thickened or contain fluid (pseudogestational sac).

Endometrioma (see Fig. 3.89)—Demonstrates high signal intensity on T1-weighted images that does not suppress with application of fat suppression. Variable brightness on T2-weighted images, but commonly intermediate to low signal intensity (shading) due to blood products. Adhesions may be present.

Functional cyst (see Fig. 3.96)—Simple fluid characteristics, thin walled. No enhancement.

Hemorrhagic cyst—Resembles functional cyst but appears bright on T1-weighted images. Variable signal intensity on T2-weighted images.

Hydrosalpinx—Tubular appearing. Contents are usually simple fluid unless complicated by hemorrhage or infection.

Metastasis (Fig. 3.186)—Thick, enhancing walls. Associated with primary malignant tumor (often GI or breast primary).

Mucinous cystadenoma—Multilocular, septated mass with variable signal intensity. May have papillary projections, although this should raise suspicion for malignancy.

Ovarian carcinoma (see Fig. 3.95)—Thick walls, papillary projections, enhancing solid elements. Look for evidence of peritoneal implants and other sites of metastasis. Ascites is often present.

Peritoneal inclusion cyst—Occurs in the presence of adhesions. No true cyst wall and may have nonspherical or irregular shape.

Sclerosing stromal tumor—Occurs in second or third decade of life. Tumor may have multilocular cystic and solid components. Solid components enhance with gadolinium.

Serous cystadenoma (see Fig. 3.97)—Typically thin-walled, unilocular. Papillary projections may be present, but should raise concern for malignancy.

Theca lutein cyst—Associated with elevated human chorionic gonadotropin levels (gestational trophoblastic disease, multiple gestations, ovarian hyperstimulation). Correlate with contents of uterus.

Tuboovarian abscess—Signs and symptoms of pelvic inflammatory disease may be present. Enlarged fallopian tubes, which may be of variable signal intensity or contain debris.

References: 41 to 43

SOLID ADNEXAL MASS

Brenner's tumor—Typically low signal intensity on T2-weighted images. May uncommonly have cystic components. Mild enhancement. Calcification often present on CT. May occur with other ovarian tumors.

Fibroma, thecoma, fibrothecoma (Fig. 3.187)—Homogeneous low signal intensity on T1- and T2-weighted images. Mimics subserosal fibroid. Enhances relatively poorly. Larger lesions may have areas of degeneration with increased

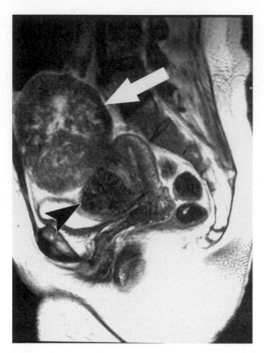

FIG. 3.187. Ovarian fibrothecoma. Sagittal T2-weighted image through the pelvis of a perimenopausal woman shows a large, predominately low signal intensity mass (*arrow*) adjacent to the uterus with some internal areas of high signal intensity. The ovaries could not be identified. Uterine fibroids were also present (*arrowhead*). This mass was initially mistaken for a subserosal leiomyoma.

signal intensity on T2-weighted images. May be associated with ascites and pleural effusion (Meigs syndrome).

Granulosa cell tumor—Vascular and often hemorrhagic. May have cystic component.

Leiomyoma (see Fig. 3.105)—Variable signal intensity and appearance but most often intermediate signal intensity on T1- and low signal intensity on T2-weighted images. May see bridging vascular structures between mass and uterus.

Lymphoma—Often bilateral. Typically homogeneous with mildly increased signal intensity on T2-weighted images. Mild enhancement with gadolinium. Ovarian follicles may be preserved.

Metastasis—May be bilateral or have cystic components. May exhibit considerable enhancement. Primary malignant tumor present.

Ovarian carcinoma—Heterogeneous, enhancing mass. Ascites often present. Evidence of peritoneal spread or hematogenous metastases may be present.

Ovarian torsion—Enlarged ovary associated with engorged vessels. Enhancement poor or absent. Ovary may be positioned in unusual location. Predisposing mass may be present.

Sclerosing stromal tumor—Occurs in second or third decade of life. Cystic component may be present. Solid components enhance.

References: 44

UTERINE MASS

Adenomyoma (see Fig. 3.82)—Manifests as focal widening of the junctional zone. Small bright internal foci may be present on T2-weighted images. Less mass effect on endometrium than fibroid. Little distortion of serosal uterine contour.

Cervical carcinoma (see Figs. 3.84, 3.209)—Enlarged irregular cervix that may disrupt cervical zonal anatomy. May extend into parametrial fat or obstruct uterus. Pelvic lymph node metastases may be present. Advanced disease commonly obstructs ureters.

Endometrial carcinoma (see Fig. 3.86)—Thickened endometrium present. Disruption of junctional zone by high signal intensity tumor on T2-weighted images suggests myometrial invasion. Tumor enhances less than uterus.

Endometrial polyp (see Figs. 3.87, 3.88)—May appear as nonspecific thickening of endometrium, or polyp may be slightly lower in signal intensity than endometrium. Enhances earlier than endometrium after gadolinium administration. May be difficult to distinguish benign from malignant polyps.

Extrauterine malignant tumors—May spread to the uterus contiguously (most common), via the peritoneal space to the serosal surface, or via hematogenous metastases. The most common extrauterine primary sites of secondary uterine malignant tumors are colon/rectum and bladder.

Gestational trophoblastic disease (Fig. 3.188)—Elevated levels of human chorionic gonadotropin present. Hydatidiform mole may appear as heterogeneous, hypervascular mass with cystic components. May contain areas of hemorrhage.

Intrauterine pregnancy—Positive pregnancy test. Fetus present.

Leiomyoma (see Figs. 3.102 to 3.106)—Most commonly intermediate signal intensity on T1-weighted images and low signal intensity on T2-weighted images. Enhances with

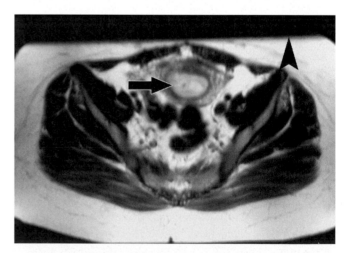

FIG. 3.188. Hydatidiform mole. Axial T2-weighted image demonstrates abnormal thickening of endometrium (*arrow*) in patient with markedly elevated human chorionic gonadotropin level. Complete molar pregnancy diagnosed at dilatation and curettage. Note use of saturation band (*arrowhead*) to reduce respiratory phase ghosting.

gadolinium unless infarcted or degenerated. Degenerated fibroids have highly variable appearance and may demonstrate cystic or hemorrhagic areas. Rarely, fatty elements may be present.

Sarcoma—Heterogeneous, irregular or poorly defined mass. May be indistinguishable from endometrial carcinoma. May invade adjacent organs. Distant metastases may be present.

References: 45 to 47

VAGINAL MASS

Bartholin gland cyst (see Fig. 3.83)—Near vaginal vestibule. Cystic on T2-weighted images, variable signal intensity on T1-weighted images. A variety of malignant lesions, including adenoid cystic carcinoma, may arise from the Bartholin gland.

Clear cell adenocarcinoma (Fig 3.189)—History of *in utero* diethylstilbestrol exposure. May be associated with T-shaped uterus.

Gartner duct cyst (see Fig. 3.91)—Occurs along anterolateral upper vagina. Simple appearing if not complicated by hemorrhage.

Hemangioma—Enhancing mass with high signal intensity on T2-weighted images.

Leiomyoma—May arise from vagina or occur as a prolapsing submucosal uterine fibroid. Appearance similar to uterine fibroids.

Local spread of extravaginal pelvic tumor—May occur with tumors of the cervix, rectum, and bladder, among others.

Melanoma—May demonstrate increased signal intensity on T1-weighted images.

Paraganglioma, pheochromocytoma (Fig. 3.190)—Typically appear very bright on T2-weighted images.

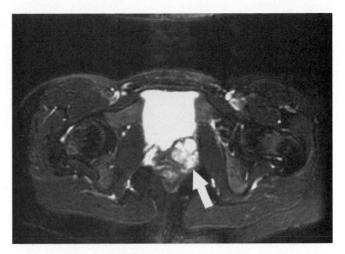

FIG. 3.190. Pheochromocytoma of vagina. Axial fat-suppressed T2-weighted image shows lobulated high signal intensity mass (*arrow*) in left wall of vagina.

Squamous cell carcinoma (Fig 3.191)—Most common primary vaginal malignant tumor. Irregular enhancing soft tissue mass. Increased signal intensity on T2-weighted images. May invade urethra, bladder, and rectum. Inguinal lymph node involvement suggests involvement of lower third of vagina.

References: 48

CYSTIC MASS OF THE MALE PELVIS

Abscess—Associated with prostatitis, Crohn disease, appendicitis, and diverticulitis. Demonstrates rim enhancement.

Benign prostatic hyperplasia (BPH)—Cysts associated with enlargement of central gland.

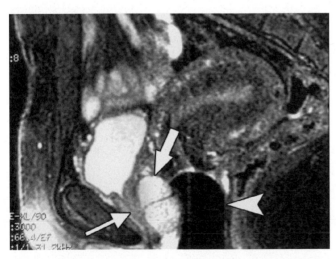

FIG. 3.189. Clear cell adenocarcinoma of vagina. Sagittal fat-suppressed T2-weighted image of pelvis performed with body coil shows high signal intensity mass (*arrow*) between coil in vagina (*arrowhead*) and urethra (*thin arrow*).

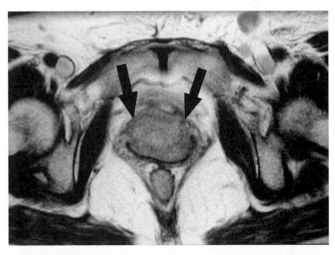

FIG. 3.191. Squamous cell carcinoma of vagina. Axial T2-weighted image through the lower pelvis demonstrates a mass (*arrows*) arising from the anterior wall of the vagina. Necrotic metastatic lymphadenopathy was present on more cephalad images of the pelvis (not shown).

Bladder diverticulum—Follows signal intensity of urine. Communicates with bladder. Stasis may lead to stone formation or, rarely, malignancy.

Cystic prostate cancer—Rare cystic lesion with irregular walls or solid components.

Ectopic ureterocele—Association with duplex kidney.

Ejaculatory duct cyst—Paramedian, intraprostatic location. May appear midline when large. High signal intensity on T2-weighted images. Variable signal intensity on T1-weighted images. Nonenhancing. May be difficult to differentiate from other types of cysts when large. Aspiration reveals spermatozoa.

Müllerian duct cyst—Midline intraprostatic cyst. Does not communicate with urethra. May contain calculi.

Seminal vesical cyst—Laterally located cystic lesion in region of seminal vesicle. Appears bright on T2-weighted images and variable on T1-weighted images. Commonly associated with ipsilateral renal agenesis. Ectopic ureterocele may rarely drain into seminal vesicle cyst.

Utricular cyst (Fig 3.192)—Midline cyst. Commonly communicates with prostatic urethra. Associated with other genitourinary anomalies (e.g., cryptorchism, hypospadias, unilateral renal agenesis, pseudohermaphroditism).

Vas deferens cyst—Paramedian in location, but may appear midline when large.

References: 49 to 52

SCROTAL MASS

Abscess—Clinical signs and symptoms of infection. Scrotal edema. Complex fluid collection of variable signal intensity with enhancing rim.

Adenomatoid tumor—Most common extratesticular neoplasm. Usually occurs in the epididymal tail, but intratesticular tumors have been described. Less intense than normal testis on T2-weighted images and enhances more than testis with intravenous gadolinium administration.

Benign testicular neoplasm (Leydig cell tumor, Sertoli cell tumor) (Fig. 3.193)—Usually homogeneous in signal intensity. Benign tumors cannot be reliably differentiated from malignant lesions of the same cell type or other testicular malignant tumors. Leydig cell tumors are more likely to be hormonally active.

Epidermoid (epidermal cyst)—Benign, sharply marginated, laminated lesion consisting of layers of keratinized material. Has a target appearance on MR images with a low signal intensity capsule. Keratinized layers appear as high signal intensity on T1- and T2-weighted images.

Epididymal cyst (Fig. 3.194)—Common, small, simple cystic lesion of epididymis.

Fibrous pseudotumor—Rare nodular fibrous lesion of the scrotum demonstrating intermediate to low signal intensity on T1-weighted and low signal intensity on T2-weighted images. Minimal enhancement with gadolinium.

Hematocele—Demonstrates variable signal intensity on T1-weighted images depending on time delay between injury and imaging. Usually has high signal intensity on T2-weighted images. History of prior trauma is helpful.

Hernia—Mass protrudes through inguinal canal. May see motion artifact due to peristalsis or evidence of gas when bowel is present. May increase in size or shift with Valsalva maneuver.

Hydrocele (Fig. 3.195)—Demonstrates simple fluid characteristics. No mass effect on testis.

Lipoma—Usually originates from spermatic cord. Parallels signal intensity of fat elsewhere on all pulse sequences.

Lymphoma—Relatively homogeneous. Isointense or hypointense on T2-weighted images.

Mesothelioma—Very rare but often malignant. May manifest as multiple nodules studding the tunica vaginalis (which is lined by mesothelial cells).

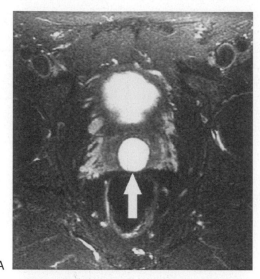

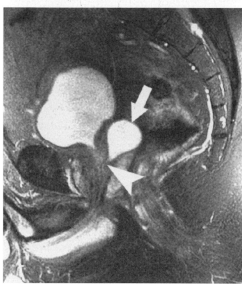

FIG. 3.192. Utricular cyst. Axial **(A)** and sagittal **(B)** fat-suppressed T2-weighted images of the pelvis show a midline cystic structure (*arrows*) posterior to bladder neck. Communication with prostatic urethra is suggested on sagittal image (*arrowhead*). (Courtesy of Christopher J. Lisanti, M.D.)

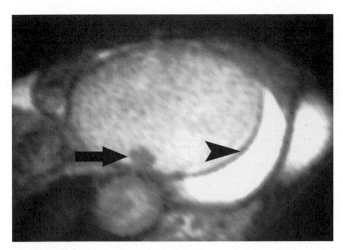

FIG. 3.193. Leydig cell tumor. Sagittal T2-weighted image demonstrates small low signal intensity mass (*arrow*) within high signal intensity testis. Note small hydrocele (*arrowhead*). (Courtesy of Neal Dalrymple, M.D.)

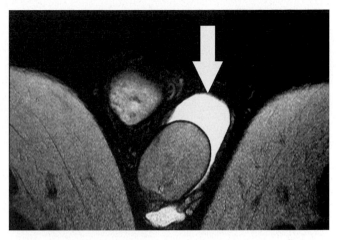

FIG. 3.195. Hydrocele. Axial T2-weighted image through the scrotum demonstrates simple hydrocele (*arrow*) that surrounds but does not displace left testis.

Sperm granuloma—Related to prior trauma (e.g., vasectomy) or inflammation.

Spermatic cord tumor—A variety of spermatic cord tumors may occur, including leiomyoma, dermoid cyst, lymphangioma, and various sarcomas.

Spermatocele—May be associated with tubular ectasia of the rete testis. Cystic mass, occurring most often in epididymal head. Common after vasectomy. Displaces testis (unlike hydrocele).

Supernumerary testis—Similar signal characteristics to normal testis.

Testicular carcinoma (Fig. 3.196)—The majority of testicular neoplasms consists of germ cell tumors. Seminomas are typically of homogeneous low signal intensity on T2-weighted images. Nonseminomatous tumors are more likely to demonstrate heterogeneity and higher signal intensity on T2-weighted images than seminomas.

Testicular cyst—Solitary or multiple. Simple fluid signal characteristics. Located near mediastinum testis.

Tubular ectasia of the rete testis (Fig. 3.197)—Often bilateral. Occurs in region of mediastinum testis. May be associated with spermatocele. Low signal intensity on T1 weighted and high signal intensity on T2-weighted images.

Varicocele—Dilatation of the veins of the pampiniform plexus associated with reversed flow in the internal spermatic vein. Characteristically appears as dilated tubular structure, often adjacent to epididymis. May demonstrate flow-related enhancement or signal void on non—contrast-enhanced sequences. Enhances with intravenous gadolinium.

References: 53, 54

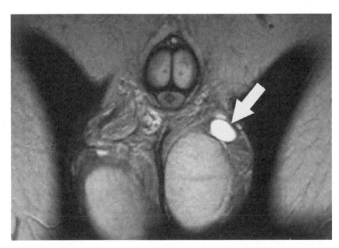

FIG. 3.194. Epididymal cyst. Coronal T2-weighted image through the scrotum demonstrates a small cyst (*arrow*) in head of epididymis.

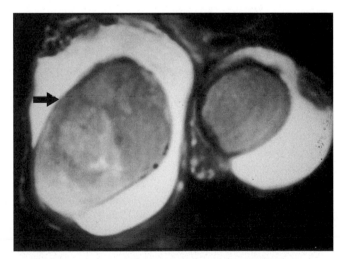

FIG. 3.196. Testicular cancer. Axial T2-weighted image through scrotum demonstrates heterogeneous enlargement of right testis (*arrow*) and bilateral hydroceles. Orchiectomy revealed seminoma. Seminomas with such high signal intensity are uncommon. (Courtesy of Neal Dalrymple, M.D.)

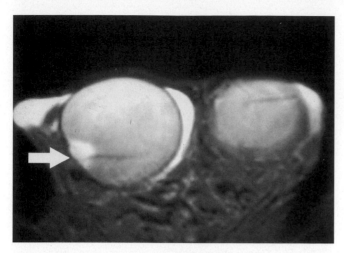

FIG. 3.197. Rete testis. Axial fat-suppressed T2-weighted image through scrotum demonstrates wedge-shaped high signal intensity region (*arrow*) corresponding to rete testis. (Courtesy of Neal Dalrymple, M.D.)

REFERENCES

1. Dodd GD III, Budzik RF Jr. Lipomatous tumors of the pelvis in women: spectrum of imaging findings. *AJR* 1990;155:317–322.
2. Outwater EK, Blasbalg R, Siegelman ES, et al. Detection of lipid in abdominal tissues with opposed-phase gradient-echo images at 1.5T: techniques and diagnostic importance. *Radiographics* 1998;18:1465–1480.
3. Neumann HP, Berger DP, Sigmund G, et al. Pheochromocytomas, multiple endocrine neoplasia type 2, and von Hippel-Lindau disease. *N Engl J Med* 1993;329:1531–1538.
4. Tattersall DJ, Moore NR. Von Hippel-Lindau disease: MRI of abdominal manifestations. *Clin Radiol* 2002;57:85–92.
5. Casper KA, Donnelly LF, Chen B, et al. Tuberous sclerosis complex: renal imaging findings. *Radiology* 2002;225:451–456.
6. Fortman BJ, Kuszyk BS, Urban BA, et al. Neurofibromatosis type 1: a diagnostic mimicker at CT. *Radiographics* 2001;21:601–612.
7. Thomsen HS, Levine E, Meilstrup JW, et al. Renal cystic diseases. *Eur Radiol* 1997;7:1267–1275.
8. Reinhold C, Hricak H, Forstner R, et al. Primary amenorrhea: evaluation with MR imaging. *Radiology* 1997;203:383–390.
9. Siegelman ES, Mitchell DG, Semelka RC. Abdominal iron deposition: metabolism, MR findings, and clinical importance. *Radiology* 1996;199:13–22.
10. Toms AP, Cash CC, Fernando B, et al. Abdominal wall hernias: a cross-sectional pictorial review. *Semin Ultrasound CT MR* 2002;23:143–155.
11. Mortelé KJ, Ros PR. Cystic focal liver lesions in the adult: differential CT and MR imaging features. *Radiographics* 2001;21:895–910.
12. Chen WP, Chen JH, Hwang JI, et al. Spectrum of transient hepatic attenuation differences in biphasic helical CT. *AJR* 1999;172:419–424.
13. Dromain C, de Baere T, Elias D, et al. Hepatic tumors treated with percutaneous radio-frequency ablation: CT and MR imaging follow-up. *Radiology* 2002;223:255–262.
14. Bartolozzi C, Lencioni R, Caramella D, et al. Treatment of hepatocellular carcinoma with percutaneous ethanol injection: evaluation with contrast-enhanced MR imaging. *AJR* 1994;162:827–831.
15. Sironi S, De Cobelli F, Livraghi T, et al. Small hepatocellular carcinoma treated with percutaneous ethanol injection: unenhanced and gadolinium-enhanced MR imaging follow-up. *Radiology* 1994;192:407–412.
16. Sironi S, Livraghi T, Meloni F, et al. Small hepatocellular carcinoma treated with percutaneous RF ablation: MR imaging follow-up. *AJR* 1999;173:1225–1229.
17. Germer C, Isbert CM, Albrecht D, et al. Laser-induced thermotherapy for the treatment of liver metastases. Correlation of gadolinium-DTPA-enhanced MRI with histomorphologic findings to determine criteria for follow-up monitoring. *Surg Endosc* 1998;12:1317–1325.
18. Hyodoh H, Hyodoh K, Takahashi K, et al. Microwave coagulation therapy on hepatomas: CT and MR appearance after therapy. *J Magn Reson Imaging* 1998;8:451–458.
19. Semelka RC, Worawattanakul S, Mauro MA, et al. Malignant hepatic tumors: changes on MRI after hepatic arterial chemoembolization—preliminary findings. *J Magn Reson Imaging* 1998;8:48–56.
20. Castrucci M, Sironi S, De Cobelli F, et al. Plain and gadolinium-DTPA-enhanced MR imaging of hepatocellular carcinoma treated with transarterial chemoembolization. *Abdom Imaging* 1996;21:488–494.
21. Kubota K, Hisa N, Nishikawa T, et al. Evaluation of hepatocellular carcinoma after treatment with transcatheter arterial chemoembolization: comparison of lipiodol-CT, power Doppler sonography, and dynamic MRI. *Abdom Imaging* 2001;26:184–190.
22. Yan F-H, Zhou K-R, Cheng J-M, et al. Role and limitation of FMPSPGR dynamic contrast scanning in the follow-up of patients with hepatocellular carcinoma treated by TACE. *World J Gastroenterol* 2002;8:658–662.
23. De Santis M, Torricelli P, Cristani A, et al. MRI of hepatocellular carcinoma before and after transcatheter chemoembolization. *J Comput Assist Tomogr* 1993;17:901–908.
24. Garra BS, Shawker TH, Chang R, et al. The ultrasound appearance of radiation-induced hepatic injury. Correlation with computed tomography and magnetic resonance imaging. *J Ultrasound Med* 1988;7:605–609.
25. Mori H, Yoshioka H, Ahmadi T, et al. Early radiation effects on the liver demonstrated on superparamagnetic iron oxide-enhanced T1-weighted MRI. *J Comput Assist Tomogr* 2000;24:648–651.
26. Onaya H, Itai Y, Yoshioka H, et al. Changes in the liver parenchyma after proton beam radiotherapy: evaluation with MR imaging. *Magn Reson Imaging* 2000;18:707–714.
27. Onaya H, Itai Y, Ahmadi T, et al. Recurrent hepatocellular carcinoma versus radiation-induced hepatic injury: differential diagnosis with MR imaging. *Magn Reson Imaging* 2001;19:41–46.
28. Padhani AR, Husband JE, Gueret Wardle D. Radiation induced liver injury detected by particulate reticuloendothelial contrast agent. *Br J Radiol* 1998;71:1089–1092.
29. Giovagnoni A, Paci E, Terilli F, et al. Quantitative MR imaging data in the evaluation of hepatic metastases during systemic chemotherapy. *J Magn Reson Imaging* 1995;5:27–32.
30. Nascimento AB, Mitchell DG, Rubin R, et al. Diffuse desmoplastic breast carcinoma metastases to the liver simulating cirrhosis at MR imaging: Report of two cases. *Radiology* 2001;221:117–121.
31. Semelka RC, Worawattanakul S, Noone TC, et al. Chemotherapy-treated liver metastases mimicking hemangiomas on MR images. *Abdom Imaging* 1999;24:378–382.
32. Yankelevitz DF, Knapp PH, Henschke CI, et al. MR appearance of radiation hepatitis. *Clin Imaging* 1992;16:89–92.
33. Kim JH, Kim MJ, Chung JJ, et al. Differential diagnosis of periampullary carcinomas at MR imaging. *Radiographics* 2002;22:1335–1352.
34. Demos TC, Posniak HV, Harmath C, et al. Cystic lesions of the pancreas. *AJR* 2002;179:1375–1388.
35. Leyendecker JR, Elsayes KM, Gratz BI, et al. MR cholangiopancreatography: spectrum of pancreatic duct abnormalities. *AJR* 2002;179:1465–1471.
36. Krebs TL, Wagner BJ. MR imaging of the adrenal gland: radiologic-pathologic correlation. *Radiographics* 1998;18:1425–1440.
37. Balci NC, Semelka RC, Patt RH, et al. Complex renal cysts: findings on MR imaging. *AJR* 1999;172:1495–1500.
38. Scialpi M, Di Maggio A, Midiri M, et al. Small renal masses: assessment of lesion characterization and vascularity on dynamic contrast-enhanced MR imaging with fat suppression. *AJR* 2000;175:751–757.
39. Negus S, Sidhu PS. MRI of retroperitoneal collections: a comparison with CT. *Br J Radiol* 2000;73:907–912.
40. Nishino M, Hayakawa K, Minami M, et al. Primary retroperitoneal neoplasms: CT and MR imaging findings with anatomic and pathologic diagnostic clues. *Radiographics* 2003;23:45–57.
41. Yamashita Y, Torashima M, Hatanaka Y, et al. Adnexal masses: accuracy of characterization with transvaginal US and precontrast and postcontrast MR imaging. *Radiology* 1995;194:557–565.
42. Kinoshita T, Ishii K, Naganuma H, et al. MR findings of ovarian tumours with cystic components. *Br J Radiol* 2000;73:333–339.

43. Jung SE, Lee JM, Rha SE, et al. CT and MR imaging of ovarian tumors with emphasis on differential diagnosis. *Radiographics* 2002;22:1305–1325.
44. Tanaka YO, Nishida M, Yamaguchi M, et al. MRI of gynaecological solid masses. *Clin Radiol* 2000;55:899–911.
45. Imaoka I, Sugimura K, Masui T, et al. Abnormal uterine cavity: differential diagnosis with MR imaging. *Magn Reson Imaging* 1999;17:1445–1455.
46. Hamm B, Kubik-Huch RA, Fleige B. MR imaging and CT of the female pelvis: radiologic-pathologic correlation. *Eur Radiol* 1999;9:3–15.
47. Metser U, Haider MA, Khalili K, et al. MR imaging findings and patterns of spread in secondary tumor involvement of the uterine body and cervix. *AJR* 2003;180:765–769.
48. Siegelman ES, Outwater EK, Banner MP, et al. High-resolution MR imaging of the vagina. *Radiographics* 1997;17:1183–1203.
49. Robert Y, Rigot JM, Rocourt N, et al. MR findings of ejaculatory duct cysts. *Acta Radiol* 1994;35:459–462.
50. Thurnher S, Hricak H, Tanagho EA. Mullerian duct cyst: diagnosis with MR imaging. *Radiology* 1988;168:25–28.
51. McDermott VG, Meakem TJ III, Stolpen AH, et al. Prostatic and periprostatic cysts: findings on MR imaging. *AJR* 1995;164:123–127.
52. Kubik-Huch RA, Hailemariam S, Hamm B. CT and MRI of the male genital tract: radiologic-pathologic correlation. *Eur Radiol* 1999;9:16–28.
53. Woodward PJ, Sohaey R, O'Donoghue MJ, et al. From the archives of the AFIP: tumors and tumorlike lesions of the testis: radiologic-pathologic correlation. *Radiographics* 2002;22:189–216.
54. Woodward PJ, Schwab CM, Sesterhenn IA. From the archives of the AFIP. Extratesticular scrotal masses: radiologic pathologic correlation. *Radiographics* 2003;23:215–240.

SECTION 3.4

What the Surgeon Needs to Know

Preoperative Assessment of Patients with Selected Tumors and Organ Transplant Candidates

This section addresses the need to keep the referring physician's interests and potential future patient management decisions in mind when interpreting an abdominal or pelvic magnetic resonance imaging (MRI) examination. For example, a surgeon referring a patient for MRI evaluation of a tumor already knows that the tumor exists and may already suspect the correct diagnosis. In this setting, the surgeon may primarily be interested in knowing if the patient is a candidate for resection and the obstacles he or she may encounter during surgery. Likewise, providing a report that states essentially "normal liver" for a living-related partial liver donor is not particularly helpful if the vascular and biliary anatomy is not specifically and carefully analyzed.

When confronted with an abdominal or pelvic tumor possibly requiring resection, an attempt should be made to answer the following general questions:

1. From what organ does the tumor originate? To answer this question, imaging in multiple planes may be necessary, and accounting for all relevant organs is critical. For example, identification of two normal-appearing ovaries dramatically reduces the likelihood that a cystic pelvic mass is of ovarian origin.
2. Does the tumor extend beyond the serosal layer or capsule of the involved organ? Infiltration or loss of surrounding fat planes or interruption of a normally low signal intensity border suggest extraserosal extension.
3. Is there evidence of invasion of adjacent organs? An intact fat plane between a tumor and an adjacent organ makes invasion unlikely.
4. Is there evidence of arterial or venous invasion or encasement? Dedicated vascular sequences may be necessary to answer this question.

5. Are there enlarged lymph nodes, and, if so, where are they located? Fat-suppressed T2-weighted images are particularly useful for identifying lymph nodes.
6. Is there evidence of distant metastases? The coronal HASTE breath-hold localizer should be scrutinized for evidence of unsuspected metastases to the spine or lung bases.
7. Are there any anatomic variants that may present a problem during surgery? Make sure that all relevant vessels or ducts are identified.
8. To achieve clear surgical margins, how much of the involved organ will need to be resected and how much will remain?

It is unrealistic to expect that a definitive answer can be provided for all of these questions in every case. If any areas of uncertainty exist, the concern can be conveyed to the referring physician with a recommendation for additional imaging (e.g., intraoperative ultrasound or angiography). Surgeons and institutions vary in their criteria for resectability of tumors. Therefore, one should avoid declarations of resectability or unresectability in the dictated report and focus instead on a detailed description of the extent of disease.

PREOPERATIVE ASSESSMENT OF LIVER TUMORS

Hepatic resection remains the best hope for cure for many patients with malignant and symptomatic benign hepatic tumors. A surgeon referring a patient for evaluation of a liver tumor is interested in the precise location of the tumor, the number and location of additional lesions by segment, the proximity of the tumor to major vascular and biliary structures, the presence of anatomic variants that may complicate

208

or preclude surgery, and whether sufficient liver mass will remain to sustain life after the tumor is resected.

Tumor location is most commonly reported by segment. The traditional segmental anatomy used by radiologists divides the liver into left and right lobes, with each lobe further subdivided into two segments. The plane separating the hepatic lobes is defined by the middle hepatic vein and the gallbladder fossa. The right hepatic lobe is divided into anterior and posterior segments by the right hepatic vein, and the left lobe is divided into medial and lateral segments by the falciform ligament. Even though this approach has the advantage of being relatively simple and reproducible, it does not correspond with the surgeon's view of hepatic anatomy. Liver surgeons view hepatic anatomy according to segments or subsegments containing specific vascular and biliary branches. This typically involves some variation of the Couinaud system (Fig. 3.198). This is a logical approach, because the sur-

geon looks for potential planes of resection between the major vascular territories upon which most segmentation systems are based.

Detection of additional lesions is critical in patients being considered for resection of hepatic metastases. Even though gadolinium chelates remain the most commonly used contrast agents for hepatic imaging, there is emerging interest in the use of alternative contrast agents such as ferumoxides for the preoperative detection of hepatic metastases (1,2).

Assessing involvement of biliary and vascular structures is critical to determining resectability of liver tumors. Successful tumor resection is generally not feasible when there is involvement of both right and left hepatic bile ducts, right and left portal veins, right and left hepatic arteries, the main portal vein, the biliary confluence, or the proper hepatic artery (Fig. 3.199). When possible, true vascular invasion or encasement (tumor directly contacts, extends along, narrows,

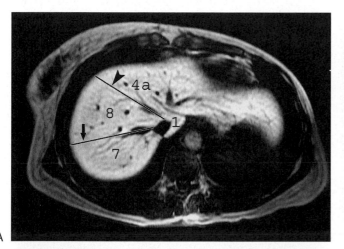
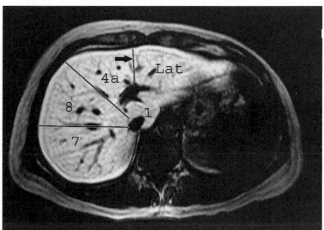

FIG. 3.198. Segmental anatomy of liver. **A:** Axial mangafodipir-enhanced T1-weighted image through upper liver shows plane of right hepatic vein (*arrow*) separating segments 7 and 8 and plane of middle hepatic vein (*arrowhead*) separating segments 8 and 4a. Segment 1 represents caudate lobe. **B:** Level slightly caudal to **(A)** at level of left portal vein shows division (*arrow*) between medial segment (4a) and lateral segment (lat) of left lobe based on position of fissure for ligamentum teres seen at different level. **C:** Axial image in same patient below level of portal vein shows segments 5 and 6 divided by right hepatic vein (*arrow*). Fissure for ligamentum teres (*arrowhead*) divides medial (4b) and lateral segments of left lobe.

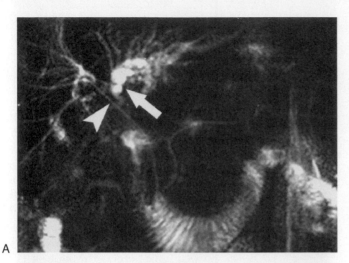

A

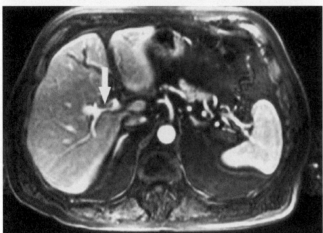

B

FIG. 3.199. Biliary and portal venous involvement with cholangiocarcinoma. **A:** Coronal thick-slab magnetic resonance cholangiopancreatography image demonstrates biliary obstruction secondary to cholangiocarcinoma that clearly involves left-sided ducts (*arrow*). Right-sided ducts are abnormal in appearance but decompressed by stent (*arrowhead*). **B:** Right-sided involvement is confirmed on fat-suppressed gadolinium-enhanced gradient echo image, which shows tumor impinging on right portal vein (*arrow*).

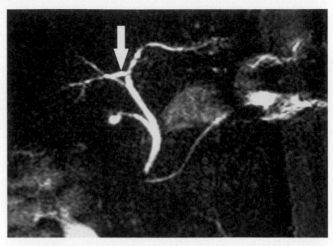

FIG. 3.200. Variant biliary anatomy. Coronal thick-slab magnetic resonance cholangiopancreatography shows right posterior bile duct draining into left hepatic duct. It is important to alert the surgeon to variant anatomy such as this to avoid interrupting biliary drainage from the right hepatic lobe during a left hepatectomy.

or extends into the vessel) should be distinguished from vessel displacement or compression due to mass effect. Identifying anatomic variants is important to avoid postoperative disruption of the vascular supply or biliary drainage of the remaining liver. For example, if a patient's right posterior bile duct drains directly into the left hepatic duct, a left hepatectomy could lead to right biliary tract obstruction if the surgeon is unaware of the anatomic variant. (Fig. 3.200). Finally, sufficient liver must remain following tumor resection to sustain life. Therefore, we often provide a volume estimate for the portion of the liver to remain following resection. It may also be useful to provide a percentage estimate of the volume to remain relative to the entire liver. The presence of imaging findings suggesting cirrhosis should be noted,

because a greater volume of residual liver may be needed for postoperative survival in this setting. In the future, three-dimensional imaging (3D) techniques will be routinely used to provide quantitative liver resection proposals allowing tumor resection to be based on a preoperative virtual surgery (3).

PREOPERATIVE ASSESSMENT OF PANCREATIC ADENOCARCINOMA

Surgery is the only treatment option with curative potential for patients with pancreatic adenocarcinoma. Therefore, it is important to accurately identify the minority of patients with pancreatic cancer who are candidates for resection. Computed tomography (CT) remains the primary imaging examination for the diagnosis and preoperative evaluation of pancreatic tumors at most centers. However, MRI may be useful in patients for whom contrast-enhanced CT is contraindicated or who require further characterization of an indeterminate CT finding. The accuracy of MRI combined with magnetic resonance cholangiopancreatography (MRCP) and magnetic resonance angiography (MRA) for differentiating benign from malignant pancreatic lesions probably approaches 90%, although the accuracy of MRI for determining tumor nonresectability is somewhat lower (4). Results with MRI for determining resectability are roughly comparable to those reported for CT, although the performance of either modality varies between studies and is likely closely linked to examination quality and interpretive expertise (5–8).

Criteria for resectability of pancreatic adenocarcinoma include absence of tumor invasion or encasement of the celiac axis, superior mesenteric artery, and common hepatic artery (Fig. 201). Tumor encasement of the superior mesenteric vein (SMV) and main portal vein are relative contraindications to surgical resection. Some surgeons perform a Whipple procedure in the setting of SMV or main portal vein involvement using a vein graft to replace the affected venous segment. Local lymph node involvement is not considered a contraindication to surgery, although it does portend a poor prognosis. Distant tumor spread, such as hepatic or peritoneal metastases, precludes curative surgical resection. (Fig. 3.201).

One particularly problematic pitfall of pancreatic cross-sectional imaging is the distinction between inflammation and neoplasia. Chronic pancreatitis is notorious for mimicking or obscuring pancreatic tumors, and acute or chronic inflammation may simulate or coexist with adenocarcinoma. For these reasons, radiologists commonly overestimate or underestimate the extent of pancreatic cancer invasion. Acknowledging this potential pitfall to the referring surgeon preoperatively may avoid future persecution at your institutional Tumor Board.

To provide the maximum amount of information to the referring surgeon about the extent of tumor, we recommend that preoperative pancreatic MRI include relatively high-resolution, fat-suppressed, dynamic contrast-enhanced images. Postcontrast images should be obtained at times approximating peak arterial enhancement, peak venous enhancement, and peak pancreatic parenchymal enhancement to maximize conspicuity of the tumor and surrounding vessels. If a thin section, 3D contrast-enhanced acquisition is performed, additional vascular sequences are usually unnecessary, because multiplanar reformations can be constructed to display the vasculature in any plane.

Fat suppression is essential to differentiate normal high signal intensity fat from infiltrating tumor and normal pancreas. A precontrast T1-weighted image without fat suppression may also demonstrate low signal intensity tumor infiltration within the high signal intensity peripancreatic fat. The addition of MRCP sequences is helpful to evaluate the ductal structures. It remains to be seen whether the contrast agent mangafodipir will offer any additional benefit for the diagnosis and staging of pancreatic cancer.

PREOPERATIVE ASSESSMENT OF PRESUMED RENAL CELL CARCINOMA

Malignant-appearing renal masses are usually treated surgically. Renal masses may be treated by open or laparoscopic removal or with ablative techniques such as radiofrequency ablation or cryotherapy. Although total nephrectomy is still considered the treatment of choice for most localized renal cell carcinomas, an increasing number of partial nephrectomies and wedge resections are being performed in suitable patients.

Determining the presence or absence of extracapsular spread (stage 2), renal vein invasion (stage 3a), lymph node involvement (stage 3b), local invasion (stage 4a), and distant metastases (stage 4b) is critical to treatment planning (Figs. 3.202, 3.203). Additionally, tumor size and location, involvement of the renal sinus, vascular anatomy, and status of the contralateral kidney may influence the choice of surgical approaches (e.g., open versus laparoscopic). Extension of intracaval tumor above the confluence of the hepatic veins may necessitate the use of cardiopulmonary bypass, so the presence and extent of intracaval extension must be elucidated (Fig. 3.204).

The evaluation of tumor thrombus in the renal vein and inferior vena cava comprises one of the more common indications for MRI in the preoperative assessment of renal cell carcinoma. For this indication, MRI has been shown to be highly sensitive and specific (9,10). Dark blood, nonenhanced bright blood, and gadolinium-enhanced MRA techniques may all be used to demonstrate the presence and extent

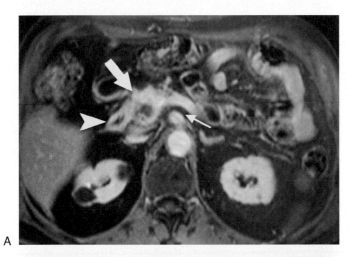

A

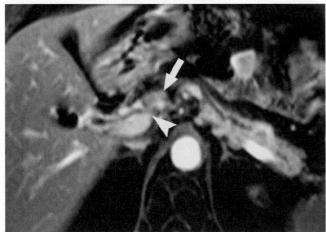

B

FIG. 3.201. Ductal adenocarcinoma of pancreas deemed unresectable at surgery. **A:** Fat-suppressed, gadolinium-enhanced T1-weighted gradient echo image of abdomen demonstrates enhancing pancreatic head mass (*arrow*). Note intact fat plane (*thin arrow*) around superior mesenteric artery. *Arrowhead* denotes duodenum. **B:** Image slightly higher than **(A)** shows tumor (*arrow*) surrounding hepatic artery and involving anterior surface of portal vein (*arrowhead*). Findings were confirmed at surgery.

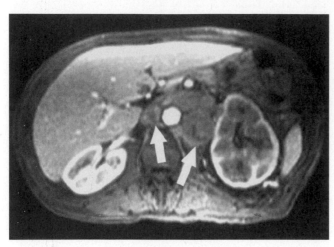

FIG. 3.202. Metastatic lymphadenopathy from renal cell carcinoma. Fat-suppressed, gadolinium-enhanced gradient echo image demonstrates extensive paraaortic lymphadenopathy (*arrows*) in patient with renal cell carcinoma.

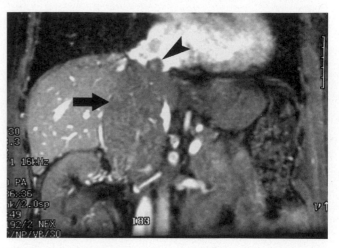

FIG. 3.204. Renal cell carcinoma with intracaval extension. Coronal fat-suppressed gradient echo image of patient with renal cell carcinoma shows expansion of intrahepatic inferior vena cava by tumor thrombus (*arrow*) that extends to level of right atrium (*arrowhead*).

of thrombus. When evaluating the renal vein for tumor, we routinely perform at least two different types of MRA sequences to confirm that the findings are reproducible and not artifactual. Intravenous contrast material is often helpful in distinguishing tumor thrombus from bland thrombus, but the enhancing tumor thrombus may become less conspicuous on venous phase images if the tumor and surrounding blood enhance to a similar degree.

The anatomy of the renal vasculature and collecting systems are well demonstrated with MR techniques and should be assessed in patients with suspected renal cell carcinoma

(11–13). The sensitivity of contrast-enhanced MRA for the detection of accessory renal arteries exceeds 90%.

MR ASSESSMENT OF PROSTATE CANCER

In patients with prostate cancer, MRI is primarily performed for local staging (14,15). The goal of prostate cancer staging is to distinguish early stage disease (T1 and T2) from more advanced disease characterized by extracapsular extension. Surgery remains an option for patients with disease confined to the prostate, whereas patients with extraprostatic disease typically undergo radiation therapy, hormonal therapy, or both.

T2-weighted sequences are critical to demonstrating the normal zonal anatomy of the prostate. The zonal anatomy of the prostate is important, because greater than 70% of adenocarcinomas of the prostate originate in the peripheral zone. On T2-weighted images, prostate carcinoma typically has low signal intensity relative to the high signal intensity peripheral zone (Fig. 3.205). When adenocarcinoma of the prostate arises from the central portion of the gland, it may be impossible to distinguish from benign prostatic hyperplasia without biopsy. The prostatic capsule appears as a hypointense rim surrounding the gland on T2-weighted images. The seminal vesicles appear as convoluted fluid-filled tubules with very bright signal on T2-weighted images. Whereas the zonal anatomy of the prostate is well demonstrated on axial images, the relationship of the prostate to the seminal vesicles is better appreciated in the sagittal and coronal planes. The use of fat suppression is generally considered unnecessary for prostate cancer staging. If fat-suppressed sequences are desired, they should be performed in addition to the routine non–fat-suppressed sequences.

The prostate is of homogeneous intermediate signal intensity on T1-weighted images. Although T1-weighted

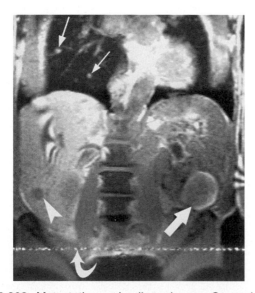

FIG. 3.203. Metastatic renal cell carcinoma. Coronal gradient echo survey image demonstrates left renal cell carcinoma (*arrow*) with liver (*arrowhead*) and lung (*thin arrows*) metastases. This illustrates importance of careful scrutiny of entire image set when staging malignant tumors. Note zipper artifact (*curved arrow*).

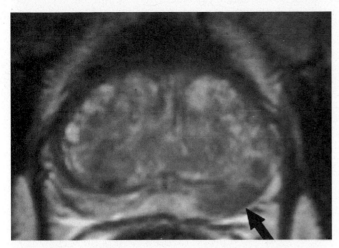

FIG. 3.205. Prostate cancer. Axial T2-weighted image through the prostate performed with an endorectal coil demonstrates low signal intensity adenocarcinoma (*arrow*) arising in peripheral zone.

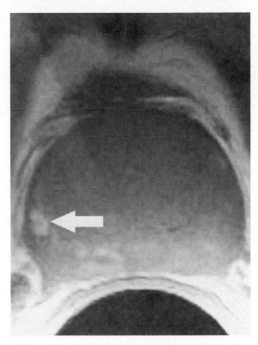

FIG. 3.206. Postbiopsy hemorrhage. Axial T1-weighted image performed with endorectal coil in patient with adenocarcinoma of the prostate involving the right neurovascular bundle shows focal area of high signal intensity (*arrow*) related to recent biopsy.

images are insensitive for the detection of prostate carcinoma, they are useful for demonstrating the neurovascular bundles, particularly in the axial plane. These structures appear as low signal intensity foci relative to the surrounding high signal intensity periprostatic fat and are located posterolaterally at approximately the five o'clock and seven o'clock positions relative to the prostate gland on an axial image. T1-weighted images are also useful for distinguishing postbiopsy hemorrhage from carcinoma, because the extracellular methemoglobin associated with hemorrhage appears bright (Fig. 3.206).

The use of intravenous contrast medium for staging prostate cancer is typically reserved for equivocal cases of extracapsular extension. Further investigation is necessary to demonstrate the benefit of dynamic imaging after gadolinium administration. Prostate carcinoma typically demonstrates early and rapidly progressive enhancement relative to the remainder of the gland following intravenous gadolinium administration (16).

Recently, 3D spectroscopic imaging of the prostate has become possible. This technique is based on differences between the ratios of choline to citrate within cancer versus normal peripheral zone tissue. Even though results are preliminary, it is likely that spectroscopic imaging will improve the accuracy of less experienced readers and reduce the variability between readers in the detection of extracapsular spread (17).

Extracapsular extension or invasion of surrounding structures is suggested on MR images by bulging, irregularity, or retraction of the prostate gland contour (Fig. 3.207). Other findings of extracapsular extension include asymmetry of the ipsilateral neurovascular bundle or seminal vesicle, loss of normal high signal intensity of the seminal vesicle on T2-weighted images, obliteration of the rectoprostatic angle, or loss of the fat plane between the prostate and inferior semi-

nal vesicle (18). The accuracy of staging varies considerably, likely because of differences in imaging technique and reporting. However, staging accuracy improves with the use of an endorectal coil and multiple imaging planes.

It is important to report involvement of the gland apex by prostate cancer, because apical involvement is associated

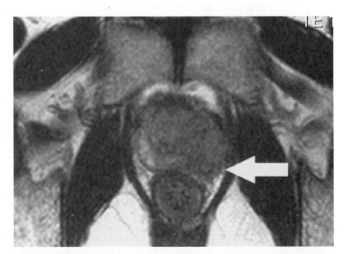

FIG. 3.207. Prostate cancer with extracapsular spread. Axial T2-weighted image obtained with pelvic coil shows extracapsular spread of tumor (*arrow*) into the neurovascular bundle and periprostatic fat. There is loss of the normal rectoprostatic angle on the left. (Courtesy of Christopher J. Lisanti, M.D.)

with a relatively high likelihood of positive surgical margins and postoperative incontinence. An estimate of tumor volume may also be useful, in that larger tumors are more likely to demonstrate extracapsular disease and lymph node metastases. The neurovascular bundles provide a pathway for the spread of prostate carcinoma where they penetrate the capsule. Their status is particularly important if nerve-sparing surgery is contemplated.

MR ASSESSMENT OF CERVICAL CARCINOMA

The appropriate choice of therapy for patients with cervical carcinoma depends on accurate tumor staging. For example, the presence of parametrial invasion by tumor typically mandates nonsurgical management such as radiation therapy. Tumor confined to the cervix (or cervix and upper vagina) may be treated with total hysterectomy, although uterus-sparing surgery may be an option in younger patients with early stage disease.

Despite the availability of new and promising imaging modalities, clinical staging of cervical carcinoma remains the standard of care. Distinguishing between surgical and nonsurgical disease remains problematic with clinical staging, however, and prognostic factors such as the presence or absence of lymphadenopathy are ignored. For these reasons, the use of MRI for staging cervical carcinoma remains an area of active research. It is reasonable to expect that imaging will come to play a greater role in cervical cancer staging (19,20).

In patients with cervical cancer, MRI provides valuable information about tumor location and size as well as extrauterine extension (21). As with much of pelvic MRI, T2-weighted images tend to provide the most useful information about staging cervical cancer. On T2-weighted images, the relatively higher signal intensity tumor can be distinguished from the relatively low signal intensity cervical stroma (Fig. 3.208). Demonstration of an intact ring of cervical stroma on T2-weighted images implies the absence of parametrial extension. With stage Ia disease, a tumor mass may not be visible with MRI, although the endocervical canal may be widened. With stage Ib disease, a mass is visible on MR images, but the entire tumor remains within the confines of the cervix. Stage IIa disease manifests as hyperintense tumor extending into the proximal, relatively low signal intensity vagina. Complete disruption of the normally hypointense cervical stroma with or without stranding in the parametrial fat indicates stage IIb disease (Fig. 3.209; see Fig. 3.84). Stage IIIa disease should be suspected when tumor extends to the lower third of the vagina or when inguinal lymphadenopathy is present. Pelvic side wall involvement (stage IIIb) manifests as ureteral obstruction or disruption of the normally hypointense pelvic musculature including the levator ani, pyriformis, or obturator internus muscles. Disruption of the fat planes normally visible between the cervix and the bladder or rectum suggests stage IVa disease. Distant metastases indicate stage IVb disease. The most critical distinction for imaging to make is between stages I to IIa disease and the more

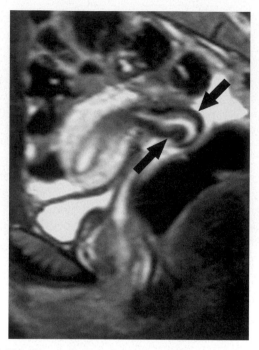

FIG. 3.208. Normal cervical stroma. Sagittal T2-weighted image through the cervix in a patient without cervical cancer demonstrates normal low signal intensity cervical stroma (*arrows*).

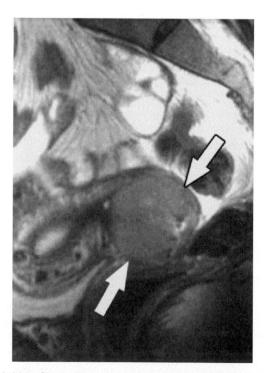

FIG. 3.209. Stage IIb cervical cancer. Sagittal T2-weighted image through the cervix demonstrates a cervical mass that obliterates the normal zonal anatomy of the cervix. The normally dark fibrous stroma is absent, consistent with parametrial invasion. (Courtesy of Hedvig Hricak, M.D., Ph.D.)

advanced stages (IIb and higher), for which curative resection is generally not feasible. The accuracy of MR for establishing the presence or absence of parametrial invasion may approach 90%.

Distention of the vagina with a viscous contrast medium before imaging is beneficial for demonstrating the normal anatomy of the cervical orifice, vaginal wall, and fornices, although the role of vaginal contrast medium for the assessment of parametrial invasion has not been established (22). Dynamic imaging following the administration of intravenous gadolinium may aid in the detection of small tumors, confirm invasion of adjacent organs, or help define fistulous tracts. However, the necessity of contrast-enhanced imaging for cervical cancer staging is still under investigation. The accuracy of MRI for evaluating pelvic lymph node metastases is similar to that of CT. Central necrosis within pelvic lymph nodes is highly predictive of metastatic disease (23).

TRANSPLANT EVALUATION

Liver Transplant Recipient Evaluation

Many transplantation centers have begun to use MRI for pretransplant imaging of patients with end-stage liver disease. MRI is useful for characterizing indeterminate hepatic lesions found by CT and can accurately depict arterial, venous, and biliary anatomy without nephrotoxic contrast material.

A pretransplant MRI study of the liver should be scrutinized for the presence of tumors and patency of the hepatic artery, portal vein, and hepatic veins. Most small hepatocellular carcinomas appear as hypervascular lesions on arterial phase images and may elude detection on other enhancement phases or noncontrast sequences. Small hypervascular lesions on arterial phase images are relatively common in cirrhotic livers, however, and many lesions less than a centimeter in diameter do not represent hepatocellular carcinoma (see Fig. 3.33) (24). Lesions too small to biopsy should be followed up with MRI. Although the optimal imaging interval for lesion follow-up remains to be defined, small (<1 cm) hepatocellular carcinomas are unlikely to progress significantly in less than 3 months. Any hypervascular lesion that increases in size between MRI examinations should be viewed as highly suspicious for hepatocellular carcinoma.

Portal vein thrombosis does not necessarily preclude transplantation, but it is important to diagnose and report to the transplant surgeon. Arterial and caval abnormalities are likewise important to convey. Liver volume provides a measure of the severity of disease and should be routinely reported. An easy way to calculate liver volume is to scan the liver with a sequence that can cover the entire organ in a single breath-hold at 10-mm increments (e.g., 8-mm slice thickness with a 2-mm gap). The liver areas (in square centimeters) determined for each slice can simply be added together to yield the liver volume in cubic centimeters. When drawing the liver volume, do not include the gallbladder or major vessels (Fig. 3.210). Table 3.1 lists the pertinent information to convey preoperatively.

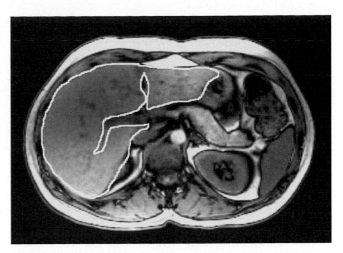

FIG. 3.210. Technique for drawing region of interest for calculation of liver volume. Note that only liver parenchyma is included in region of interest. Major vascular structures and gallbladder should be omitted.

MRI is well-suited for the evaluation of posttransplant complications such as vascular thrombosis or stenosis, pseudoaneurysm formation, intrahepatic or extrahepatic bile duct obstruction, hepatic infarction, and the development of postoperative fluid collections. (Figs. 3.211, 3.212). The detection of intrahepatic biliary strictures suggests hepatic ischemia and should prompt a search for hepatic artery abnormalities. Although increased periportal signal intensity on T2-weighted images is a nonspecific finding that may be seen relatively soon after liver transplantation, expansion of the periportal space with replacement of the periportal fat after the acute period may be a sign of posttransplant lymphoproliferative disorder. MRI alone cannot reliably diagnose graft rejection.

Living-Related Organ Donation

As the demand for donor organs exceeds the supply of cadaveric organs, living-related organ donation is becoming increasingly common. Both the kidney and liver may be transplanted successfully from one living individual to another. As the demand for this type of surgery increases, requests for preoperative assessment of the donor anatomy and health will increase. Therefore, it is important for radiologists to familiarize themselves with the exclusion criteria for organ donation and other information critical to surgical planning.

TABLE 3.1. *Pertinent information for preliver transplantation evaluation with MRI*

Liver volume
Presence and location of tumors
Patency of the hepatic artery, portal and mesenteric veins, and hepatic veins
Vascular anomalies
Extrahepatic biliary abnormalities
Presence and location of varices

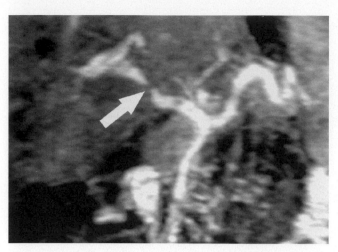

FIG. 3.211. Anastomotic stenosis of portal vein in transplant recipient. Coronal three-dimensional gadolinium-enhanced MR portogram demonstrates severe stenosis of portal anastomosis (*arrow*) following liver transplantation. Stenosis was successfully treated with transhepatic angioplasty.

Living-Related Kidney Donation

The arterial and venous anatomy, presence of vascular and ureteric anomalies, size and position of the kidneys, and presence of parenchymal abnormalities are of great importance to the transplant surgeon evaluating a potential donor (Figs. 3.213, 3.214). Preoperative assessment of anatomy is particularly important before laparoscopic donor nephrectomy, because variations in anatomy may be more difficult to appreciate intraoperatively with this technique. State-of-the-art CT and MRI are both capable of providing all of this information in a single examination with similar results (25,26). However, MRI is not associated with contrast-induced nephropathy and does not expose the patient to ionizing radiation. MRA achieves a sensitivity of at least 90% for detection of accessory renal arteries.

To provide relevant anatomic information and exclude disease, parenchymal imaging should be combined with MRA and MR urography. Standard noncontrast MR images may be obtained in the axial plane. By acquiring multiple appropriately timed coronal 3D gradient echo sequences, the arterial, venous, nephrogram, and excretory phases can all be imaged. If a test dose (commonly 2 mL) of gadolinium is administered to determine proper timing, the predynamic 3D gradient echo sequence may serve the purpose of the MR urogram, because there is typically excretion of contrast into the collecting system by the time the dynamic sequence is ready to be performed (a delay of approximately 5 minutes works well). A delayed 3D gradient echo sequence performed soon after the full diagnostic dose of gadolinium may be performed as an additional MR urogram, although furosemide administration or intravenous hydration may be necessary to prevent signal loss due to the T2 shortening effects of the contrast agent. The predynamic 3D gradient echo image data may be subtracted from the arterial phase scan as a means of improving vessel conspicuity as long as there is no significant spatial misregistration between the two data sets. Similarly, if the arterial phase is free of venous contamination, it may be subtracted from the venous phase images to provide a pure venous image. When interpreting images, it is critical to study the source data in addition to the reconstructed images. This is particularly important when looking for small accessory arteries that may be obscured by background signal on thick maximum intensity projections. It is also important not to confuse overlapping lumbar or mesenteric vessels with accessory renal arteries on reconstructed images.

When interpreting a living-related donor study, look for and report the information provided in Table 3.2. The presence of an anomaly or abnormality on the MR examination does not necessarily exclude a patient as a potential donor. However, these findings may influence which kidney is donated or the operative approach (laparoscopic or open) for donor nephrectomy.

Living-Related Hemiliver Donation

Pretransplant imaging evaluation of a potential liver donor is critical to reduce the potential for complications and exclude unsuitable candidates. The goals of imaging are to map the vascular and biliary anatomy, identify parenchymal abnormalities, and estimate the respective volumes of the portion of liver to be donated and the portion that is to remain. MRI is ideally suited for such an evaluation and may someday eliminate the need for more invasive preoperative imaging procedures such as catheter angiography and endoscopic retrograde cholangiopancreatography (27).

FIG. 3.212. Multiple complications in transplant recipient. **A:** Coronal maximum intensity projection of three-dimensional (3D) gadolinium-enhanced magnetic resonance angiography (MRA) performed to evaluate abnormal hepatic artery waveforms on sonogram performed after liver transplantation. Note patent hepatic artery (*arrow*). **B:** Sagittal view of same data set as **(A)** shows unsuspected severe stenosis of recipient's native celiac artery origin (*arrow*), which was repaired surgically. **C:** Three months later, patient was reexamined with magnetic resonance cholangiopancreatography (MRCP) to evaluate abnormal liver function tests. Coronal thick-slab MRCP revealed anastomotic bile duct stricture (*arrow*) and small bowel obstruction (*arrowhead*). On a thin section MRCP image (not shown), an abnormal cystic lesion was detected in region of pancreas. Arterial phase **(D)** and portal venous phase **(E)** 3D gadolinium-enhanced MRA performed to evaluate cystic lesion revealed hepatic artery thrombosis (*arrow*) **(D)** and pseudoaneurysm of the hepatic artery anastomosis (*arrow*) **(E)**. Note area of hepatic infarction (*arrowhead*) **(E)**.

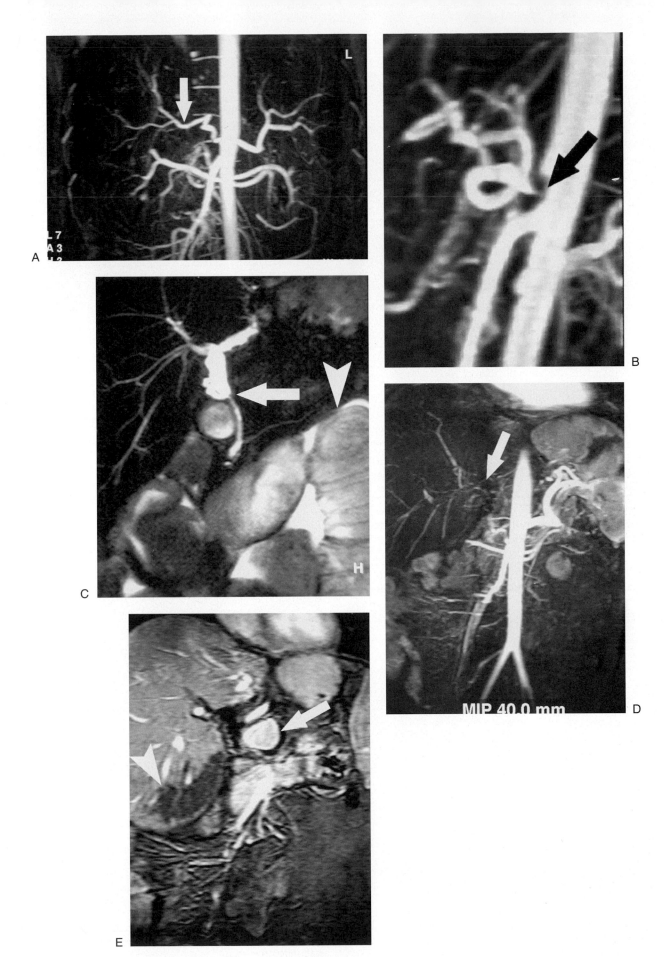

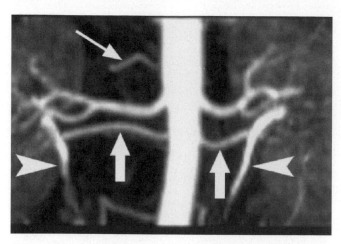

FIG. 3.213. Accessory renal arteries. Coronal maximum intensity projection image from three-dimensional gadolinium-enhanced renal magnetic resonance angiography demonstrates bilateral accessory renal arteries (*arrows*). Note ureters (*arrowheads*). Care must be taken not to confuse lumbar arteries (*thin arrow*) with accessory renal arteries.

Typically, adult-to-adult liver transplantation involves donation of the right hepatic lobe. To ensure that the recipient can be sustained by the donated hemiliver, the estimated mass of the donated liver should be at least 1% of the recipient's body mass. For this reason, separate liver volumes must be calculated for the right and left lobes. The usual resection plane is 1 cm lateral to the middle hepatic vein, which divides the liver into right and left lobes, and extends to the portal bifurcation.

Our current living-donor protocol consists of axial in-phase and opposed-phase T1-weighted images to assess for fatty infiltration, axial fat-suppressed T2-weighted images to screen for and characterize parenchymal abnormalities, and an ax-

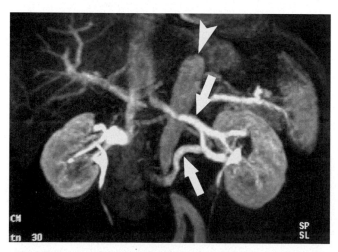

FIG. 3.214. Circumaortic left renal vein. Partial volume coronal maximum intensity projection image acquired during the venous phase shows circumaortic left renal vein (*arrows*) surrounding aorta (*arrowhead*).

TABLE 3.2. *Pertinent information for living-related renal donor MR examinations*

Renal size and location
Congenital renal anomalies
Renal parenchymal abnormalities
Number of renal arteries supplying each kidney
Early renal artery branching
Location of main and accessory renal artery origins
Renal artery stenosis or fibromuscular dysplasia
Venous anomalies (e.g., circumaortic or retroaortic renal vein, inferior vena cava anomalies)
Ureteral anomalies or abnormalities
Incidental abnormalities that may endanger the life of the donor or recipient

ial dynamic gadolinium-enhanced T1-weighted 3D gradient echo sequence to further screen for parenchymal abnormalities and assess the vasculature. Precontrast, arterial, portal venous, and equilibrium phases are acquired. The biliary system is assessed with heavily T2-weighted MRCP sequences in multiple planes. An appropriately timed 3D gadolinium-enhanced dynamic sequence in the axial plane can be reformatted in multiple planes to better demonstrate vascular anatomy, and vessel conspicuity may be improved by subtracting the precontrast scan from the various vascular phase images. If the vascular anatomy is not sufficiently clear on the axial dynamic enhanced scans, a dedicated MRA sequence is performed in the coronal plane with a second injection of

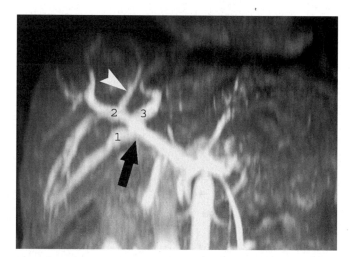

FIG. 3.215. Portal trifurcation in living-related right hemiliver donor. Preoperative oblique coronal maximum intensity projection reconstruction of axially acquired three-dimensional gadolinium-enhanced gradient echo sequence shows portal vein trifurcation (*arrow*) into right posterior segment (1), right anterior segment (2), and left (3) portal branches. This complicated graft harvest necessitated additional bench surgery at time of transplantation to facilitate portal anastomosis in recipient. A large portal branch (*arrowhead*) appeared to be supplying segment 4a on conventional catheter portography (not shown). However, axial MR source images confirmed that this branch was confined to the right hepatic lobe, allowing donation to proceed.

gadolinium (not to exceed the maximum allowable dose) using a larger flip angle for greater background suppression. Alternatively, we have occasionally found a 3D phase-contrast MRA to be useful in lieu of a second contrast-enhanced sequence. In patients with poorly visualized bile ducts on standard T2-weighted MRCP sequences, contrast-enhanced MRCP using a hepatobiliary agent (e.g., mangafodipir) may be beneficial for demonstrating the nondistended bile ducts.

Some vascular or biliary anatomic variants are not contraindications to liver donation, but they may alter the surgical approach (Figs. 3.215, 3.216). For example, if a right posterior segment bile duct arises from the left common bile duct, the surgeon must create two separate biliary anastomoses in the recipient. An accessory left hepatic bile duct arising from the right side may exclude a patient from donating. Large accessory right hepatic veins or large branches of the middle hepatic vein draining the right lobe may need to

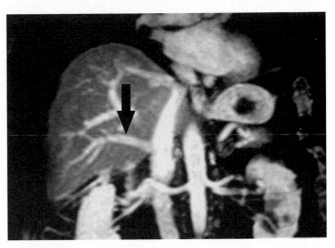

FIG. 3.217. Accessory right hepatic vein. Coronal partial volume maximum intensity projection image from gadolinium-enhanced T1-weighted gradient echo sequence demonstrates large accessory right hepatic vein (*arrow*). A vessel this large would necessitate reimplantation in recipient receiving right hemiliver graft.

be reimplanted in the recipient (Fig. 3.217). Sacrificing such veins can adversely affect the vascular outflow of the liver graft, leading to congestion and failure. A portal trifurcation or dual right lobe arterial supply necessitates additional back table graft preparation to facilitate anastomosis in the recipient. It is helpful to identify replaced or accessory hepatic arteries, and critical to describe a segment IV artery or portal vein arising from the right side, creating a potential problem for right hemiliver donation.

Because surgical expertise in living donor liver transplantation varies among institutions, radiologists should check with their own transplant surgeons regarding their list of relative and absolute contraindications to hemiliver donation. In addition, it is useful to review the relevant findings on preoperative MRI examinations directly with the transplant surgeon. When beginning to evaluate living donors with MRI, we suggest also obtaining other standard imaging examinations until the accuracy of MRI has been established at the particular institution. Correlation of MRI examinations with intraoperative findings is critical to establishing the validity of the technique and interpretation.

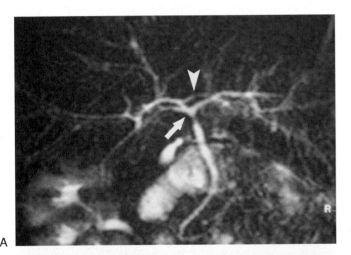

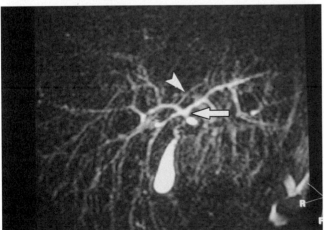

FIG. 3.216. Biliary variant in potential living-related donor. Coronal **(A)** and oblique axial **(B)** thick-slab magnetic resonance cholangiopancreatography images demonstrate a near triple confluence (*arrows*) of the left, right anterior, and right posterior ducts. In addition, a small left-sided accessory duct (*arrowheads*) drains into the right posterior duct.

REFERENCES

1. Matsuo M, Kanematsu M, Itoh K, et al. Detection of malignant hepatic tumors: comparison of gadolinium- and ferumoxide-enhanced MR imaging. *AJR* 2001;177:637–643.
2. del Frate D, Bazzocchi M, Mortele KJ, et al. Detection of liver metastases: comparison of gadobenate dimeglumine-enhanced and ferumoxides-enhanced MR imaging examinations. *Radiology* 2002;225:766–772.
3. Glombitza G, Lamade W, Demiris AM, et al. Virtual planning of liver resections: image processing, visualization and volumetric evaluation. *Int J Med Inf* 1999;53:225–237.
4. Lopez Hänninen E, Amthauer H, Hosten N, et al. Prospective evaluation of pancreatic tumors: accuracy of MR imaging with MR cholangiopancreatography and MR angiography. *Radiology* 2002;224:34–41.

5. Trede M, Rumstadt B, Wendl K, et al. Ultrafast magnetic resonance imaging improves the staging of pancreatic tumors. *Ann Surg* 1997;226:393–405.
6. Sheridan MB, Ward J, Guthrie JA, et al. Dynamic contrast-enhanced MR imaging and dual phase helical CT in the preoperative assessment of suspected pancreatic cancer: a comparative study with receiver operating characteristic analysis. *AJR* 1999;173:583–590.
7. Nishiharu T, Yamashita Y, Abe Y, et al. Local extension of pancreatic carcinoma: assessment with thin-section helical CT versus with breath-hold fast MR Imaging-ROC analysis. *Radiology* 1999;212:445–452.
8. Arslan A, Buanes T, Geitung JT. Pancreatic carcinoma: MR, MR angiography and dynamic helical CT in the evaluation of vascular invasion. *Eur J Radiol* 2001;38:151–159.
9. Laissy JP, Menegazzo D, Debray MP, et al. Renal carcinoma: diagnosis of venous invasion with Gd-enhanced MR venography. *Eur Radiol* 2000;10:1138–1143.
10. Aslam Sohaib SA, Teh J, Nargund VH, et al. Assessment of tumor invasion of the vena caval wall in renal cell carcinoma cases by magnetic resonance imaging. *J Urol* 2002;167:1271–1275.
11. Choyke PL, Walther MM, Wagner JR, et al. Renal cancer: preoperative evaluation with dual-phase three-dimensional MR angiography. *Radiology* 1997;205:767–771.
12. Hany TF, Leung DA, Pfammatter T, et al. Contrast-enhanced magnetic resonance angiography of the renal arteries. Original investigation. *Invest Radiol* 1998;33:653–659.
13. Papachristopoulos G, Bis KG, Shetty AN, et al. Breath-hold 3D MR angiography of the renal vasculature using a contrast-enhanced Multiecho gradient-echo technique. *Invest Radiol* 1999;34:731–738.
14. Bartolozzi C, Crocetti L, Menchi I, et al. Endorectal magnetic resonance imaging in local staging of prostate carcinoma. *Abdom Imaging* 2001;26:111–122.
15. Engelbrecht MR, Jager GJ, Laheij RJ, et al. Local staging of prostate cancer using magnetic resonance imaging: a meta-analysis. *Eur Radiol* 2002;12:2294–2302.
16. Jager GJ, Ruijter ET, van der Kaa CA, et al. Dynamic TurboFLASH subtraction technique for contrast-enhanced MR imaging of the prostate: correlation with histopathologic results. *Radiology* 1997;203:645–652.
17. Yu KK, Scheidler J, Hricak H, et al. Prostate cancer: prediction of extracapsular extension with endorectal MR imaging and three-dimensional proton MR spectroscopic imaging. *Radiology* 1999;213:481–488.
18. Yu KK, Hricak H, Alagappan R, et al. Detection of extracapsular extension of prostate carcinoma with endorectal and phased-array coil MR imaging: multivariate feature analysis. *Radiology* 1997;202:697–702.
19. Boss EA, Barentsz JO, Massuger LF, et al. The role of MR imaging in invasive cervical carcinoma. *Eur Radiol* 2000;10:256–270.
20. Nicolet V, Carignan L, Bourdon F, et al. MR imaging of cervical carcinoma: a practical staging approach. *Radiographics* 2000;20:1539–1549.
21. Hricak H, Lacey CG, Sandles LG, et al. Invasive cervical carcinoma: comparison of MR imaging and surgical findings. *Radiology* 1988;166:623–631.
22. Van Hoe L, Vanbeckevoort D, Oyen R, et al. Cervical carcinoma: optimized local staging with intravaginal contrast-enhanced MR imaging—preliminary results. *Radiology* 1999;213:608–611.
23. Yang WT, Lam WW, Yu MY, et al. Comparison of dynamic helical CT and dynamic MR imaging in the evaluation of pelvic lymph nodes in cervical carcinoma. *AJR* 2000;175:759–766.
24. Jeong YY, Mitchell DG, Kamishima T. Small (<20 mm) enhancing hepatic nodules seen on arterial phase MR imaging of the cirrhotic liver: clinical implications. *AJR* 2002;178:1327–1334.
25. Halpern EJ, Mitchell DG, Wechsler RJ, et al. Preoperative evaluation of living related renal donors: comparison of CT angiography and MR angiography. *Radiology* 2000:216;434–439.
26. Rankin SC, Jan W, Koffman CG. Noninvasive imaging of living related kidney donors: evaluation with CT angiography and gadolinium-enhanced MR angiography. *AJR* 2001;177;349–355.
27. Fulcher AS, Szucs RA, Bassignani MJ, et al. Right lobe living donor liver transplantation: preoperative evaluation of the donor with MR imaging. *AJR* 2001;176(6):1483–1491.

SECTION 4

Additional Useful Information

Atlas of Abdominal and Pelvic Magnetic Resonance Imaging Anatomy

ORGANS OF THE UPPER ABDOMEN
(Figs. 4.1, 4.2, 4.3)

On T1-weighted images, the normal liver has intermediate signal intensity, but is brighter than the spleen. On T2-weighted images, the spleen normally appears considerably higher in signal intensity than the liver, particularly with fat suppression applied. The division between the right and left hepatic lobes is marked externally by the interlobar fissure. The position of this fissure is best identified on cross-sectional images by a line extending from the gallbladder fossa to the middle hepatic vein. The right hepatic lobe is separated into anterior and posterior segments by the right hepatic vein. The left hepatic lobe is divided into medial and lateral segments by the fissure for the ligamentum teres. The caudate lobe is positioned between the inferior vena cava and the portal vein. A third fissure, the fissure for the ligamentum venosum, extends into the liver anterior to the caudate lobe. The venous drainage of the caudate lobe into the inferior vena cava is independent of the main hepatic veins.

The liver may be further divided into eight numbered (often by Roman numerals) segments based on blood supply and biliary drainage (see Fig. 3.198). The caudate lobe represents segment 1. The left lateral segment consists of segments 2 and 3. The division between segments 2 and 3 is somewhat controversial (left hepatic vein versus left portal vein) but not of great clinical importance, in that resections involving the left lateral segment routinely include both segments 2 and 3. The left portal vein divides the medial left lobe into segments 4a (superior) and 4b (inferior). The right hepatic lobe is divided by the right hepatic and portal veins into four segments arranged clockwise as viewed from the right lateral approach (Fig. 4.4). Segment 5 is anterior to the right hepatic vein and inferior to the right portal vein. Segment 6 is posterior to the right hepatic vein and inferior to the right portal vein. Segment 7 is posterior to the right hepatic vein and superior to the right portal vein, and segment 8 is anterior to the right hepatic vein and superior to the right portal vein.

The pancreas, adrenal glands, and kidneys are retroperitoneal structures. The pancreas normally appears relatively bright on T1-weighted images, particularly when fat suppression is applied (see Fig. 4.1C). The pancreatic head is bordered by the duodenum and is traversed by the distal common bile duct. The uncinate process comes to a point dorsal to the superior mesenteric vein. The splenic vein runs along the dorsal surface of the pancreatic body and tail, which are typically 1 to 2 cm thick. The adrenal glands are linear or triangular shaped structures positioned superomedially to the kidneys. The limbs of the adrenal glands typically measure less than 1 cm thick. The kidneys are relatively bright structures on fat-suppressed T2-weighted images and typically demonstrate clearly defined corticomedullary differentiation on fat-suppressed T1-weighted images.

Lymph nodes appear on magnetic resonance (MR) images as round or oval structures distributed adjacent to the blood vessels (after which they are typically named). Lymph nodes demonstrate decreased signal intensity relative to surrounding fat on T1-weighted images and high signal intensity on fat-suppressed T2-weighted images, and they appear as enhancing bright structures on fat-suppressed T1-weighted images after administration of intravenous gadolinium.

BILIARY AND PANCREATIC DUCTAL ANATOMY
(Fig. 4.5)

The intrahepatic bile ducts normally join to form three major ducts that are visualized in the majority of patients by magnetic resonance cholangiopancreatography (MRCP)—the right posterior segment duct, the right anterior segment duct (which follows a more craniocaudal course than the posterior segment duct), and the left hepatic duct. The right posterior segment duct (draining segments 6 and 7) and the right anterior duct (draining segments 5 and 8) join to form the right hepatic duct. The right and the left hepatic ducts join to form the common hepatic duct. The cystic duct joins the common

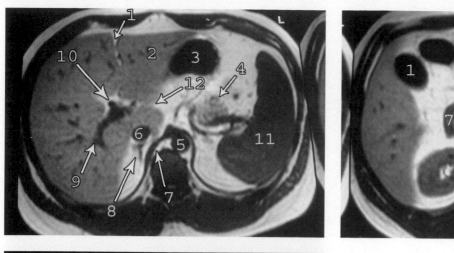

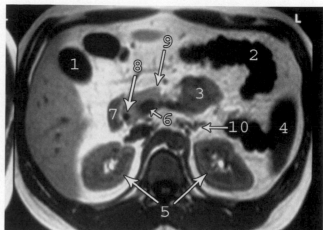

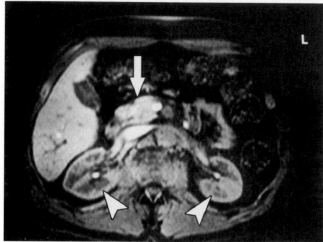

FIG. 4.1. Axial T1-weighted anatomy of abdomen. **A:** 1, fissure for ligamentum teres; 2, lateral segment left lobe liver; 3, stomach; 4, tail of pancreas; 5, aorta; 6, inferior vena cava; 7, right crus of diaphragm; 8, right adrenal gland; 9, right posterior segment branch portal vein; 10, common hepatic duct; 11, spleen; 12, fissure for ligamentum venosum. **B:** 1, gallbladder; 2, splenic flexure of colon; 3, small bowel; 4, spleen; 5, kidneys; 6, portal confluence; 7, duodenum, 8, common bile duct; 9, pancreas; 10, left adrenal gland. **C:** Unenhanced, fat-suppressed T1-weighted image of the abdomen shows relatively high signal intensity of normal pancreas (*arrow*) and normal corticomedullary differentiation of kidneys (*arrowheads*).

hepatic duct to form the common bile duct. The common bile duct enters the pancreatic head and joins the pancreatic duct near the ampulla. The caudate lobe has its own variable biliary drainage via the right or left hepatic ducts.

A wide variety of biliary variants may occur. The most common variant is drainage of the right posterior duct into the distal left hepatic duct (see Fig. 3.200). Also relatively common is a triple confluence, which occurs when the right anterior, right posterior, and left hepatic ducts converge at a single confluence to form the common hepatic duct. In this situation, the right hepatic duct is absent. A large number of other variants may occur, including but not limited to variable insertion of the cystic duct, the right posterior duct draining into the common hepatic duct, cystic duct, or right side of the right anterior duct, and accessory right and left hepatic ducts with variable drainage.

The normal pancreatic duct is less than 4 mm in diameter and joins the distal common bile duct at the ampulla. Occasionally, a small dorsal duct (Santorini) can be seen draining via the minor papilla. Pancreatic duct variants include pancreas divisum, which consists of separate dorsal and ventral ducts draining into the minor papilla and ampulla, respectively, and annular pancreas.

VASCULAR ANATOMY OF THE ABDOMEN (Figs. 4.6, 4.7)

The aorta gives off several major branches in the abdomen that are clearly demonstrated with magnetic resonance angiography (MRA): the celiac artery (supplies the liver, spleen, stomach, and portions of the duodenum and pancreas), superior mesenteric artery (supplies the jejunum,

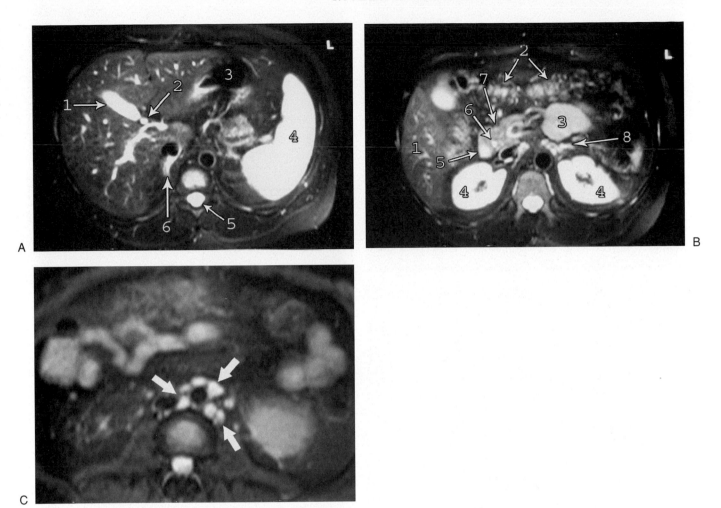

FIG. 4.2. Axial fat-suppressed T2-weighted anatomy of abdomen. **A:** 1, gallbladder; 2, common hepatic duct; 3, stomach; 4, spleen; 5, spinal canal; 6, right adrenal gland. **B:** 1, caudal right lobe liver; 2, transverse colon; 3, small bowel; 4, kidneys; 5, duodenum; 6, common bile duct; 7, pancreas; 8, left adrenal gland. **C:** Lymph nodes are typically very bright on fat-suppressed T2-weighted images as shown in this case of paraaortic lymphadenopathy (*arrows*).

ileum, cecum, ascending colon, and a portion of the transverse colon), inferior mesenteric artery (supplies the remainder of the transverse colon, descending colon, sigmoid colon, and superior rectum), and renal arteries (supply the kidneys). The aorta divides into right and left common iliac arteries, which further bifurcate into internal iliac arteries (predominantly supply the pelvic organs and musculature) and external iliac arteries (predominantly supply the lower extremities).

The celiac artery typically divides into common hepatic, splenic, and left gastric arteries, although variants are common. The common hepatic artery gives off the gastroduodenal artery (supplies the stomach, duodenum, and pancreas) to become the proper hepatic artery. The proper hepatic artery typically divides into right and left hepatic arteries near the liver hilum. The two most common variants of hepatic artery anatomy are the replaced or accessory right hepatic artery arising from the superior mesenteric artery and the replaced

or accessory left hepatic artery arising from the left gastric artery. The former artery is easily recognized on axial images by its characteristic course between the portal vein and inferior vena cava. The latter variant is recognized on axial images as an artery traveling in the fissure for the ligamentum venosum.

The liver has a dual blood supply provided by the portal vein and hepatic artery. The bile ducts course with these blood vessels to form the portal triads. The portal vein is formed by the confluence of the splenic and superior mesenteric veins and divides into right and left portal veins near the liver hilum. These portal branches further divide into the right anterior and posterior and left medial and lateral segmental veins. The inferior mesenteric vein usually drains into the splenic or superior mesenteric vein near the portal confluence. The right, middle, and left hepatic veins follow a separate superomedial course from the portal veins to drain into the inferior vena cava near the right atrium. Frequently, accessory hepatic veins

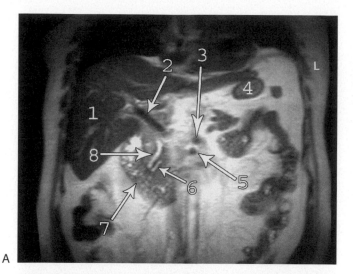

A

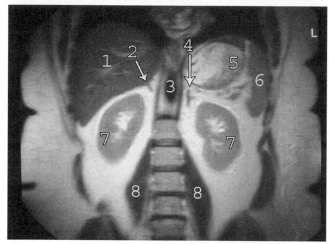

B

FIG. 4.3. Coronal anatomy of abdomen. **A:** Coronal HASTE image of anterior abdomen. 1, right hepatic lobe; 2, main portal vein; 3, celiac artery; 4, stomach; 5, superior mesenteric artery; 6, pancreatic duct; 7, duodenum; 8, common bile duct. **B:** Coronal HASTE image of posterior abdomen. 1, Right hepatic lobe; 2, right adrenal gland; 3, aorta; 4, left adrenal gland; 5, stomach; 6, spleen; 7, kidneys; 8, psoas muscles.

(see Fig. 3.217) are present that drain independently into the inferior vena cava.

PORTOSYSTEMIC COLLATERALS (Fig. 4.8)

Portosystemic collaterals (varices) are frequently encountered in the setting of portal hypertension. On axial images, one or more vessels may be seen originating from the left portal vein and coursing in or adjacent to the fissure for the ligamentum teres. These recanalized paraumbilical veins typically communicate with the systemic venous system via epigastric or internal mammary veins. The left gastric (coronary) vein may flow retrograde from the region of the portal confluence to the azygous venous system, producing gas-

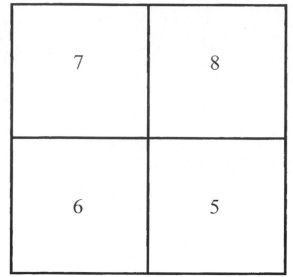

FIG. 4.4. Segmental anatomy of the right hepatic lobe as viewed from the right side. The horizontal line represents the right portal vein. The vertical line represents the right hepatic vein.

troesophageal varices. Varices supplied by the short gastric veins (or other veins that typically drain into the splenic vein) often drain into the left renal vein, producing spontaneous splenorenal or gastrorenal shunts. The inferior mesenteric vein commonly flows retrograde in the setting of portal hypertension to communicate with the systemic venous system via the retroperitoneal (gonadal, renal, and lumbar) veins

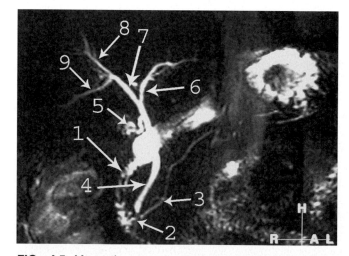

FIG. 4.5. Magnetic resonance cholangiopancreatography anatomy. 1, duodenum; 2, ampulla; 3, pancreatic duct; 4, common bile duct; 5, cystic duct; 6, left hepatic duct, 7, right hepatic duct; 8, right anterior segment duct; 9, right posterior segment duct. Gallbladder has been removed.

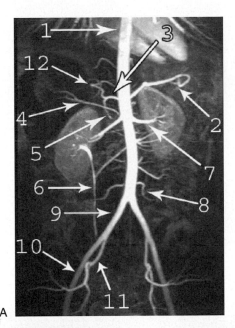

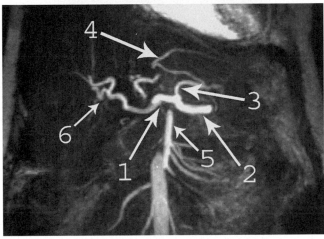

FIG. 4.6. Arterial anatomy of the abdomen. A: Coronal maximum intensity projection arterial image. 1, aorta; 2, splenic artery; 3, common hepatic artery; 4, replaced right hepatic artery from superior mesenteric artery (normal variant); 5, gastroduodenal artery; 6, ureter; 7, left renal artery; 8, lumbar artery; 9, right common iliac artery; 10, right external iliac artery; 11, right internal iliac artery, 12, left hepatic artery. B: Partial volume coronal maximum intensity projection image. 1, common hepatic artery; 2, splenic artery; 3, left gastric artery, 4, accessory left hepatic artery arising from left gastric artery (normal variant); 5, superior mesenteric artery; 6, right hepatic artery.

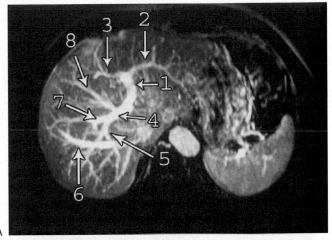

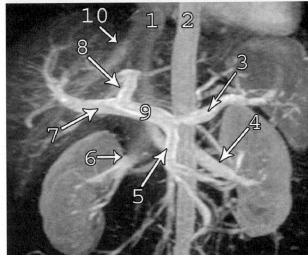

FIG. 4.7. Venous anatomy of the abdomen. A: Axial maximum intensity projection of portal and hepatic venous anatomy. 1, left portal vein; 2, lateral segment portal branch; 3, medial segment portal branch; 4, right portal vein; 5, posterior segment portal branch; 6, right hepatic vein (overlaps portal branches); 7, anterior segment portal branch, 8, middle hepatic vein (overlaps portal branches). B: Coronal maximum intensity projection venous image. 1, inferior vena cava; 2, aorta; 3, splenic vein; 4, left renal vein; 5, superior mesenteric vein; 6, right renal vein; 7, right portal vein; 8, left portal vein; 9, main portal vein; 10, hepatic vein.

or hemorrhoidal veins. Splenic vein thrombosis produces characteristic enlargement of gastroepiploic veins along the greater curvature of the stomach, although these veins typically drain back into the superior mesenteric vein rather than the systemic venous system. Numerous other potential collateral pathways exist, which can best be elucidated by scrolling through images in multiple planes on a workstation.

FEMALE PELVIC ANATOMY (Figs. 4.9, 4.10)

The uterus consists of the cervix and uterine corpus, both of which demonstrate multiple zones of distinctly different signal intensity on T2-weighted images. Following administration of intravenous gadolinium, the myometrium enhances rapidly and brightly, while the endometrium enhances in a more delayed manner. The ovaries of premenopausal women contain multiple follicles, which are best demonstrated on T2-weighted images. Occasionally, intense ring-enhancement of a corpus luteum cyst may be seen following administration of intravenous gadolinium.

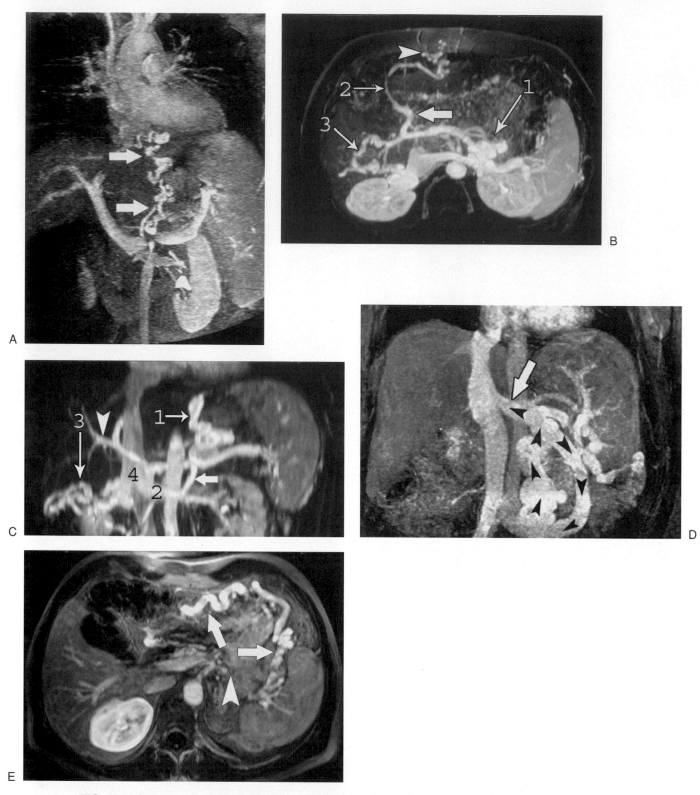

FIG. 4.8. Common venous collateral pathways in portal hypertension demonstrated with three-dimensional gadolinium enhanced magnetic resonance angiography. **A:** Coronal maximum intensity projection (MIP) image of gastroesophageal varices (*arrows*). These are supplied primarily by left gastric (coronary) and accessory left gastric veins and drain to azygous system. Left gastric vein usually arises near portal confluence. **B:** Axial MIP images of three different collateral pathways in one patient. 1, gastrorenal varices connect the splenic and left renal veins via the short gastric veins; 2, recanalized paraumbilical vein connects left portal vein (*large arrow*) with systemic venous system via either internal mammary veins (*arrowhead*) or epigastric veins; 3, varices draining from gastrocolic trunk of superior mesenteric vein to right renal vein.

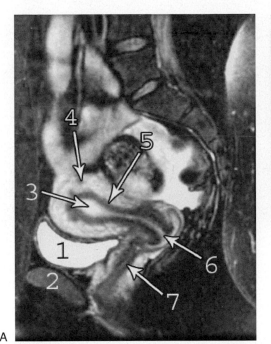

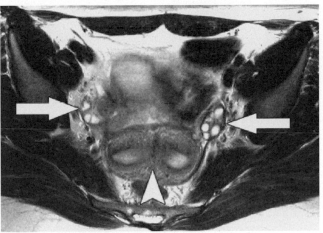

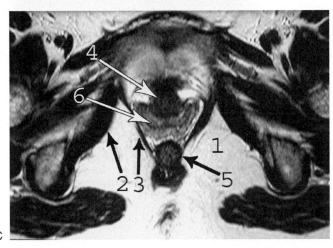

FIG. 4.9. Female pelvic anatomy. **A:** Sagittal T2-weighted anatomy of uterus. 1, urinary bladder; 2, pubic symphysis; 3, endometrium; 4, myometrium; 5, junctional zone; 6, cervix; 7, vagina. **B:** Ovaries with follicles (*arrows*). Note septate uterus (*arrowhead*). **C:** Axial T2-weighted anatomy of perineum. 1, ischiorectal fossa; 2, obturator internus muscle; 3, levator ani muscle; 4, urethra; 5, rectum; 6, vagina.

FIG. 4.8. (*Continued*) **C:** Coronal MIP projection of same patient as in **(B)**. 1, gastrorenal varices (*large arrow* shows communication with left renal vein); 2, left renal vein; 3, superior mesenteric to right renal varices; 4, inferior vena cava. *Arrowhead* shows right portal vein. Recanalized paraumbilical vein is not included in this reconstruction volume. **D:** Varices connecting enlarged inferior mesenteric vein (IMV) with left renal vein (*arrow*) via gonadal vein. Direction of flow is indicated by *arrowheads*. Origin of IMV overlaps left renal vein on this projection. IMV also frequently communicates with retroperitoneal veins and with internal iliac veins via hemorrhoidal veins (not shown). **E:** Axial MIP image of enlarged gastroepiploic vein (*arrows*) secondary to splenic vein thrombosis. Presence of this enlarged collateral vein should immediately arouse suspicion for splenic vein thrombosis. *Arrowhead* marks position where splenic vein should be visualized when patent.

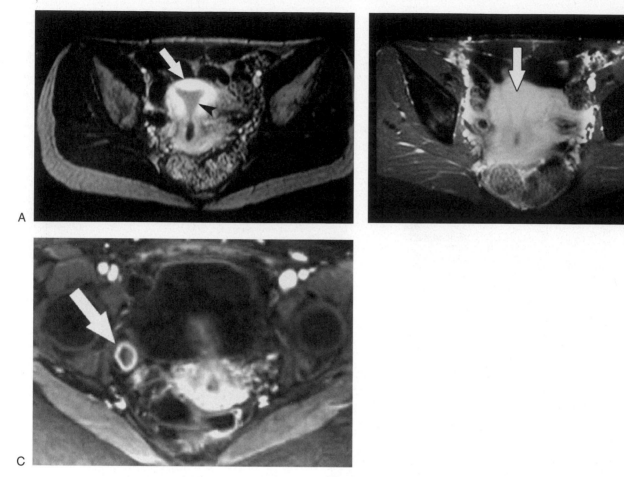

FIG. 4.10. Enhancement of female pelvic organs with contrast. **A:** Axial fat-suppressed T1-weighted image through pelvis performed shortly after administration of gadolinium demonstrates enhancement of myometrium (*arrow*) to a greater extent than endometrium (*arrowhead*). **B:** Delayed fat-suppressed T1-weighted image demonstrates normal delayed enhancement of endometrium (*arrow*). **C:** Post-gadolinium fat-suppressed T1-weighted image shows normal wall enhancement of corpus luteum cyst (*arrow*).

Two common uterine anomalies are bicornuate uterus and septate uterus (Fig. 4.11). These can be distinguished on MRI, because in the case of bicornuate uterus, the uterine horns are considerably divergent and a fundal cleft is present between the horns. Other uterine anomalies include unicornuate uterus (single uterine horn) and uterus didelphys (two cervices present with variable presence of vaginal septum). A rudimentary uterine horn may be present with unicornuate uterus.

Some of the pelvic muscles frequently encountered during pelvic imaging are demonstrated in Figure 4.12.

MALE PELVIC ANATOMY (Figs. 4.13, 4.14)

Anatomically, the prostate is divided into the peripheral zone, from which most prostate cancers arise, the central zone, the transitional zone, and the anterior fibromuscular stroma. The internal anatomy of the prostate is best shown on axial T2-weighted images, which demonstrate the high signal intensity peripheral zone surrounding the relatively hypointense central gland consisting of the central and transitional zones. The paired neurovascular bundles can be found on axial T1-weighted images along the posterolateral aspect of the gland. The paired seminal vesicles lie above the prostate and normally exhibit low signal intensity on T1-weighted images and high signal intensity on T2-weighted images.

The normal testes are of intermediate signal intensity (isointense to skeletal muscle) on T1-weighted images and are relatively bright on T2-weighted images. The mediastinum testis appears as a low signal intensity band on T2-weighted images. The epididymis has relatively lower signal intensity than the testis on T2-weighted images but enhances to a greater extent than the testis after gadolinium administration. Following gadolinium administration, the normal testis demonstrates gradual, progressive enhancement.

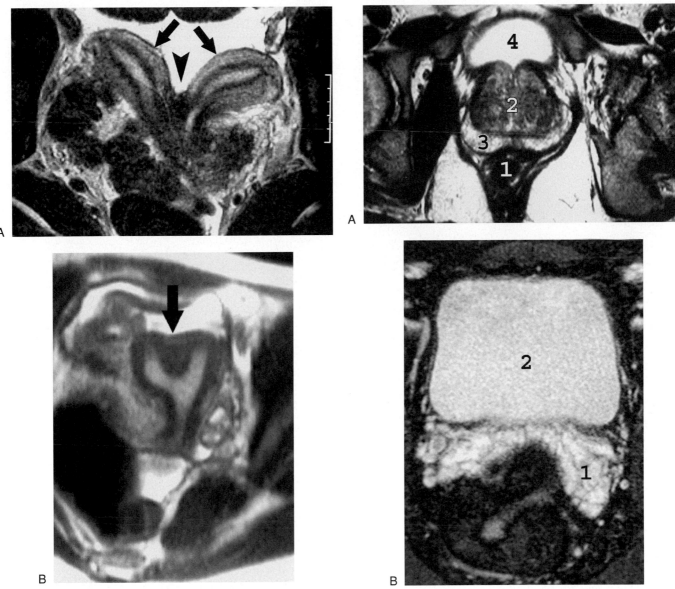

FIG. 4.11. Uterine variants. A: Bicornuate uterus. Note large separation between uterine horns (*arrows*) and deep fundal cleft (*arrowhead*). B: Subseptate uterus. Note lack of fundal cleft (*arrow*) at site of thick septum.

FIG. 4.13. Male pelvic anatomy. A: Axial T2-weighted image through prostate. 1, rectum; 2, central gland (with benign prostatic hypertrophy); 3, peripheral zone; 4, bladder. Left obturator internus muscle is absent. B: Axial fat-suppressed T2-weighted image through seminal vesicles. 1, seminal vesicle; 2, bladder.

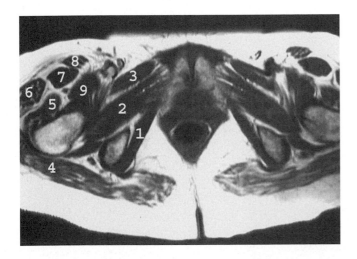

FIG. 4.12. Muscles visualized on MRI of pelvis. 1, obturator internus, 2, obturator externus; 3, pectineus; 4, gluteus maximus; 5, vastus lateralis; 6, tensor fascia lata; 7, rectus femoris; 8, sartorius; 9, iliopsoas.

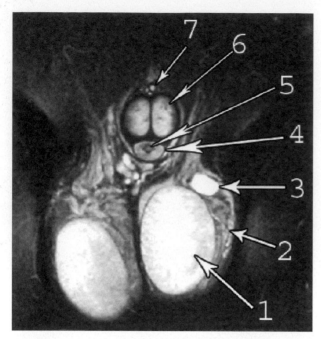

FIG. 4.14. Coronal T2-weighted image of normal scrotal and penile anatomy. 1, testis; 2, epididymis; 3, epididymal cyst; 4, corpus spongiosum; 5, urethra; 6, corpora cavernosa; 7, dorsal vessels.

SUGGESTED READINGS

Dohke M, Watanabe Y, Okumura A, et al. Anomalies and anatomic variants of the biliary tree revealed by MR cholangiopancreatography. *AJR* 1999;173:1251–1254.

Kim M, Mitchell DG, Ito K. Portosystemic collaterals of the upper abdomen: review of anatomy and demonstration on MR imaging. *Abdom Imaging* 2000;25:462–470.

Mortelé KJ, Ros PR. Anatomic variants of the biliary tree: MR cholangiographic findings and clinical applications. *AJR* 2001:177;389–394.

Nunes LW, Schiebler MS, Rauschning W, et al. The normal prostate and periprostatic structures: correlation between MR images made with an endorectal coil and cadaveric microtome sections. *AJR* 1995;164:923–927.

Stoker J, Halligan S, Bartram CI. Pelvic floor imaging. *Radiology* 2001;218:621–641.

Tan IL, Stoker J, Zwamborn AW, et al. Female pelvic floor: endovaginal MR imaging of normal anatomy. *Radiology* 1998;206:777–783.

SECTION 4.2

Frequently Asked Questions

When is MRI preferable to CT for imaging the liver, kidneys, or pancreas?

Many patients in whom iodinated contrast agents are contraindicated are referred for magnetic resonance imaging (MRI) instead of computed tomography (CT) for cross-sectional imaging. The usual contraindications to iodinated contrast agents include renal insufficiency or a history of a prior moderate-to-severe allergic reaction to these agents. Patients may also be diverted from CT to MRI when residual barium from a prior gastrointestinal study remains in the bowel. Barium can cause severe artifacts on a CT scan but produces little or no distortion on abdominal MR images. MRI is also preferable to CT for assessing iron-deposition disorders and fatty infiltration or sparing of the liver or pancreas. With the widespread availability of high-quality magnetic resonance cholangiopancreatography (MRCP) sequences, MRI offers superior evaluation of biliary and pancreatic duct disease.

The currently available gadolinium chelates have biodistribution properties that are almost identical to iodinated contrast agents. Like iodinated agents, they are distributed in the extracellular fluid space and are eliminated primarily via glomerular filtration. For this reason, a dynamic multiphase MRI examination is unlikely to yield more information than a dynamic multiphase CT scan in terms of lesion enhancement characteristics. The advantage of MRI over CT is the ability to further characterize tissue with chemical shift imaging or T1 and T2 relaxation times.

MRI requires a greater degree of patient cooperation than CT, and severely ill patients may not tolerate the longer imaging times of MRI. Local expertise is another factor in determining whether a patient should be referred for CT or MRI. In most cases, a well-performed and expertly interpreted CT scan is preferable to a poorly performed and interpreted MR scan.

Which is better, CTA or MRA?

Computed tomography angiography (CTA) and magnetic resonance angiography (MRA) are equally efficacious in assessing many vascular abnormalities of the abdomen and pelvis. When choosing between these techniques, one should consider several factors. These include the availability of equipment and expertise, history of contrast allergy, renal insufficiency, or claustrophobia, the size of the patient, and the presence of implanted devices, which might cause the patient harm or result in unacceptable image artifact.

MRA has the advantage of potentially providing quantitative flow data, although this is not widely used. If performed at a standard clinical dose (0.1 mmol/kg), contrast-enhanced MRA may be repeated, if necessary, without fear of nephrotoxicity. Noncontrast-enhanced MRA techniques can be repeated as often as necessary to obtain an efficacious result.

When should patients be kept NPO before performing abdominal MRI?

It is not necessary to keep patients NPO (given nothing by mouth) for most MRI examinations. Nausea and vomiting are rarely encountered with gadolinium administration, and intestinal contents rarely interfere with diagnosis. Limiting oral intake before MRCP may be helpful to reduce gastric and small bowel signal, which may interfere with thick-slab images of the biliary and pancreatic ducts. However, creative scan plane acquisition can also be used to overcome this problem. Intestinal contents are frequently bright on three-dimensional (3D) gradient echo sequences used for MRA and may degrade the quality of 3D reconstructions. Although dietary restrictions may reduce this signal, much of this signal can also be eliminated with subtraction techniques. A few MRI techniques, such as MR colonography, do require dietary restrictions, but they are not widely performed.

Is it useful to administer glucagon for abdominal MRI?

Some experts recommend administration of glucagon for imaging the bowel and peritoneum. As MR sequences become faster, the need for glucagon even in these settings will likely diminish. The only situation in which we routinely administer glucagon is when imaging with an endorectal coil. In this case, 1 mg of glucagon injected intravenously just before imaging reduces rectal contractions that can seriously degrade image quality.

Which sequence is most sensitive for lesion detection in the liver?

No single sequence is 100% sensitive for the detection of liver lesions. In addition, the sensitivity of some sequences may be enhanced with the use of intravenous contrast agents. In the case of routine imaging, dynamic gadolinium-enhanced fat-suppressed T1-weighted images are currently the most sensitive. However, other sequences may occasionally demonstrate lesions not seen on the dynamic series. The sensitivity of T2-weighted sequences varies greatly. A respiratory-triggered fat-suppressed T2-weighted fast spin echo sequence in a cooperative patient detects more lesions than a breath-hold fast spin echo sequence in an uncooperative patient. In addition, sensitivity depends in part on the type of lesion imaged. For example, HASTE sequences have very high sensitivity for detecting benign lesions such as cysts and hemangiomas. However, the sensitivity for detecting malignant tumors with these techniques is considerably less. Finally, the sensitivity of T1-weighted and T2-weighted imaging can be enhanced for some lesions with the addition of mangafodipir and ferumoxides respectively, although these agents are only used selectively at most centers.

What is the best T2-weighted sequence for abdominal and pelvic MRI?

A variety of T2-weighted sequences can be used to evaluate the abdomen and pelvis. Most centers use a T2-weighted fast spin echo sequence for routine imaging. However, these sequences typically have scan times of several minutes. As a result, they cannot be performed during suspended respiration without significant modification, and image quality may be poor in uncooperative patients. HASTE sequences perform well when motion is a problem, in the presence of ascites, and when imaging fluid-containing structures (e.g., for MRCP and MR urography). In addition, these sequences are relatively resistant to susceptibility artifact. However, image blurring and a relatively low signal-to-noise ratio limit these sequences. In addition, many MR practitioners have noted subjectively decreased solid tumor conspicuity with these sequences.

Preliminary evidence suggests GRASE imaging performs similarly to fast spin echo imaging in the abdomen, although clinical experience with this sequence is limited. Scan times tend to be shorter with GRASE. This sequence has the additional advantage of reducing the specific absorption rate compared with fast spin echo, an important benefit when imaging at field strengths greater than 1.5 T. Steady-state gradient echo sequences, such as trueFISP or balanced FFE, allow for rapid production of images that appear T2-weighted, although the actual image contrast is T2/T1-weighted.

Can T2-weighted imaging be performed after gadolinium administration?

In most instances, the answer is yes. Structures that concentrate gadolinium, such as the renal collecting systems, demonstrate signal loss resulting from the T2 shortening effects of gadolinium. However, most structures and organs do not concentrate gadolinium chelate sufficiently for this effect to be of significant concern. There is some evidence that the conspicuity of solid liver lesions improves on T2-weighted images performed *after* the administration of intravenous gadolinium (1).

Should I be using 2D or 3D dynamic contrast-enhanced imaging of the abdomen?

In general, stick with what works best on a particular scanner. A well-executed dynamic two-dimensional (2D) scan is clearly preferable to a poor quality 3D scan. In general, though, there is a steady trend toward 3D dynamic imaging for most abdominal and pelvic applications. There are three main advantages of 3D acquisitions: (1) the thin effective slice thickness (2 to 3 mm) improves through-plane resolution; (2) isotropic or near-isotropic voxels facilitate multiplanar reconstruction in any plane; and (3) arterial and venous phase images provide an excellent depiction of the abdominal and pelvic vasculature.

Should I use a gradient echo or spin echo technique for T1-weighted imaging of the abdomen and pelvis?

Gradient echo imaging is preferable any time breath-hold imaging is advantageous. As a result, gradient echo imaging has largely replaced spin echo imaging for most abdominal applications. Spin echo and fast spin echo imaging are used more commonly in the pelvis where respiratory motion is not as problematic. In addition, these latter sequences provide for higher resolution imaging with improved signal-to-noise ratio.

If an adrenal mass is indeterminate on noncontrast CT, what is the likelihood that MRI will be diagnostic for adenoma?

In-phase and opposed-phase MRI and noncontrast CT rely on the same histologic feature to characterize adrenal masses (2). With both techniques, detection of a significant concentration of intracellular lipid leads to a diagnosis of adenoma. Adrenal masses with insignificant intracellular lipid are considered to represent other types of adrenal masses or lipid-poor adenomas. Therefore, it is unlikely that an MRI study will be helpful if the noncontrast CT scan is indeterminate. However, the answer depends partly on the Hounsfield threshold used to characterize the adrenal mass with CT. If one sets the CT threshold low (e.g., less than 10 HU), some adrenal masses considered indeterminate by CT may demonstrate signal loss on opposed-phase images.

Does an entire adrenal mass need to lose signal on opposed-phase imaging to call it an adenoma?

Although most adrenal adenomas demonstrate homogeneous signal loss on opposed-phase images, some do not. Heterogeneous signal loss can occur when some portions of an adenoma contain more lipid than others. In addition, adenomas complicated by hemorrhage can contain areas that do not "drop out" on opposed-phase images (Fig. 4.15).

There is an entity, referred to as a *collision tumor*, in which a metastatic focus exists in or is contiguous with an adrenal

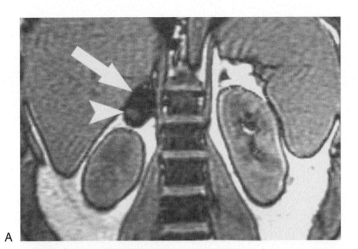

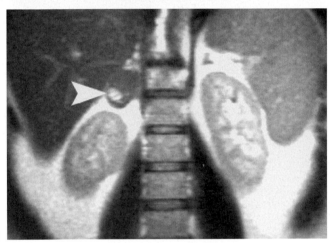

FIG. 4.15. Adrenal adenoma with hemorrhage. **A:** Coronal opposed-phase gradient echo image through right adrenal mass (*arrow*) demonstrates small focus (*arrowhead*) that failed to lose signal relative to the in-phase image (not shown). The remainder of adrenal mass demonstrated signal dropout on opposed-phase image typical of adenoma. **(B).** Same focal area (*arrowhead*) shows increased signal intensity on corresponding coronal T2-weighted HASTE image. At surgery, right adrenal adenoma with focal hemorrhage was found.

adenoma (Fig. 4.16) (3). This is a very unusual finding and is considerably less common than an adenoma with hemorrhage or variable lipid content. However, any area of heterogeneity that appears masslike should be viewed with suspicion, particularly if the patient has a known malignant tumor. Sometimes comparison with prior examinations reveals that the mass has either grown over time or remained stable for several years, improving diagnostic confidence.

Is it necessary to use an endorectal coil for prostate imaging?

An endorectal coil is recommended for prostate imaging. At 1.5 T, we are willing to accept some level of patient discomfort for the benefit of improved resolution and signal-to-noise ratio. There is some speculation that the prostate can

be satisfactorily imaged at 3 T using only an external pelvic coil, but this has not yet been thoroughly investigated.

Are low-to-mid field strength (<1 T) magnets adequate for abdominal and pelvic imaging?

The primary limitation of low field strength systems is reduced signal-to-noise ratio. In many cases, this limits the potential for breath-hold imaging and increases acquisition times significantly. Even so, some imaging centers are performing basic abdominal and pelvic MRI at field strengths less than 1 T. In many cases, this is done to accommodate severely claustrophobic patients in an open scanner who might otherwise forego a needed examination. In other cases, a higher field strength system may not be available. In our experience, most attempts at low field strength abdominal and pelvic MRI result in inferior image quality compared to high field strength imaging. However, when other options are not available, imaging at low field strength may successfully address some basic diagnostic issues. As new ways are found to overcome the problems of low signal-to-noise ratio and long acquisition times, lower field strength scanners may eventually become more capable of performing abdominal and pelvic examinations.

Are there potential advantages to using very high field strength MR systems (≥3 T) for abdominal and pelvic imaging?

Imaging at 3 T is not necessarily twice as good as imaging at 1.5 T. However, higher field strength systems offer some definite advantages, such as improvements in the signal-to-noise ratio, which can be used to increase temporal and spatial resolution. Spectroscopic resolution is also improved on 3 T systems, which also have the potential for multinuclear imaging. However, some artifacts such as chemical shift and magnetic susceptibility are increased. The specific absorption rate (SAR), which is a measure of the energy deposition within the patient, increases significantly with field strength. As a result, patients may experience more heating during MRI examinations, and protocols may need to be altered to maintain the SAR within acceptable limits. Additionally, T1 relaxation times are increased, and T2 relaxation times are slightly reduced at 3 T compared with lower field strengths.

Ultimately, it is likely that many of the disadvantages of high field strength imaging will be minimized through new hardware and protocol innovations. As a result, the improved spatial and temporal resolution of these systems will become the prevailing force driving the integration of high field strength MR into the abdominal and pelvic imaging armamentarium. The combination of high field strength and parallel imaging (e.g., SENSE, SMASH) will be particularly beneficial in this regard.

Are timing runs necessary before dynamic enhanced imaging of the abdomen, or can a fixed scan delay be used for most patients and indications?

Although the arrival time of contrast agent within a specific organ or vascular structure can vary greatly between patients, most patients fall within a reasonably narrow range.

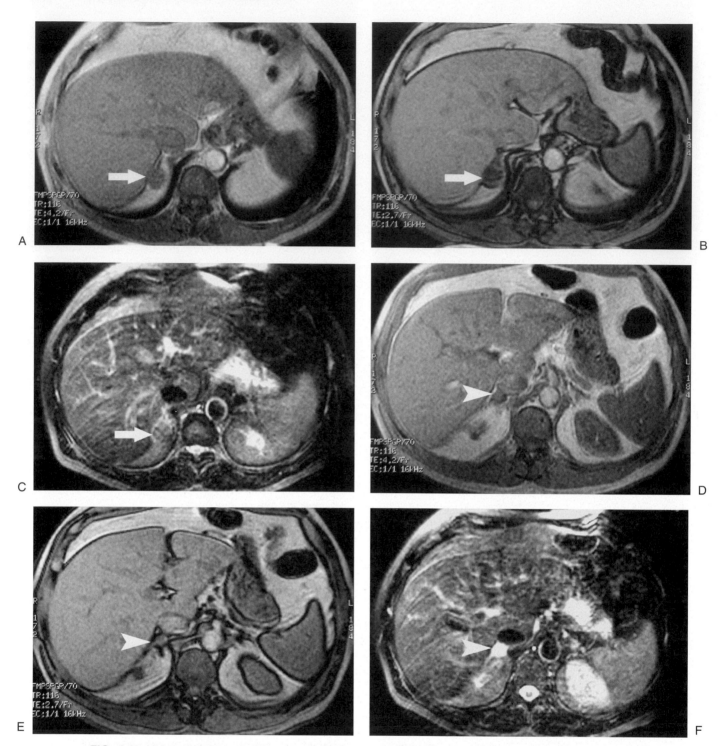

FIG. 4.16. Adrenal adenoma and metastasis (collision tumor). In-phase **(A)** and opposed-phase **(B)** gradient echo and T2-weighted fast spin echo **(C)** images of right adrenal gland demonstrate a small adenoma (*arrows*) that exhibits typical signal loss on opposed-phase image. In-phase **(D)** and opposed-phase **(E)** images at a slightly different level in the same patient demonstrate a second right adrenal mass (*arrowheads*) that does not lose signal on opposed-phase images. **F:** T2-weighted image shows mass (*arrowhead*) to be much higher in signal intensity than adenoma in **(C)**. Biopsy of smaller mass revealed lung cancer metastasis.

Therefore, a standard delay can be used for many routine indications. This strategy has worked well at many institutions for CT scanning. Timing runs (or other means of precisely determining the appropriate scan delay) are recommended whenever precision timing is required or when a patient's cardiovascular status falls outside of the normal range. If a standard scan delay determined for a typical injection rate from an antecubital intravenous line is chosen, then the delay must be modified to accommodate injection through a central line or hand/foot vein or if a nonstandard injection rate is used.

Can dynamic enhanced MRI and MRA be performed even without a power injector?

Power injectors are tremendously convenient and facilitate more accurate and consistent timing of MR data acquisition after injection of contrast material. However, high-quality contrast-enhanced MRI and MRA examinations can be performed without a power injector. A common approach is to use a three-way stopcock connected to the patient, a syringe of contrast material, and a syringe of saline flush. Successful hand-injected studies require coordination between the person injecting the contrast material and the MR technologist performing the image acquisition.

Which intravenous contrast agent should I use for liver imaging?

Gadolinium is generally considered the intravenous contrast agent of choice for most abdominal and pelvic applications, despite the existence of alternative liver imaging agents. Gadolinium chelates have the distinct advantage of being safe to administer as a rapid intravenous bolus. However, mangafodipir may be useful to detect metastases or differentiate between metastases and hepatocellular lesions. Mangafodipir has also been used successfully to image the biliary system. Ferumoxides may add sensitivity for the detection of focal hepatic lesions or aid in characterizing lesions containing Kupffer cells such as focal nodular hyperplasia. Gadolinium-based hepatobiliary agents have shown promise in clinical trials, but have not yet been approved for clinical use in the United States.

Is Mangafodipir useful for pancreatic imaging?

Although originally developed and approved for hepatic imaging, intravenous mangafodipir produces considerable pancreatic enhancement as well. Preliminary studies have shown that mangafodipir may be useful in demonstrating focal pancreatic lesions (Fig. 4.17) (4,5). There is also some evidence to suggest that mangafodipir-enhanced MRI is comparable to contrast-enhanced helical CT for the diagnosis and staging of pancreatic cancer (6). However, there is currently insufficient data to advocate that mangafodipir replace gadolinium for evaluation of most pancreatic disorders. In addition, mangafodipir cannot be safely administered as a rapid bolus, limiting its potential for evaluating the peripancreatic vasculature.

Do malignant tumors ever take up mangafodipir or superparamagnetic iron oxide?

Mangafodipir uptake has been well documented in hepatocellular carcinoma and appears to correlate with histo-

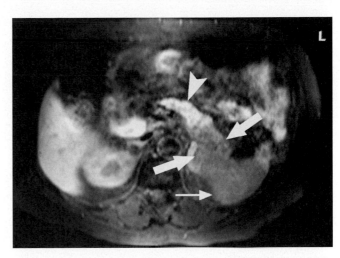

FIG. 4.17. Pancreatic adenocarcinoma. Fat-suppressed T1-weighted image performed through pancreatic tail following administration of intravenous mangafodipir demonstrates mass in tail of pancreas (*arrows*) that enhances to lesser degree than normal pancreatic tissue (*arrowhead*). Note lack of splenic enhancement (*thin arrow*).

logic differentiation (well-differentiated tumors tend to take up more of the agent) (7). Mangafodipir uptake has also been documented in some liver metastases of nonhepatocellular origin (8). However, most metastases do not enhance with mangafodipir.

Some well-differentiated hepatocellular carcinomas may also take up ferumoxides, likely related to the presence of Kupffer cells (9).

Can patients with renal insufficiency receive gadolinium?

We routinely use extracellular gadolinium chelates in patients with renal insufficiency. These agents have not been shown to adversely affect renal function (10,11).

Can gadolinium be administered safely to patients on dialysis?

All of the currently approved gadolinium-chelates are dialyzable, although several dialysis sessions are necessary to remove the drug completely (12,13). We use gadolinium chelates in patients on hemodialysis with the recommendation that patients be dialyzed within 24 to 48 hours after receiving the contrast (i.e., patients are counseled not to miss their next scheduled dialysis appointment). Gadolinium chelates can also be safely administered to patients on peritoneal dialysis. In patients with severe renal insufficiency, we are careful to use the minimum amount of contrast necessary to perform a diagnostic study.

Can patients breast-feed after receiving gadolinium?

There is no convincing evidence to suggest that maternal gadolinium administration in approved doses poses a significant threat to the breast-feeding infant (14,15). Gadolinium is excreted only in small amounts in human breast milk. Of the gadolinium ingested by a breast-feeding infant, only a small amount is believed to be absorbed. Most of the gadolinium absorbed by an infant's gastrointestinal tract is rapidly excreted by the kidneys. As a result, the amount of free gadolinium that an infant is exposed to through breast-feeding is exceedingly small. Despite lack of supporting evidence, it is common practice to suspend breast-feeding for a period of time (usually about 24 hours) after maternal gadolinium administration.

Is it possible to scan patients with intravascular stents or IVC filters? Do they create much artifact?

We routinely image patients with inferior vena cava (IVC) filters and intravascular stents (16). However, a waiting period for certain devices is recommended before subjecting the device to a strong magnetic field. Before imaging a patient with an IVC filter or intravascular stent, we recommend confirming the specific type of device present and the date of implantation. When in doubt, one should check with the device manufacturer regarding any recommended waiting period before imaging. A 4- to 6-week waiting period after stent or filter implantation has been used by many MR practitioners for stainless steel devices. There is no evidence to support a waiting period before undergoing MRI at 1.5 T for devices made entirely of titanium, nitinol, tantalum or other nonferromagnetic materials.

In general, the more ferromagnetic the device, the greater the artifact it produces on an MR image, although prosthetic design also influences the amount of artifact created (17). Stainless steel devices typically obliterate all signal in the immediate vicinity of the device (Fig. 4.18). Therefore, the vessel lumen in which a stainless steel filter or stent is placed cannot be imaged (at the level of the device) with current MRA techniques. Nitinol devices produce considerably less signal loss than stainless steel devices. Some evidence suggests tantalum stents may be best suited for imaging with MRA techniques, producing relatively little artifact.

Is there a role for MR spectroscopy or diffusion imaging in the abdomen and pelvis?

MR spectroscopy applications in the abdomen and pelvis are largely investigational. Most of the research in this area has focused on MR spectroscopy of prostate cancer, and this will likely be one of the first applications to gain clinical acceptance. For diagnosing extracapsular spread of prostate cancer, MR spectroscopy has been shown to reduce interobserver variability and improve the accuracy of inexperienced readers when compared with standard endorectal coil imaging (18). MR spectroscopy has also been investigated for the evaluation of chronic liver disease, characterization of liver tumors and adrenal masses, solid organ transplant evaluation, and detection and characterization of cervical carcinoma and other female pelvic tumors.

Diffusion refers to random molecular motion. Diffusion imaging in the abdomen and pelvis is also investigational. As with spectroscopy, it is hoped that diffusion-weighted imaging and diffusion coefficients will aid in the characterization of abdominal and pelvic masses and inflammatory processes (19).

Largely as a result of the neuroimaging applications of MR spectroscopy and diffusion imaging, many newer MR scanners are equipped to perform these functions. It is likely only a matter of time before their clinical utility is reproducibly demonstrated for specific abdominal and pelvic applications.

When I go to meetings or read textbooks, many of the MRI images shown appear to be smooth and sharp. However, when I look at my images, they don't seem as polished. What am I doing wrong?

Chances are good that you are doing nothing wrong. Many promotional images are postprocessed with software that smoothes the images to make them look more presentable. This does not add to the diagnostic value of the images but does tend to instill feelings of inadequacy in the reader.

REFERENCES

1. Jeong YY, Mitchell DG, Holland GA. Liver lesion conspicuity: T2-weighted breath-hold fast spin-echo MR imaging before and after gadolinium enhancement—initial experience. *Radiology* 2001;219:455–460.
2. Outwater EK, Siegelman ES, Huang AB, et al. Adrenal masses: correlation between CT attenuation value and chemical shift ratio at MR imaging with in-phase and opposed-phase sequences. *Radiology* 1996;200:749–752.
3. Schwartz LH, Macari M, Huvos AG, et al. Collision tumors of the adrenal gland: demonstration and characterization at MR imaging. *Radiology* 1996;201:757–760.
4. Gehl HB, Urhahn R, Bohndorf K, et al. Mn-DPDP in MR imaging of pancreatic adenocarcinoma: initial clinical experience. *Radiology* 1993;186:795–798.
5. Diehl SJ, Lehmann KJ, Gaa J, et al. MR imaging of pancreatic lesions. Comparison of manganese-DPDP and gadolinium chelate. *Invest Radiol* 1999;34:589–595.
6. Schima W, Fugger R, Schober E, et al. Diagnosis and staging of pancreatic cancer: comparison of mangafodipir trisodium-enhanced MR imaging and contrast-enhanced helical hydro CT. *AJR* 2002;179:717–724.
7. Murakami T, Baron RL, Peterson MS, et al. Hepatocellular carcinoma: MR imaging with mangafodipir trisodium (Mn-DPDP). *Radiology* 1996;200:69–77.

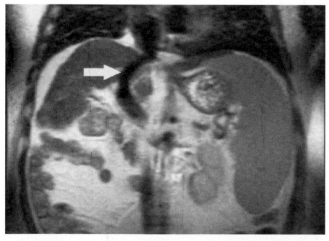

FIG. 4.18. Transjugular intrahepatic portosystemic shunt (TIPS) artifact. Coronal HASTE image in patient with prior TIPS placement using stainless steel endoprosthesis. Note signal void (*arrow*) is localized to immediate vicinity of stent without compromising remainder of image.

8. Wang C, Ahlstrom H, Eriksson B. Uptake of mangafodipir trisodium in liver metastases from endocrine tumors. *J Magn Reson Imaging* 1998;8:682–686.

9. Lim JH, Choi D, Cho SK, et al. Conspicuity of hepatocellular nodular lesions in cirrhotic livers at ferumoxides-enhanced MR imaging: importance of Kupffer cell number. *Radiology* 2001;220:669–676.

10. Prince MR, Arnoldus C, Frisoli JK. Nephrotoxicity of high-dose gadolinium compared with iodinated contrast. *J Magn Reson Imaging* 1996;6:162–166.

11. Tombach B, Bremer C, Reimer P, et al. Renal tolerance of a neutral gadolinium chelate (gadobutrol) in patients with chronic renal failure: results of a randomized study. *Radiology* 2001;18:651–657.

12. Joffe P, Thomsen HS, Meusel M. Pharmacokinetics of gadodiamide injection in patients with severe renal insufficiency and patients undergoing hemodialysis or continuous ambulatory peritoneal dialysis. *Acad Radiol* 1998;5:491–502.

13. Okada S, Katagiri K, Kumazaki T, et al. Safety of gadolinium contrast agent in hemodialysis patients. *Acta Radiol* 2001;42:339–341.

14. Hylton NM. Suspension of breast-feeding following gadopentetate dimeglumine administration. *Radiology* 2000;216:325–326.

15. Kubik-Huch RA, Gottstein-Aalame NM, Frenzel T, et al. Gadopentetate dimeglumine excretion into human breast milk during lactation. *Radiology* 2000;216:555–558.

16. Shellock FG. Magnetic resonance safety update 2002: implants and devices. *J Magn Reson Imaging* 2002;16:485–496.

17. Cavagna F, Berletti R, Schiavon F. In vivo evaluation of intravascular stents at three-dimensional MR angiography. *Eur Radiol* 2001;11:2531–2535.

18. Yu KK, Scheidler J, Hricak H, et al. Prostate cancer: prediction of extracapsular extension with endorectal MR imaging and three-dimensional proton MR spectroscopic imaging. *Radiology* 1999;213:481–488.

19. Ichikawa T, Haradome H, Hachiya J, et al. Diffusion-weighted MR imaging with single-shot echo-planar imaging in the upper abdomen: preliminary clinical experience in 61 patients. *Abdom Imaging* 1999;24:456–461.

SECTION 4.3

Modifying Sequence Parameters

This section describes the effects of modifying many of the user-defined parameters commonly encountered in abdominal and pelvic MRI. The primary (but not only) role of each parameter is listed, along with the effects of changing it in isolation. Although the effects of each parameter change described are typical, there are exceptions. For example, increasing the repetition time (TR) generally increases scan time. However, increasing the TR also allows data for more slices to be acquired during a multislice acquisition. This may eliminate the need for a second acquisition and, therefore, shorten overall scan time. Also, changing a scan parameter does not necessarily simultaneously result in all the effects described. For example, increasing slice thickness may result in increased anatomic coverage for the same scan time or the same anatomic coverage at decreased scan time.

REPETITION TIME

Primary effect: controls T1 contrast.
Increasing the TR:
    Decreases T1 contrast.
    Increases scan time.
    Improves signal-to-noise ratio.
    Increases the number of slices possible during a multislice
        acquisition.
Decreasing the TR has the opposite effect.

Note: For a gradient echo acquisition, T1 contrast is controlled by a combination of the TR and the flip angle.

ECHO TIME (see Figs. 1.7, 1.8)

Primary effect: controls T2 contrast.
Increasing the echo time (TE):
    Increases T2 contrast (to a point).
    Decreases signal-to-noise ratio.
    Decreases the number of slices that can be obtained during
        a given TR.
Decreasing the TE has the opposite effect.

Note: Signal-to-noise decreases with increases in TE, because a longer TE allows more time for proton dephasing to occur. This results in a smaller net transverse magnetization vector and, therefore, less signal. For a gradient echo acquisition, the TE determines whether an in-phase or an opposed-phase image is produced.

INVERSION TIME

The effect of altering the inversion time (TI) for an inversion recovery sequence is not as straightforward as changing some of the other parameters discussed herein. For an inversion recovery sequence, a specific TI must be chosen to create the desired image contrast or to null signal from a specific tissue (e.g., fat). Increasing or decreasing the TI away from this value usually produces an undesirable result. For example, a short tau inversion recovery (STIR) sequence uses a specific TI (which depends on field strength) to null the signal from fat. Increasing this value may result in a water-suppressed image (because water has a longer T1 than fat and recovers through the null point at a later time). Decreasing the TI results in suppression of neither fat nor water.

FLIP ANGLE (Fig. 4.19)

Primary effect: controls image contrast.
Increasing the flip angle:
    May result in more saturation of longitudinal magnetization (less signal).
    Results in creation of more transverse magnetization (more
        signal).
Decreasing the flip angle has the opposite effect.

Note: Because of the opposing effects on signal resulting from increases in the flip angle, one can assume that there is a particular flip angle for each combination of T1 and TR for which maximal signal is generated. This angle is referred to as the *Ernst angle*. In imaging, however, we are more interested in the flip angle that gives us the best contrast

240

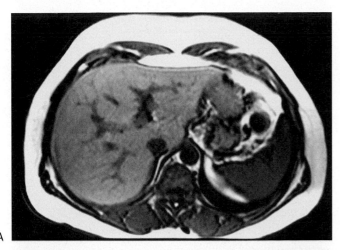

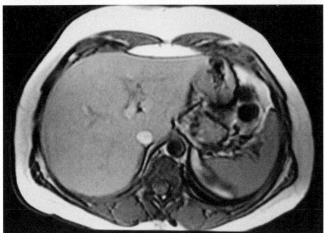

FIG. 4.19. Effect on image contrast of changing flip angle from 80 to 30 degrees. **A:** T1-weighted spoiled gradient echo image of upper abdomen performed with flip angle of 80 degrees demonstrates excellent T1-weighted contrast with significant signal intensity difference between liver and spleen. **B:** Same sequence as **(A)** repeated with 30-degree flip angle demonstrates reduced image contrast.

between tissues for a given application. Because partial flip angles are predominately used for T1-weighted imaging, we focus on the effects of flip angle on T1 contrast at a given TR. If the TR is relatively long and the flip angle is small, all tissues will have plenty of time to recover full longitudinal magnetization before the next excitation pulse regardless of T1 value. This results in poor image contrast. If the TR is relatively short and the flip angle is large, even tissues with a relatively short T1 will not have sufficient time to recover longitudinal magnetization before the next excitation. This also results in poor image contrast. Therefore, decreases in flip angle are usually accompanied by decreases in TR in order to maintain adequate T1 contrast (and vice versa). In the case of magnetic resonance angiography (MRA), however, saturation of the background tissues is desirable. Therefore, a larger flip angle is often used for MRA than for routine T1-weighted imaging.

SLICE THICKNESS (Fig. 4.20)

Primary effect: controls through-plane (perpendicular to the imaging plane) spatial resolution.

Increasing slice thickness:

Decreases through-plane spatial resolution.

Increases anatomic coverage or reduces scan time for the same coverage.

Increases signal-to-noise ratio.

Increases partial volume effects.

Decreasing the slice thickness has the opposite effect.

Note: Signal-to-noise ratio improves with increased slice thickness, because the resulting larger voxels contain more protons contributing to the overall signal.

INTERSLICE GAP

Primary effect: controls crosstalk.
Increasing the interslice gap:

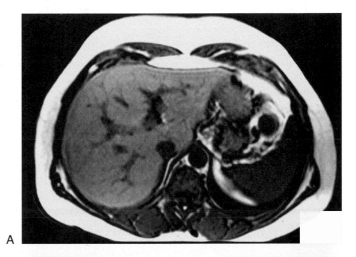

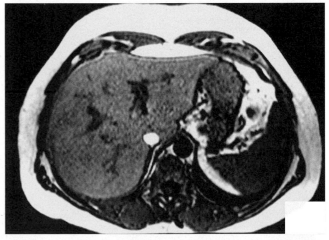

FIG. 4.20. Effect of changing slice thickness. **A:** T1-weighted spoiled gradient echo image of upper abdomen performed with 10-mm slice thickness. **B:** Same sequence as **(A)** repeated with 4-mm slice thickness. Image sharpness and through plane resolution are improved, but image signal-to-noise ratio is reduced.

Reduces crosstalk.

Improves signal-to-noise ratio (due to reduced crosstalk).

Increases anatomic coverage.

Degrades multiplanar and three-dimensional (3D) reconstructions.

Decreasing the gap has the opposite effect.

Note: Radiofrequency (RF) excitation of one slice during an MR pulse sequence has an effect on adjacent slices if no spatial gap exists between slices. This interference between slices is referred to as *crosstalk* and may degrade image quality. An alternative method of reducing crosstalk is to use an interleaved slice acquisition.

MATRIX

Primary effect: controls in-plane spatial resolution.

Increasing the number of frequency-encoding samples (assuming field of view [FOV] remains unchanged):

Increases spatial resolution.

Decreases signal-to-noise ratio.

Increasing the number of phase-encoding steps (assuming FOV remains unchanged):

Increases spatial resolution.

Decreases signal-to-noise ratio.

Increases scan time.

Reduces truncation artifact in the phase-encoding direction.

Decreasing the matrix has the opposite effect.

Note: Signal-to-noise ratio decreases with increasing matrix because the resulting smaller voxels contain fewer protons contributing to the overall signal. Also note that

increases in frequency encoding have no effect on scan time.

FIELD OF VIEW (Fig. 4.21)

Primary effect: controls in-plane anatomic coverage.

Increasing the FOV:

Increases anatomic coverage.

Decreases spatial resolution.

Increases signal-to-noise ratio.

Reduces wrap-around artifact.

Decreasing the FOV has the opposite effect.

Note: Signal-to-noise ratio increases with increasing FOV, because the resulting larger voxels contain more protons contributing to the overall signal.

Most MR manufacturers offer an option referred to as *rectangular FOV* (or RFOV). This allows for a reduction in the number of phase-encoding steps (and thus a reduction in scan

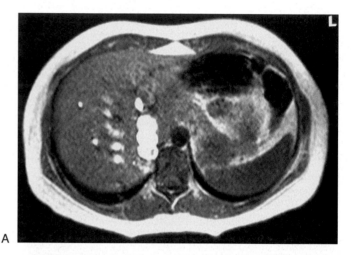

A

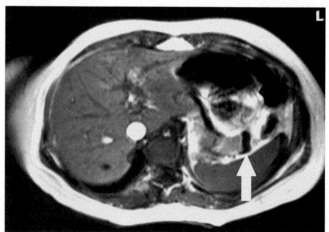

B

FIG. 4.22. Effect of changing receiver bandwidth. **A:** T1-weighted spoiled gradient echo image obtained with high sampling frequency (low water-fat shift) shows considerable image noise. **B:** Image repeated with low sampling frequency (high water-fat shift) has considerably less noise than **(A)** but chemical shift artifact (*arrow*) is much more apparent.

FIG. 4.21. Effect of reducing field-of-view (FOV). T1-weighted spoiled gradient echo image in same patient as in Figure 4.19 demonstrates wraparound artifact caused by reducing FOV without oversampling in the phase-encoding direction (anterior to posterior).

time) along the narrower dimension of the anatomy of interest. In general, the resulting time savings more than compensates for the reduction in signal-to-noise ratio. Therefore, the use of a rectangular FOV is routine for abdominal and pelvic MRI at most centers.

SIGNAL AVERAGES (NEX, NSA, ACQUISITIONS)

Primary effect: controls signal-to-noise ratio.
Increasing the number of signal averages:
  Increases signal-to-noise ratio.
  Reduces the effects of motion.
  Increases image blurring (smooths the image).
  Increases scan time.
Decreasing the number of signal averages has the opposite effect.

Note: Doubling the number of signal averages does not double the signal-to-noise ratio, but rather increases the signal-to-noise ratio by the square root of 2 (approximately a factor of 1.4). However, doubling the number of signal averages increases the scan time by a factor of 2.

ECHO TRAIN LENGTH (TURBO FACTOR)

Primary effect: controls scan time.
Increasing the echo train length (ETL):
  Shortens scan time.
  Increases image blurring.
Decreasing the ETL has the opposite effect.

Note: Because forming and sampling an echo takes time, only a finite number of echoes can be sampled during a given TR. At some point, the TR must be increased to accommodate more echoes.

RECEIVER BANDWIDTH (SAMPLING FREQUENCY) (Fig. 4.22)

Primary effect: controls image noise.
Increasing the receiver bandwidth:
  Decreases signal-to-noise ratio.
  Decreases chemical shift artifact.
  Decreases TE (thereby decreasing scan time).
Decreasing the receiver bandwidth has the opposite effect.

SECTION 4.4

Magnetic Resonance Imaging Acronyms and Abbreviations

To many radiologists, the world of magnetic resonance imaging (MRI) is like a secret society, consisting of a few radiologists, physicists, and equipment manufacturers who converse in their own incomprehensible language consisting of nonintuitive abbreviations and acronyms. It seems that the proliferation of acronyms and abbreviations has impeded rather than enhanced the dissemination of MR knowledge and created an air of intimidation and frustration surrounding abdominal and pelvic MRI.

We have found that MRI of the abdomen and pelvis becomes much less intimidating to our residents when we remind them that most of the available MR pulse sequences are designed to create one of two things—a T1-weighted image or a T2-weighted image (intermediate-weighted or proton density images are rarely used in abdominal and pelvic imaging). Furthermore, most pulse sequences generate these images using either a spin echo or gradient echo. Therefore, no matter what they are called, most abdominal and pelvic MR sequences are one of four basic types: spin echo T1-weighted, spin echo T2-weighted, gradient echo T1-weighted, or gradient echo T2-weighted (this latter sequence is more correctly referred to as T2*-weighted, because gradient refocusing fails to correct for magnetic field heterogeneities). As an additional modification, MR sequences may involve measuring a single echo per excitation (e.g., standard spin echo or gradient echo), multiple echoes per excitation (e.g., fast spin echo or echo planar), or all necessary echoes per excitation (single shot) (Fig. 4.23).

All pulse sequences are not available on all scanners. This is a source of endless frustration for radiologists desiring to apply sequences described in the literature to their own practice. Some sequences must be purchased (at a premium) from the scanner manufacturer. Others are only made available to beta test sites, or they require special hardware such as unique surface coils or high-performance gradients.

This section presents the more commonly encountered vendor-specific acronyms and abbreviations related to abdominal and pelvic MRI. Despite the large number of MR acronyms and abbreviations, certain generalizations can be made that may help one interpret a vendor-specific term. For example, *G, GR, GE, or GRE* usually refers to gradient echo. *Field echo* (FE) is another term for gradient echo. In general, the terms *fast* and *turbo* imply a rapid sequence that reduces scan time through a multishot technique. The letters *IR* in a term imply the use of an inversion recovery pre-pulse.

ASSET: Array spatial sensitivity encoding technique See SENSE.

BALANCED FFE: Balanced fast field echo See FISP/trueFISP.

DRIVE: Driven equilibrium

Driven equilibrium techniques use a 90-degree radiofrequency (RF) pulse combined with a gradient refocusing pulse and a spoiling gradient to force magnetization from the transverse back into the longitudinal plane. DRIVE allows the TR to be reduced for echo train spin echo sequences by shortening the T1 relaxation time of fluid (which reduces the waiting period before the next excitation pulse). The shorter TR results in shorter imaging times without compromising the high signal intensity of fluids. DRIVE is primarily used for three-dimensional (3D) fast/turbo spin echo imaging.

EPI: Echo planar imaging

EPI acquires multiple gradient echoes per excitation. EPI can be performed as a single-shot or multishot technique but requires high-performance gradients (not available on some systems). Several EPI acquisition schemes exist, all of which allow for extremely rapid imaging. However, EPI may be limited by artifacts (e.g., susceptibility). EPI is currently seldom used for abdominal and pelvic imaging, although new abdominal and pelvic applications are being developed.

FIESTA: Fast imaging employing steady-state acquisition See FISP/TrueFISP

FISP/TrueFISP: Fast imaging with steady-state precession (Fig. 4.24)

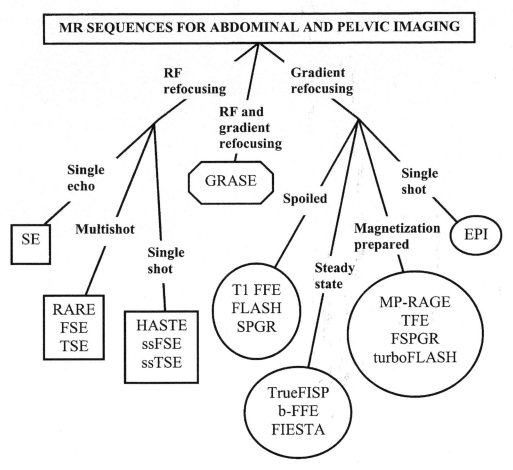

FIG. 4.23. Sequences for abdominal and pelvic MRI. This figure illustrates the differences between various MR sequences that are likely to be encountered in abdominal and pelvic MRI and the relationships between different acronyms and abbreviations.

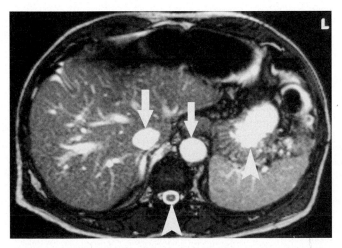

FIG. 4.24. Axial image of upper abdomen obtained with balanced-fast field echo sequence (b-FFE, FIESTA, true-FISP). Note bright vessels (*arrows*) and fluid (*arrowheads*).

A steady-state gradient echo sequence, FISP samples the free induction decay signal. No spoiling is applied, allowing both longitudinal and transverse components of magnetization to persist in a steady state. This original sequence is seldom used in abdominal and pelvic imaging. Similar sequences are GRASS, FAST, and FFE. In trueFISP imaging, the free induction decay signal and spin echo/stimulated echo signal are collected simultaneously, resulting in a predominately T2/T1-weighted image. Fluid and intravascular blood appear bright and tissue interfaces are sharp with this sequence. Flow artifacts seen with HASTE may be eliminated with trueFISP. These sequences are useful for imaging fluid-filled structures, such as the biliary tract, pancreatic duct, and urinary collecting system, as well as for vascular and fetal imaging. TrueFISP is similar to balanced FFE and FIESTA.

FLASH: Fast low-angle shot (Fig. 4.25).

FLASH is a gradient echo technique in which RF spoiling is used to eliminate residual transverse magnetization at the end of each cycle. The sequence combines a partial flip angle with a relatively short repetition time (TR) (compared with spin echo) to create T1-weighted images. T2*-weighted images can be acquired by increasing the TR and echo time

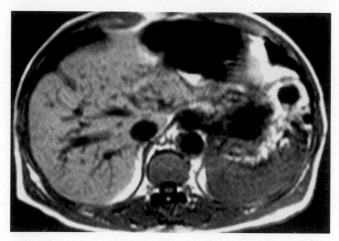

FIG. 4.25. Axial image of upper abdomen obtained with T1-weighted spoiled gradient echo sequence (FFE, FLASH, SPGR).

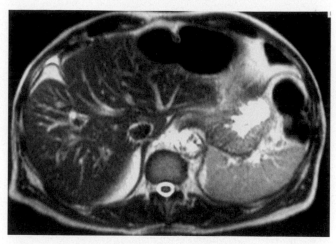

FIG. 4.27. Axial image of upper abdomen obtained with half-Fourier single-shot echo train spin sequence (ssFSE, ssTSE, HASTE). Fat suppression was not applied.

(TE). The main advantage of this technique is its ability to perform breath-hold T1-weighted imaging. FLASH-type sequences have replaced spin echo T1-weighted techniques for many abdominal applications, including dynamic contrast-enhanced imaging. FLASH techniques are also useful for chemical shift imaging. Similar sequences include T1 FFE (also referred to as FFE, potentially creating confusion with the unspoiled version) and SPGR.

FFE: Fast field echo
See FLASH (spoiled) and FISP (steady state).
FSE: Fast spin echo
See RARE
GraSE: Gradient and spin echo (Fig. 4.26)
GraSE (also written GRASE) is a hybrid technique combining elements of gradient echo and spin echo imaging to preserve the benefits of each sequence type while reducing

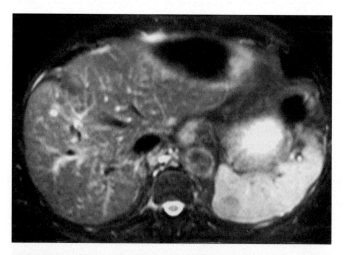

FIG. 4.26. Axial image of upper abdomen obtained with fat-suppressed GraSE sequence. Fat-suppression was accomplished with spectral presaturation inversion recovery.

their limitations. T1- or T2-weighted contrast is possible. Abdominal and pelvic applications are similar to those for TSE, although GraSE is not widely used at 1.5 T. However, its use is likely to increase at field strengths of 3 T and higher because GraSE causes less tissue heating (specific absorption rate) than comparable TSE sequences.

GRASS: Gradient recalled acquisition in the steady state. See FISP.

HASTE: Half-Fourier acquisition single-shot turbo spin echo (Fig. 4.27)

HASTE is a single-shot echo train spin echo sequence that exploits the symmetry of k-space to reduce scan times. As a single-shot technique, all phase-encoding steps are performed following a single 90-degree excitation pulse. Half-Fourier techniques reduce acquisition times by acquiring only slightly more than half of k-space data. The symmetry of k-space allows interpolation of the remaining data to create an image. Scan time is reduced proportionally to the reduction in phase-encoding steps. Images are usually T2-weighted. HASTE sequences are resistant to physiologic motion because of their short acquisition times. The use of multiple refocusing pulses minimizes susceptibility artifacts. However flow artifacts are common. HASTE excels at imaging fluid, but lesion conspicuity in solid organs may be reduced compared with other techniques. HASTE is commonly used for MR cholangiopancreatography (MRCP), MR urography, fetal imaging, and gastrointestinal imaging. HASTE scans are also widely used as breath-hold localizers. Similar to ssFSE and ssTSE using half-Fourier acquisition.

MP-RAGE: Magnetization-prepared rapid acquisition gradient echo

MP-RAGE is a rapid gradient echo technique using a 180-degree inversion pre-pulse to improve T1 contrast. These are very fast acquisitions, which are resistant to breathing artifacts. Images tend to have relatively low signal-to-noise ratios. They can be performed as a single-shot or multishot

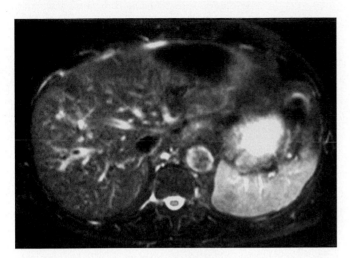

FIG. 4.28. Axial image of upper abdomen obtained with fat-suppressed echo train spin echo sequence (FSE, TSE). Fat suppression was accomplished with spectral presaturation inversion recovery.

acquisition and are similar to TurboFLASH and TFE using an inversion pre-pulse.

RARE: Rapid acquisition with relaxation enhancement (Fig. 4.28)

RARE is an echo train (or multishot) spin echo (SE) sequence in which each 90-degree excitation is followed by numerous 180-degree refocusing pulses. This results in considerable time savings compared to conventional SE. Images can be T1- or T2-weighted. Examples of RARE techniques include FSE and TSE. RARE techniques have essentially replaced conventional spin echo T2-weighted sequences for non–breath-hold abdominal and pelvic imaging. RARE techniques are also widely used for MRCP and MR urography.

SE: Spin echo

The first sequence to gain widespread clinical application, conventional SE (sometimes referred to as CSE) is a single-echo technique consisting of a 90-degree excitation pulse followed by a 180-degree refocusing pulse. It can be T1-, T2-, or intermediate-weighted. Signal-to-noise ratio is high but imaging times are long. Although T2-weighted conventional spin echo imaging is rarely used in the abdomen and pelvis, the SE pulse sequence is still used occasionally for non–breath-hold T1-weighted imaging.

SENSE: Sensitivity encoding

One of a family of parallel scanning techniques (see also SMASH), SENSE makes use of an array of multiple receiver coils, which are used in parallel to reduce scan time. This technique works by collecting data with a reduced field of view (by increasing the distance between lines in k-space while maintaining maximum k-values or overall size of k-space), thereby creating an aliased image. Because of local differences in coil sensitivities, which are determined in advance, a full field-of-view image can be created from these

data (a process referred to as *unfolding*). SENSE is similar to ASSET.

SGE: Spoiled gradient echo
See FLASH.

SMASH: Simultaneous acquisition of spatial harmonics

SMASH is a rapid imaging technique allowing some MR data points to be acquired in parallel rather than sequentially. In other words, multiple lines of data are acquired simultaneously by using an array of RF coils having different spatial sensitivities. Since multiple additional k-space lines are filled for each application of the phase-encoding gradient, imaging time is significantly reduced. This technique can be used to accelerate most rapid imaging sequences but requires an appropriate multicoil array and a sufficient number of receiver channels. Like SENSE and ASSET, SMASH is a parallel imaging technique.

SPGR: Spoiled gradient recalled echo (spoiled GRASS)
See FLASH.

SPIR: Spectral presaturation inversion recovery (see Figs. 4.26, 4.28)

SPIR is a method of fat suppression that uses a 180-degree inversion pre-pulse. This technique differs from STIR, in that the pre-pulse in SPIR is frequency-selective to invert only fat protons. This difference allows SPIR to be used with paramagnetic contrast agents such as gadolinium.

ssFSE: Single-shot fast spin echo
See HASTE.

ssTSE: Single-shot turbo spin echo
See HASTE.

STIR: Short tau inversion recovery.

STIR is a method of fat suppression that uses a 180-degree inversion pre-pulse. Unlike SPIR, the pre-pulse is not selective for fat. Imaging begins when the longitudinal magnetization of fat crosses the null point. This technique is not dependent on the homogeneity of the magnetic field, resulting in excellent, uniform fat suppression. However, because all short-T1 entities are suppressed, this technique should not be used for fat-suppressed T1-weighted imaging after administration of a paramagnetic contrast agent.

TFE: Turbo field echo
See MP-RAGE.

TurboFLASH:
See MP-RAGE.

TurboSTIR: Turbo short tau inversion recovery

TurboSTIR combines the fat suppression technique of STIR with a long echo train spin echo sequence (TSE or FSE). This technique provides uniform fat suppression, but signal-to-noise ratio is often sacrificed to shorten scan time. Contrast is primarily T2-weighted. Most often used for breath-hold imaging of the upper abdomen.

VIBE: Volume interpolated breath-hold examination.

VIBE is a three-dimensional, T1-weighted gradient echo sequence that uses zero fill interpolation to increase spatial resolution without a significant time penalty. This allows rapid, high-resolution imaging during a breath-hold. A time-efficient form of fat saturation is typically applied. This sequence is very similar to that used for contrast-enhanced MRA (VIBE uses a lower flip angle, however) and is often used for dynamic contrast-enhanced imaging of the abdomen and pelvis.

SUGGESTED READINGS

Brown MA, Semelka RC. MR imaging abbreviations, definitions, and descriptions: a review. *Radiology* 1999;213:647–662.

Elster AD. Gradient-echo MR imaging: Techniques and acronyms. *Radiology* 1993;186:1–8.

Mugler JP. Overview of MR imaging pulse sequences. *Magn Reson Imaging Clin N Am* 1999;7:661–697.

Nitz WR. MR imaging: acronyms and clinical applications. *Eur Radiol* 1999;9:979–997.

Oshio K, Feinberg DA. GRASE (gradient- and spin-echo) imaging: a novel fast MRI technique. *Magn Reson Med* 1991;20:344–349.

Pruessmann KP, Weiger M, Scheidegger MB, et al. SENSE: sensitivity encoding for fast MRI. *Magn Reson Med* 1999;42:952–962.

Rofsky NM, Lee VS, Laub G, et al. Abdominal MR imaging with a volumetric interpolated breath-hold examination. *Radiology* 1999;212:876–884.

Sodickson DK, Manning WJ. Simultaneous acquisition of spatial harmonics (SMASH): fast imaging with radiofrequency coil arrays. *Magn Reson Med* 1997;38:591–603.

Glossary of Magnetic Resonance Imaging Terms

Aliasing: Sometimes used to refer to wraparound artifact, which results when portions of the body outside of the field of view are spatially mismapped to the contralateral side of the image. In phase-contrast magnetic resonance angiography (MRA), aliasing refers to the representation of rapid flow as slow flow in the opposite direction due to setting an inappropriately low velocity encoding parameter.

Acquisition: An acquired MR data set sufficient to create an image.

Background projection: An artifact of maximum intensity projection. Background projection occurs when high signal intensity voxels resulting from random noise are projected as pixels on the image. The probability of these high signal intensity noise voxels being encountered by a projection ray increases with reconstructed volume thickness. As a result, thick reconstructions tend to have a higher signal intensity background.

Bandwidth: See sampling bandwidth.

Body coil: The permanent transmit and receive coil built into the scanner was originally referred to as the body coil. The term is also used to refer to a surface coil used for body imaging applications (e.g., phased-array body coil, quadrature body coil).

Centric ordered: A sequence designed to acquire the central lines of k-space before the peripheral lines. This type of acquisition is necessary for contrast-enhanced sequences triggered automatically or manually using real-time bolus tracking.

Chemical shift: The difference in resonant frequency between protons in different substances or environments. This difference increases with field strength. Chemical shift may be expressed independent of field strength as parts per million.

Coil: Refers to any scanner element designed to generate a magnetic field gradient (e.g., gradient coil), detect an MR signal (e.g., receive coil), or generate a radiofrequency (RF) pulse (e.g., transmit coil).

Crosstalk: When an imaging slice is excited with an RF pulse, some tissue on either side of the slice is excited due to the imperfect slice profile of the RF pulse. When adjacent slices are acquired sequentially without an intervening gap, this phenomenon results in signal loss in the final image.

Decay: Loss of net magnetization.

Dephasing: Loss of phase coherence of precessing protons.

Diffusion: Random movement of molecules or small particles as a result of Brownian (thermal) motion.

Diffusion imaging: An MR imaging (MRI) technique that creates image contrast from differences in the diffusion characteristics of tissues.

Echo: The signal measured as a result of transverse magnetization rephasing.

Echo train: Multiple echoes produced as a result of multiple refocusing steps after a single excitation.

Effective TE: The time from the excitation pulse to the echo created during application of the zero phase-encoding step of an echo train MR acquisition.

Fat suppression: Selective elimination of signal from fat through one of a variety of methods.

Fat saturation: A method of fat suppression. A common method of fat saturation uses a fat-selective RF pulse to tip the net magnetization vector of fat into the transverse plane. This transverse magnetization is then rapidly spoiled (dephased).

Ferromagnetic: Substances with a large positive magnetic susceptibility are referred to as ferromagnetic. These substances become permanently magnetized when exposed to an external magnetic field.

Flip angle: The degree (often displayed using a rotating frame of reference) to which the net magnetization vector is tipped by an RF pulse from its initial longitudinal orientation. The flip angle is controlled by the amplitude and duration of the RF pulse.

Flow compensation: See gradient moment nulling.

Fold-over suppression: See phase oversampling.

Fourier transform: The mathematic operation performed on a set of digitized MRI data to create an image. The Fourier transform extracts spatial information from the phase and frequency data obtained during an MR acquisition.

Fractional echo: A method of reducing scan time by sampling only a portion of the echo during readout. The inherent symmetry of k-space allows interpolation of the remaining data necessary to create an image. Similar to partial echo, half-echo, and asymmetric echo.

Free induction decay: The rapidly decaying signal (net transverse magnetization) produced immediately after an RF excitation.

Frequency encoding: The process of spatially encoding the MR signal along one axis through the application of a magnetic field gradient. The frequency-encoding gradient is typically applied during creation of the echo and, unlike the phase encoding gradient, remains constant for each echo.

Ghost: A faint duplicate image of a structure resulting from spatial misregistration of some of the signal from that structure. Ghosts typically occur along the phase-encoding axis and are most often the result of phase errors induced by periodic motion.

Gradient: A variation, typically linear, in magnetic field strength over distance. The hardware producing this variation is also commonly referred to as a gradient or gradient coil.

Gradient echo: Signal or echo produced after an excitation by using gradient reversal to reestablish phase coherence.

Gradient moment nulling: Also known as flow compensation, gradient moment nulling refers to modifications of the imaging gradient profiles to correct for phase shifts created by motion. Theoretically, this correction can be performed for higher orders of motion, such as acceleration, but it is typically performed only for constant velocity flow.

Half-Fourier: A technique for reducing image acquisition time by sampling just over half the total number of phase-encoding steps necessary to create an image. The inherent symmetry of k-space allows for extrapolation of the remaining data. The use of half-Fourier reduces scan time by slightly less than 50%. Similar to halfscan and $^{1}/_{2}$ NEX.

Halfscan: See half-Fourier.

In-phase image: Image produced when the net magnetization vectors of water and fat are in-phase. This requires use of a specific echo time (TE) that differs depending on magnetic field strength.

Intermediate weighted: Image contrast that is neither T1-weighted nor T2-weighted, but mainly reflects differences in tissue proton densities. This is accomplished with a sufficiently long TR to allow longitudinal magnetization of tissues to recover nearly completely (minimizing T1-weighted contrast) and a sufficiently short TE to reduce image contrast based on differences in T2-relaxation between tissues (minimizing T2-weighted contrast). These images are sometimes referred to as proton density weighted.

Inversion pulse: A 180-degree RF pre-pulse given before the excitation pulse of an imaging sequence. Varying the time between the inversion pulse and the excitation pulse controls image contrast.

Inversion time (TI): The time between an inversion pulse and an excitation pulse.

Isotropic: A voxel with equal dimensions along each axis is said to be isotropic. Motion that is uniform in all three dimensions is likewise isotropic.

k-space: The single most reviled term in MRI. K-space is a digital representation of the phase and frequency data inherent in the analog signal, or echo, collected during each phase-encoding step. (The frequency-encoding gradient is applied during the echo sampling. Therefore, frequency encoding also occurs during each phase-encoding step.) The raw MR data points are sampled in k-space and converted into image data via the Fourier transform.

Larmor equation: The relationship between resonance frequency and field strength is represented by the Larmor equation, which states that the precessional frequency of a nucleus is proportional to the externally applied magnetic field. Specifically, the precessional frequency equals the gyromagnetic ratio multiplied by the magnetic field strength. The gyromagnetic ratio is a constant for each type of nucleus.

Larmor frequency: Also known as the resonance frequency. This is the precessional frequency of protons at a given magnetic field strength as predicted by the Larmor equation. In acquiring an MR image, the frequency of the RF pulses must match the Larmor frequency of the protons of interest.

Longitudinal magnetization: Net magnetization component aligned with the main magnetic field.

Magnetization transfer: The transfer of magnetization between relatively immobile protons in macromolecules, which have a relatively broad range of resonant frequencies, and free water protons. This effect is used to suppress background signal intensity in MRA by saturating large macromolecules with an off-resonance RF pulse. The subsequent exchange of magnetization between water protons and the macromolecules results in signal loss within parenchymal tissue, but not within flowing blood. Magnetization transfer may also be used to alter image contrast for other applications, although it is not widely used in abdominal and pelvic imaging.

MIP (maximum intensity projection): An image reconstruction technique that projects only the highest signal intensity voxel along each projection ray through a volume of data as a pixel on the final image. This is currently the standard image processing technique used to create projection images ("angiograms") from MRA source data.

Multishot acquisition: A means of reducing scan times by creating and collecting more than one echo after each excitation pulse. Each echo corresponds to a different phase-encoding step. As a result, multiple phase-encoding steps are performed during each repetition time (TR) interval. Spin echo or gradient echo pulse sequences can be designed as multishot sequences. Echo train spin echo (fast/turbo spin echo) and echo planar sequences are examples of multishot techniques.

Multislice acquisition: A means of improving imaging efficiency by acquiring data from more than one imaging slice during the "down time" of an imaging cycle. Additional slices can be excited during the time interval between collection of the echo and the next excitation pulse for a given slice. By increasing the TR, more slices can be acquired during a multislice acquisition. To avoid crosstalk, slices should be excited in an interleaved (noncontiguous) manner.

Null point: The time when a substance recovers to the point of zero longitudinal magnetization following a 180-degree inversion pulse.

Opposed-phase image: An image in which the data are acquired at a time when water and fat protons are approximately 180 degrees out of phase. Opposed-phase images are usually acquired using a T1-weighted gradient echo sequence with an appropriate TE value.

Paramagnetic: Describes a material that contains magnetic moments that can be aligned with an external magnetic field, thereby amplifying the field strength. In contrast to ferromagnetic materials, paramagnetic materials do not retain permanent magnetization when they are removed from the external magnetic field. Examples of paramagnetic materials include mangafodipir and the extracellular gadolinium chelates used as MR contrast agents.

Partial volume effect: An artifact of cross-sectional imaging, this effect results from averaging of the signal intensity of different tissues within a voxel. As a result, the tissue interfaces within that voxel cannot be resolved. Therefore, a voxel that bridges an interface between high and low signal intensity structures displays intermediate signal intensity. This effect becomes more apparent as slice thickness increases.

Phase-contrast angiography: A type of MR angiography based on the phase shifts experienced by protons moving (as in flowing blood) relative to a magnetic field gradient.

Phase encoding: The process of spatially encoding MR data along an axis by inducing varying amounts of phase difference along that axis. This phase difference is created by application of a gradient (phase-encoding gradient) before collection of the echo. The process of phase encoding must be repeated multiple times to allow localization of the signal sources along the phase-encoding axis.

Phase oversampling: A method of eliminating wraparound artifact in the phase-encoding direction by acquiring and discarding additional data outside the field of view. Similar to no-phase-wrap and fold-over suppression.

Phased array coil: A surface coil system consisting of multiple independent surface coils that function as an array of independent receivers. Phased-array coils are commonly used for abdominal and pelvic applications because they combine an increase in signal-to-noise ratio (SNR) with a large field of view.

Pixel (picture element): The smallest discrete unit of a digital image. A digital image consists of multiple pixels.

Each pixel represents one voxel of tissue on the final image and is of uniform signal intensity.

Proton density: Refers to the number of protons in a given voxel available to contribute to the MR signal. A proton density–weighted image is one in which the contributions to image contrast from differences in T1 and T2 relaxation times have been minimized.

Quadrature coil: An RF receiver coil consisting of two elements arranged perpendicularly with a 90-degree phase shift between them. This configuration significantly improves SNR.

Radiofrequency pulse: A magnetic field created by the transmit coil that oscillates or rotates at the Larmor frequency of hydrogen protons (in the RF range) at a particular field strength. RF pulses are used to excite, rephase, or saturate tissue.

Readout gradient: Frequency-encoding gradient. The readout gradient is so called because it is turned on during collection of the echo.

Receiver coil: The hardware apparatus consisting of conducting wire that detects the MR signal (net transverse magnetization).

Rectangular FOV: A method of shortening scan time by reducing the number of phase-encoding steps, typically along the shorter dimension of the body. By simultaneously reducing the field of view and the matrix size along the phase-encoding axis, image resolution is maintained.

Sampling bandwidth: The rate at which the analog MR signal or echo is sampled in the process of converting it to digital data.

Saturation: The loss of net longitudinal magnetization within tissue resulting from the application of repeated RF pulses with a relatively short repetition interval compared to the tissue T1 value.

Saturation band: An RF pulse applied in the presence of a spoiler gradient over a slab of tissue designed to selectively eliminate signal from that tissue. Saturation bands are used in time-of-flight MRA to allow selective visualization of the arterial or venous system. They are also commonly placed over the subcutaneous fat of the anterior abdominal wall to minimize phase encoding artifacts caused by respiratory motion.

Sensitivity encoding: A technique used to reduce scan time by using the sensitivities of phased-array coil elements (determined through a calibration process) to unwrap an image acquired with an intentionally reduced field of view. (The reduced field of view creates the image wrap that is subsequently mathematically unwrapped). This reduced field of view requires fewer phase-encoding steps to acquire, thus decreasing scan time.

Shimming: The process of adjusting the main magnetic field to maximize its homogeneity. Successful MRI requires a relatively homogeneous magnetic field. When a patient is placed in the scanner, small magnetic field heterogeneities are created. These field heterogeneities can be corrected using shim coils, which generate magnetic field gradients that compensate for irregularities in the main field. Activation of the shim coils is called *active shimming*. This is particularly important when using a technique, such as fat saturation, that relies on precisely defined resonant frequencies of protons within fatty and nonfatty tissues. Passive shimming refers to the use of metal plates permanently installed in the scanner to create a homogeneous magnetic field.

Signal-to-noise ratio (SNR): The SNR is one of the most important determinants of image quality. Simply stated, SNR is a ratio of the desirable signal generated with MRI to the background noise from all sources. Many factors determine the SNR, including field strength (and other properties of the scanner hardware), pulse sequence, voxel size, sampling frequency, and the source of the signal.

Single-shot: Single-shot refers to the use of a single excitation pulse to generate an image. This implies that all the necessary phase-encoding steps to create an image occur after a single excitation. The TR for a single-shot sequence is, therefore, infinite.

Slew rate: The slew rate of a scanner is the maximum gradient amplitude divided by the time it takes to reach maximum amplitude (rise time). Units for slew rate are Tesla/meter-second. The minimum TR achievable is determined in part by the slew rate.

Spin echo: The signal generated by application of an RF refocusing pulse after an RF excitation pulse. Spin echo sequences typically use a 90-degree excitation pulse and one or more 180-degree refocusing pulses.

Spiral imaging: A spiral acquisition uses two oscillating gradients during readout to fill k-space in a spiral configuration beginning with the central (high image contrast) data. This type of imaging is not yet widely available, because high performance gradients and complex reconstruction methods are required.

Spoiled: A sequence is said to be spoiled when the residual transverse magnetization remaining after collection of the echo is actively destroyed through dephasing, typically by applying an additional gradient (referred to as a *spoiler gradient*).

Steady-state sequence: If a spoiler gradient is not applied between successive RF pulses in a gradient echo sequence, and the TR is sufficiently shorter than the tissue T2 value, the residual transverse magnetization reaches a steady state and is sustained between RF pulses. A portion of this residual transverse magnetization gets converted to longitudinal magnetization with each subsequent RF pulse. Sequences in which the phase coherence of transverse magnetization is sustained are referred to as steady-state free precession sequences.

Surface coil: A receiver coil, used to detect the MR signal, that is placed directly on the structure of interest. Surface coils are used primarily to improve the SNR.

Susceptibility: The magnetic susceptibility of a substance determines how it interacts with and the degree to which it becomes magnetized by an external magnetic field. The

mathematical definition of magnetic susceptibility is the ratio of magnetization induced in a material divided by the field to which it is exposed.

Diamagnetic substances tend to disperse the local magnetic field, resulting in a slight reduction in local field strength. Paramagnetic substances, which contain unpaired electrons, concentrate or enhance the local magnetic field. These effects are present only as long as the substance is exposed to an extrinsic magnetic field. Ferromagnetic substances maintain residual magnetization even after the extrinsic magnetic field is turned off. Magnetic susceptibility artifact is caused by magnetic field distortion created at the interface between substances of differing magnetic susceptibility.

T1 relaxation: Also known as spin-lattice relaxation, T1 relaxation refers to the regrowth of longitudinal magnetization resulting from energy transfer from protons to their local environment. The time constant, T1, can be approximated as the time required for longitudinal magnetization to regrow to 63% of its original value after a 90-degree excitation.

T1-weighted: Image contrast based predominantly on differences in the T1 relaxation times of tissues. T1-weighting is often accomplished by using relatively short TR and TE values. The short TR maximizes the effect of differences in tissue T1 values, whereas the short TE minimizes the effect of differences in tissue T2 values on image contrast.

T2 relaxation: Also known as spin-spin relaxation, T2 relaxation refers to the decay of transverse magnetization resulting from the loss of phase coherence due to intrinsic causes such as magnetic field fluctuations in the local environment of the proton. T2 decay is the result of interactions at the molecular and atomic level and is irreversible. The time constant, T2, can be approximated as the time required for the net transverse magnetization to decay to 37% of its original value as a result of spin-spin interactions (not resulting from magnetic field heterogeneity that contributes to T2* decay).

T2* relaxation: The rate of transverse magnetization decay (represented by free induction decay) resulting from reversible and irreversible causes of proton dephasing. T2* relaxation combines the effects of irreversible T2 decay and reversible proton dephasing from extrinsic magnetic field heterogeneity. T2* decay is considerably more rapid than T2 decay.

T2-weighted: Image contrast based predominantly on differences in the T2 relaxation times of tissues. T2-weighting is often accomplished by using relatively long TE and TR values. The long TR minimizes the contribution of differences in T1 relaxation times, whereas the long TE maximizes the effect of differences in tissue T2 values on image contrast.

TE (echo time): Time between the center of the excitation pulse and the center of the echo.

TR (repetition time): Time between successive RF excitation pulses.

Transverse magnetization: The component of the rotating magnetization vector within the transverse plane. It occurs after an RF excitation pulse converts longitudinal (z) magnetization completely or partially into x-y magnetization. The transverse component of magnetization is measured to produce an MR image.

Truncation artifact: An artifact created by applying a Fourier transform to an undersampled data set (i.e., the data set is truncated). Truncation is most apparent at high-contrast interfaces and often manifests as multiple lines paralleling these interfaces. This artifact is reduced by increasing the matrix size (collecting more data).

Venc or VENC: Abbreviation for velocity-encoding parameter.

Velocity-encoding parameter: A parameter (cm/s) that must be specified in advance when performing phase-contrast MRA. The number chosen controls the bipolar gradient strength, thereby specifying the velocity of flow that will result in a 180-degree phase shift. The velocity-encoding pa-rameter should be selected to be slightly higher than the maximum velocity of flow one wishes to image and can be selected for a single direction or for all three axes. Setting this parameter too high results in poor signal from the vessel of interest. Selecting a parameter that is too low results in rapid flow (experiencing a greater than 180-degree phase shift) being misrepresented as slow flow in the opposite direction.

Voxel (volume element): A volume of tissue with a defined location in three-dimensional space. The signal derived from a voxel is represented by a pixel on the MR image.

Zero fill interpolation: A means of improving the apparent resolution of an MRI examination by collecting an incomplete data set and filling the unfilled portions of k-space with zeros, allowing a fast Fourier transform to be performed on the data. This allows a reduction in scan time or an improvement in spacial resolution for the same scan time.

Subject Index

Note: Page numbers followed by f *indicate figures; those followed by* t *indicate tables.*